T0408447

# The Aynho Cartulary and its Documentary Culture

## Medieval Documentary Cultures

SERIES EDITORS

Laura L. Gathagan (Associate Professor of History, State University of New York College at Cortland)

Charles Insley (Senior Lecturer in Medieval History, University of Manchester)

This series provides a home for investigations into all aspects of documentary culture in the Middle Ages, both secular and ecclesiastical; documents are here understood in their widest possible form, as manuscripts, books, and other material sources, including but not limited to cartularies, charters, letters, and seals. Its aim is to engage and embrace multiple and intersecting fields of study, among them the commissioning, production and dissemination of documents, material culture, gender, lay and monastic literacy, and the creation of memory. Both monographs and strongly-focussed essay collections are welcomed.

Proposals/preliminary enquiries may be sent to the editors and/or publisher at the addresses below.

laura.gathagan@cortland.edu
charles.insley@manchester.ac.uk
cpalmer@boydell.co.uk

PREVIOUSLY PUBLISHED

*Forgeries and Historical Writing in England, France, and Flanders, 900–1200*, Robert F. Berkhofer III

# The Aynho Cartulary and its Documentary Culture

## Study, Text, and Translation

*Richard Allen and Benjamin Pohl*

THE BOYDELL PRESS

© Richard Allen and Benjamin Pohl 2025

*All Rights Reserved.* Except as permitted under current legislation
no part of this work may be photocopied, stored in a retrieval system,
published, performed in public, adapted, broadcast,
transmitted, recorded or reproduced in any form or by any means,
without the prior permission of the copyright owner

The right of Richard Allen and Benjamin Pohl to be identified as
the authors of this work has been asserted in accordance with
sections 77 and 78 of the Copyright, Designs and Patents Act 1988

First published 2025
The Boydell Press, Woodbridge

ISBN 978 1 83765 179 5

The Boydell Press is an imprint of Boydell & Brewer Ltd
PO Box 9, Woodbridge, Suffolk IP12 3DF, UK
and of Boydell & Brewer Inc.
668 Mt Hope Avenue, Rochester, NY 14620–2731, USA
website: www.boydellandbrewer.com

A CIP catalogue record for this book is available
from the British Library

The publisher has no responsibility for the continued existence or accuracy of URLs
for external or third-party internet websites referred to in this book, and does not
guarantee that any content on such websites is, or will remain, accurate or appropriate

*For Mikal, Leah, and Anneli.*

# CONTENTS

# ILLUSTRATIONS

## FIGURES



## TABLES

## GENEALOGIES



The authors and publisher are grateful to all the institutions and individuals listed for permission to reproduce the materials in which they hold copyright. Every effort has been made to trace the copyright holders; apologies are offered for any omission, and the publisher will be pleased to add any necessary acknowledgement in subsequent editions.

# ACKNOWLEDGEMENTS

Researching and writing this book together has been a voyage of discovery, one that took us into unfamiliar and often uncharted – though certainly not un*chartere*d – territory. Just like any adventure, ours was enabled and supported in various ways (financially, logistically, intellectually, emotionally, etc.) by a multitude of patrons, sponsors, collaborators, colleagues, friends, and family. Those who deserve to be singled out here for special mention include the British Academy, which generously financed our research with a grant from the Neil Ker Memorial Fund in 2021–2 (NK22\220013), as well as our respective employers, Magdalen College, Oxford, and the University of Bristol. At Magdalen, we have benefited from the assistance and support of several people, but especially Lucy Gwynn, Anne Chesher, and Emily Jennings. The President and Fellows of Magdalen are also to be thanked for their permission to reproduce the images of the Aynho material which are to be found below. At Bristol, those who offered their help and expertise especially include Brendan Smith, Simon Parsons, and Mark Hailwood. We would like to thank the Oxford Conservation Consortium, particularly Emma Skinner, for kindly helping us to produce the high-quality images of the Aynho Cartulary reproduced in Part II of this book, as well as the Bibliothèque patrimoniale d'Avranches, especially Étienne Baptiste, for supplying the image for Fig. 4.3 and giving us permission for its reproduction. Others who readily gave their time and knowledge in support of this research are Liesbeth van Houts, Sethina Watson, the anonymous reviewer of our initial book proposal, the no-longer anonymous reader of the final manuscript, Kathryn Dutton (whose own book-length study and edition of a thirteenth-century cartulary is forthcoming), the series co-editors of *Medieval Documentary Cultures*, Laura Gathagan and Charles Insley, and Boydell and Brewer's own Caroline Palmer. They were each instrumental in the successful development of this book, from inception to completion, and for this we wish to express our deepest thanks to them. Last but not least, we owe our single greatest debt to our two amazing wives, Mikal and Leah, as well as, in Ben's case, to his wonderful and ever-curious daughter, Anneli. It is to them that this book is dedicated.

# ABBREVIATIONS

| | |
|---|---|
| *ANS* | *Anglo-Norman Studies* |
| Baker | G. Baker, *The History and Antiquities of the County of Northampton* (2 vols, London, 1822–41) |
| *BF* | H.C. Maxwell-Lyte (ed.), *Liber Feodorum. The Book of Fees, Commonly Called Testa de Nevill. Reformed from the Earliest MSS. by the Deputy keeper of the Records* (3 vols, London, 1920–31) |
| BL | London, British Library |
| *Cartularies* | G.R.C. Davis, *Medieval Cartularies of Great Britain and Ireland*, rev. C. Breay et al. (London, 2010) |
| *CBMLC* | R. Sharpe et al. (eds), *Corpus of British Medieval Library Catalogues* (16 vols, London, 1990–) |
| *CChR* | *Calendar of Charter Rolls preserved in the Public Record Office* (6 vols, London, 1903–27) |
| *CCR* | *Calendar of the Close Rolls preserved in the Public Record Office. Henry III* (14 vols, London, 1902–38); *Calendar of the Close Rolls preserved in the Public Record Office. Edward I* (5 vols, London, 1900–08) |
| *CFR* | *Calendar of the Fine Rolls preserved in the Public Record Office* (22 vols, London, 1911–62) |
| *CIPM* | *Calendar of Inquisitions Post Mortem and other analogous Documents, 1236–1307* (4 vols, London, 1904–13) |
| Cooper | N. Cooper, *Aynho: A Northamptonshire Village* (Banbury, 1984) |
| *CPL* | *Calendar of Entries in the Papal Register Relating to Great Britain and Ireland: Papal Letters* (23 vols, London, 1893–) |

| | |
|---|---|
| *CPR* | H.C. Maxwell-Lyte (ed.), *Calendar of the Patent Rolls preserved in the Public Record Office. Henry III* (6 vols, London, 1901–13); H.C. Maxwell-Lyte (ed.), *Calendar of the Patent Rolls preserved in the Public Record Office. Edward I* (4 vols, London, 1893–1901) |
| *CR* | *Close Rolls of the Reign of Henry III preserved in the Public Record Office, 1227–1272* (14 vols, London, 1902–38) |
| *CRR* | *Curia regis rolls … preserved in the Public Record Office* (20 vols, London, 1920–2006) |
| *Domesday* | J. Morris (ed.), *Domesday Book* (35 vols, Chichester, 1973–86) |
| Dugdale, *Monasticon* | W. Dugdale, *Monasticon Anglicanum*, new edn by H. Ellise and B. Bandinel (6 vols, London, 1817–30) |
| *Early Ches. Charts.* | G. Barraclough (ed.), *Facsimiles of Early Cheshire Charters* (Preston, 1957) |
| *EEA* | *English Episcopal Acta* (47 vols, Oxford, 1980–) |
| *EHR* | *English Historical Review* |
| *EPNS* | English Place-Name Society, *Survey of English Place-Names* (151 vols, Cambridge, 1924–) |
| *Fasti* | J. Le Neve, *Fasti Ecclesiae Anglicanae 1066–1300*, new edn D.E. Greenway (11 vols, London, 1968–) |
| Hall, *England* | D. Hall, *The Open Fields of England* (Oxford, 2014) |
| Hall, *Northamptonshire* | D. Hall, *The Open Fields of Northamptonshire* (Northampton, 1995) |
| Hoskin (ed.), *Grosseteste* | P. Hoskin (ed.), *Robert Grosseteste as Bishop of Lincoln: The Episcopal Rolls, 1235–1253* (Woodbridge, 2015) |
| *JMH* | *Journal of Medieval History* |
| Keats-Rohan (ed.), *Domesday People* | K.S.B. Keats-Rohan (ed.), *Domesday People: A Prosopography of Persons occurring in English Documents, 1066–1166. 1: Domesday Book* (Woodbridge, 1999) |
| Keats-Rohan (ed.), *Domesday Descendants* | K.S.B. Keats-Rohan (ed.), *Domesday Descendants: A Prosopography of Persons occurring in English Documents 1066–1166. 2. Pipe Rolls to Cartae Baronum* (Woodbridge, 2002) |

| | |
|---|---|
| *Lexicon* | J.F. Niermeyer and C. van de Kieft (eds), *Mediae Latinitatis lexicon minus*, rev. ed. (2 vols, Leiden, 2002) |
| MCA | Magdalen College Archives |
| *MRB* | *Monastic Research Bulletin* |
| *ODNB* | *Oxford Dictionary of National Biography* |
| *PR* | *Pipe Rolls*, published by the Pipe Roll Society |
| *Rolls of Sutton* | R.M.T. Hill (ed.), *The Rolls and Register of Bishop Oliver Sutton* (8 vols, Woodbridge, 1948–) |
| *Rot. Chart.* | T.D. Hardy (ed.), *Rotuli chartarum in Turri londinensi asservati* (London, 1837) |
| *Rot. de Dominabus* | J.H. Round (ed.), *Rotuli de dominabus et pueris et puellis de XII comitatibus (1185)* (London, 1913) |
| *Rot. Fin.* | T.D. Hardy (ed.), *Rotuli de oblatis et finibus in Turri Londinensi asservati, tempore regis Johannis* (London, 1835) |
| *Rot. Gravesend* | F.N. Davis et al. (eds), *Rotuli Ricardi Gravesend diocesis Lincolniensis* (Oxford, 1925) |
| *Rot. Litt. Claus.* | T.D. Hardy (ed.), *Rotuli litterarum clausarum in turri Londinensi asservati* (2 vols, London, 1833–4) |
| *Rot. Litt. Pat.* | T.D. Hardy (ed.), *Rotuli litterarum patentium in Turri londinensi asservati* (London, 1835) |
| *Rot. Welles* | W. Phillimore and F.N. Davis (eds), *Rotuli Hugonis de Welles, Episcopi Lincolniensis A.D. MCCIX–MCCXXXV* (3 vols, Lincoln, 1912–14) |
| *TMR* | *The Medieval Review* |
| TNA | Kew, The National Archives |
| VCH | Victoria County History |
| Vincent (ed.), *Henry II* | N. Vincent (ed.), *The Letters and Charters of Henry II, King of England, 1154–1189* (7 vols, Oxford, 2021–4) |
| *Word-List* | R.E. Latham (ed.), *Revised Medieval Latin Word-List from British and Irish Sources* (London, 1965) |

# NOTE ON THE TEXT

Some preliminary words of explanation are required regarding the rendering of personal/place names, currencies, measurements, percentages, etc., in the book's individual chapters, in the edition/translation of the Aynho Cartulary, and in the transcriptions of Aynho charters in the Appendix. Proper names are rendered in keeping with anglophone conventions (e.g., Stephen rather than Étienne; Ralph rather than Raoul or Radulf/Rodulf; etc.), with toponymics of French/Norman origin given in their francophone forms using 'de/le/la' rather than 'of/the' (e.g., Guy de la Haye, Baldwin de Boulogne, Robert de Beaumont, etc.), except for those conventionally anglicised in the scholarship (e.g., Robert of Mortain). Surnames of French/Norman origin are also given in their francophone forms (e.g., Richard le Machun, Henry le Gras, etc.), except when there is a common English cognate (e.g., William le Chamberlayn = William Chamberlain; Thomas le Neuman = Thomas Newman, etc.). Toponyms and toponymic surnames that cannot be identified definitively are rendered as they appear in the sources using italics (e.g., *Sefneacres*, *Langeford'*, *Stanihulle/Stanille*, etc.; Warin de *Verineto*, William de *Adles*, etc.), although these have been standardised when a toponym has more than one form (e.g., *Verineto/Vireneto/Vireni/Virineto* is thus consistently rendered as de *Verineto*). Surnames have also been standardised when there is more than one form (e.g., Neirenuit/Neirenut/Neirnut/Neyrnut is always rendered as Neirenuit). Names of identifiable settlements, counties, regions, and administrative sub-divisions like hundreds and parishes have been normalised (e.g., Northamptonshire, King's Sutton, Croughton, etc.). All currencies are given as they appear in the sources without conversion, using digits and the conventional symbols/abbreviations for pounds, shillings, and pence (e.g., £1 13s 5d), with Latin *marca/-ae* translated as 'mark/-s'.[1] Units of land and land-related taxation are given in acres (one acre = four roods), virgates (one virgate = thirty acres), and hides (one hide = four virgates = 120 acres), with numbers smaller than 100 spelled out except for fractions (e.g., 1 ½ acres, 1.8 virgates, etc.).[2] All measurements have been

[1] This is in keeping with other recent work on thirteenth-century England such as D. Carpenter, *Henry III: Reform, Rebellion, Civil War, Settlement, 1258–1272* (New Haven, CT, 2023), p. xiv.

[2] For further reference, see the glossary in Hall, *England*, pp. 344–6.

converted to the modern metric system for ease of reference and are given in digits (i.e., 2 mm, 5.4 cm, 30 m, 85.8 km, etc.). Percentages are given in digits followed by the conventional symbol (e.g., 10.4%). Consecutive date ranges such as regnal years, episcopacies, and terms of office are indicated by an en dash (e.g., 1160–1200), while non-consecutive or unconfirmed periods with a *terminus a quo* and a *terminus ad quem* are designated by a multiplication sign (e.g., *c.*1296 × *c.*1310). Throughout the book, references to individual acts in the Aynho Cartulary are made in brackets citing the numbers assigned to them in the edition and using boldface (e.g., no. **5**, nos. **13–17**, etc.). Depending on context, these numbers can therefore refer to both original acts and copies thereof in the cartulary. Meanwhile, original Aynho deeds *not* copied in the cartulary are referenced with the alphanumerical sigla established in the Appendix (e.g., no. **A1**, nos. **A11–A12**, etc.) to facilitate both cross-reference within the present study and future citation of these important but hitherto unedited/unpublished documents. Aynho deeds later than the cartulary's period of composition (i.e., post-*c.*1280) and therefore absent from the Appendix are cited by their archival reference numbers, assigned at the beginning of the seventeenth century, in the muniments of Magdalen College, Oxford (i.e., Aynho 5, Aynho 60–1, etc.). All URLs cited in this book were last accessed in May 2024.

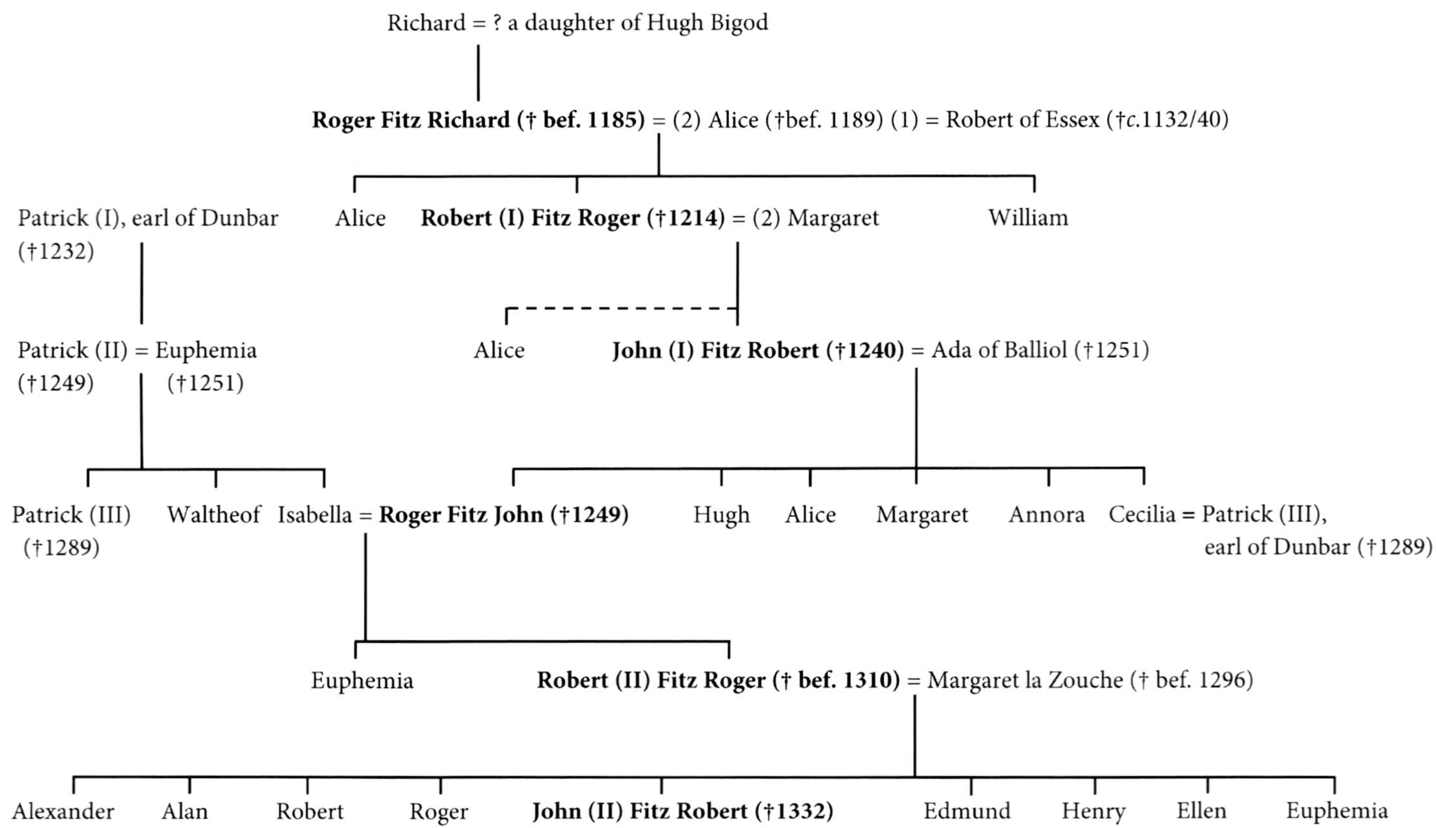


Genealogy 1. The descent of Roger Fitz Richard.

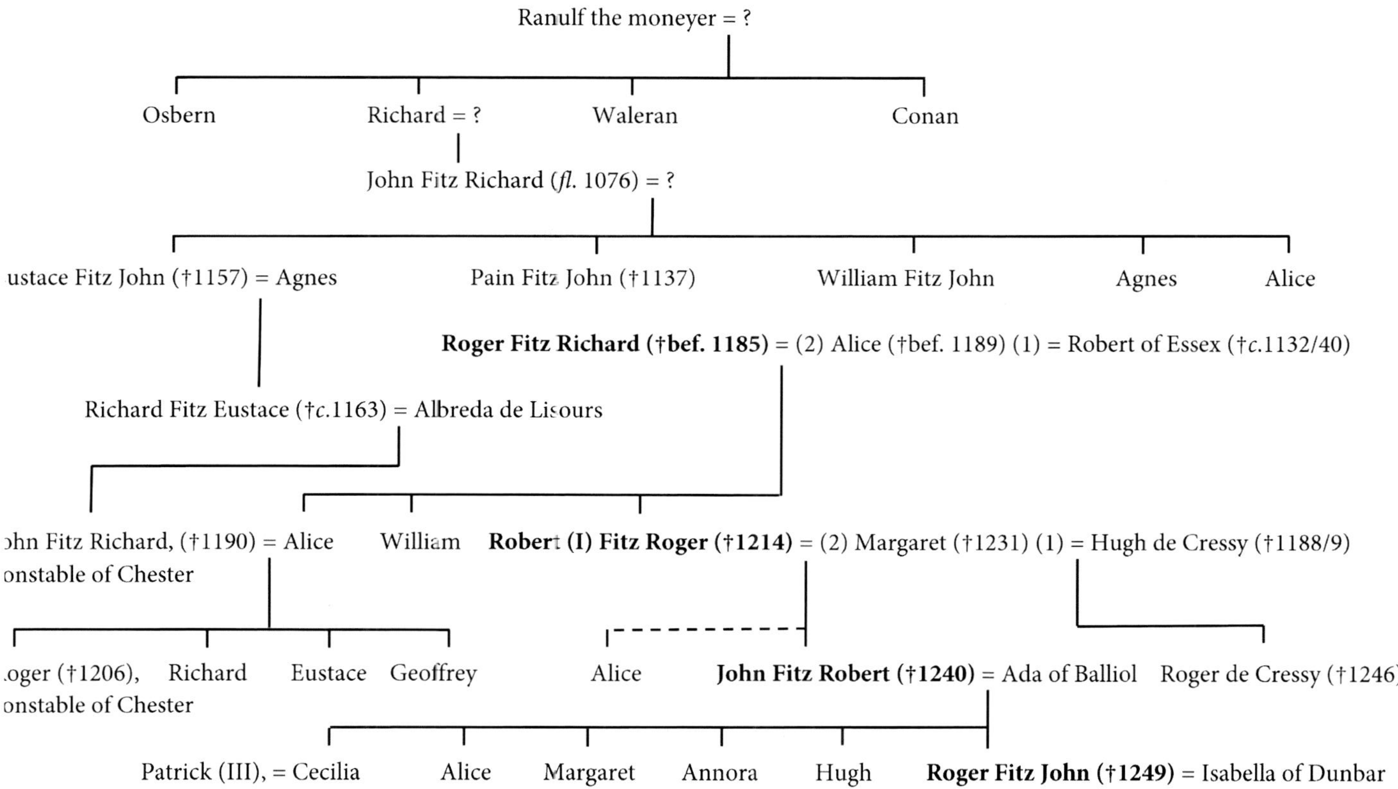


Genealogy 2. The descent of Roger Fitz Richard and the constables of Chester.

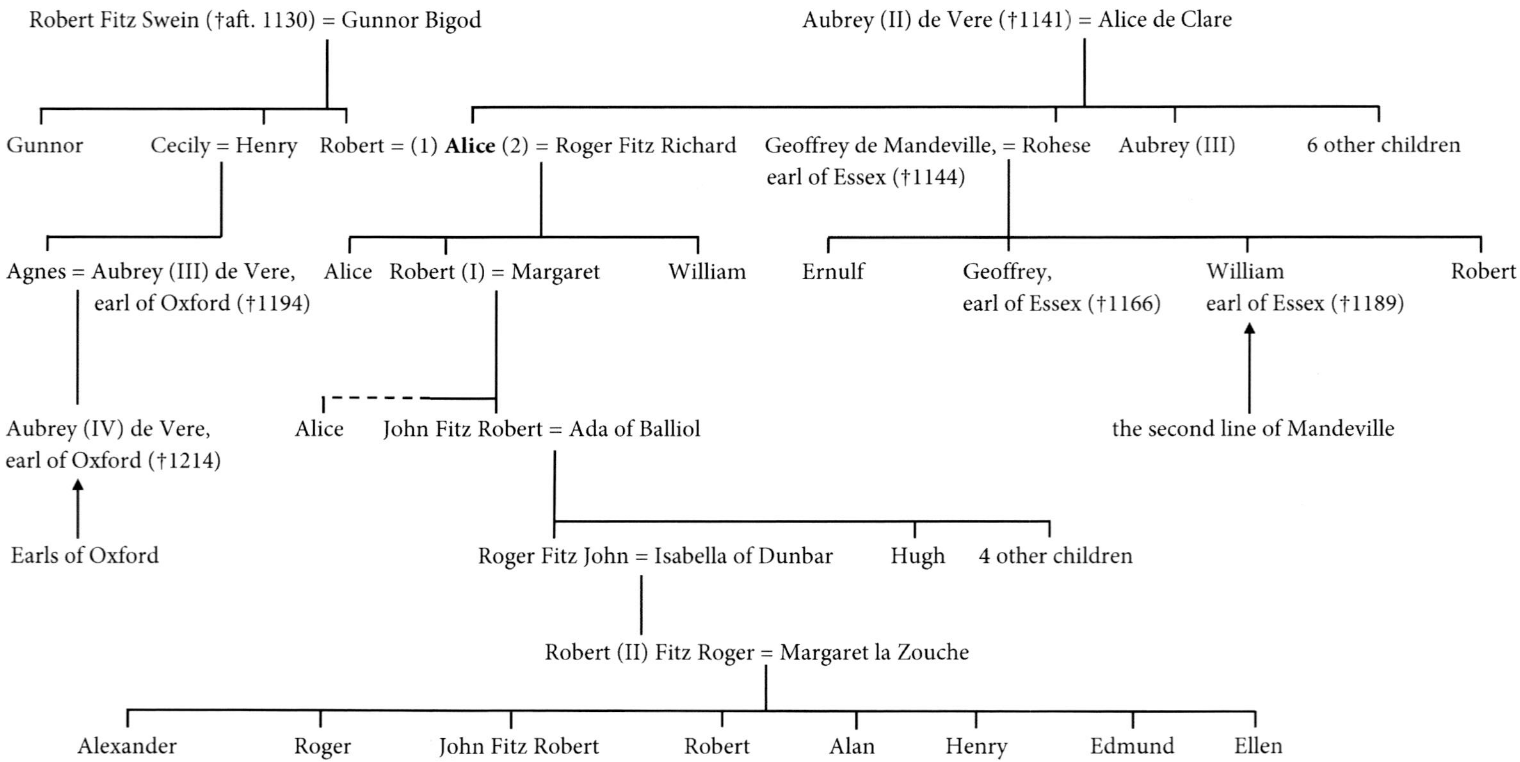


Genealogy 3. The descent of Alice of Essex and the earls of Oxford and Essex.

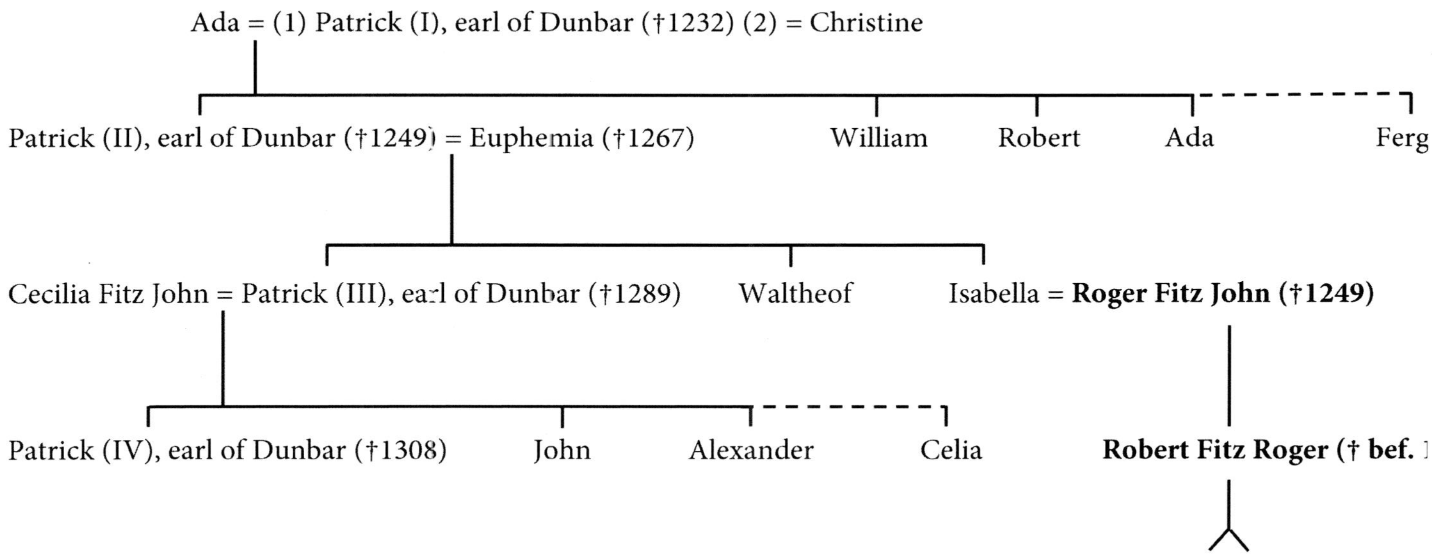


Genealogy 4. The earls of Dunbar and the descent of Roger Fitz John.

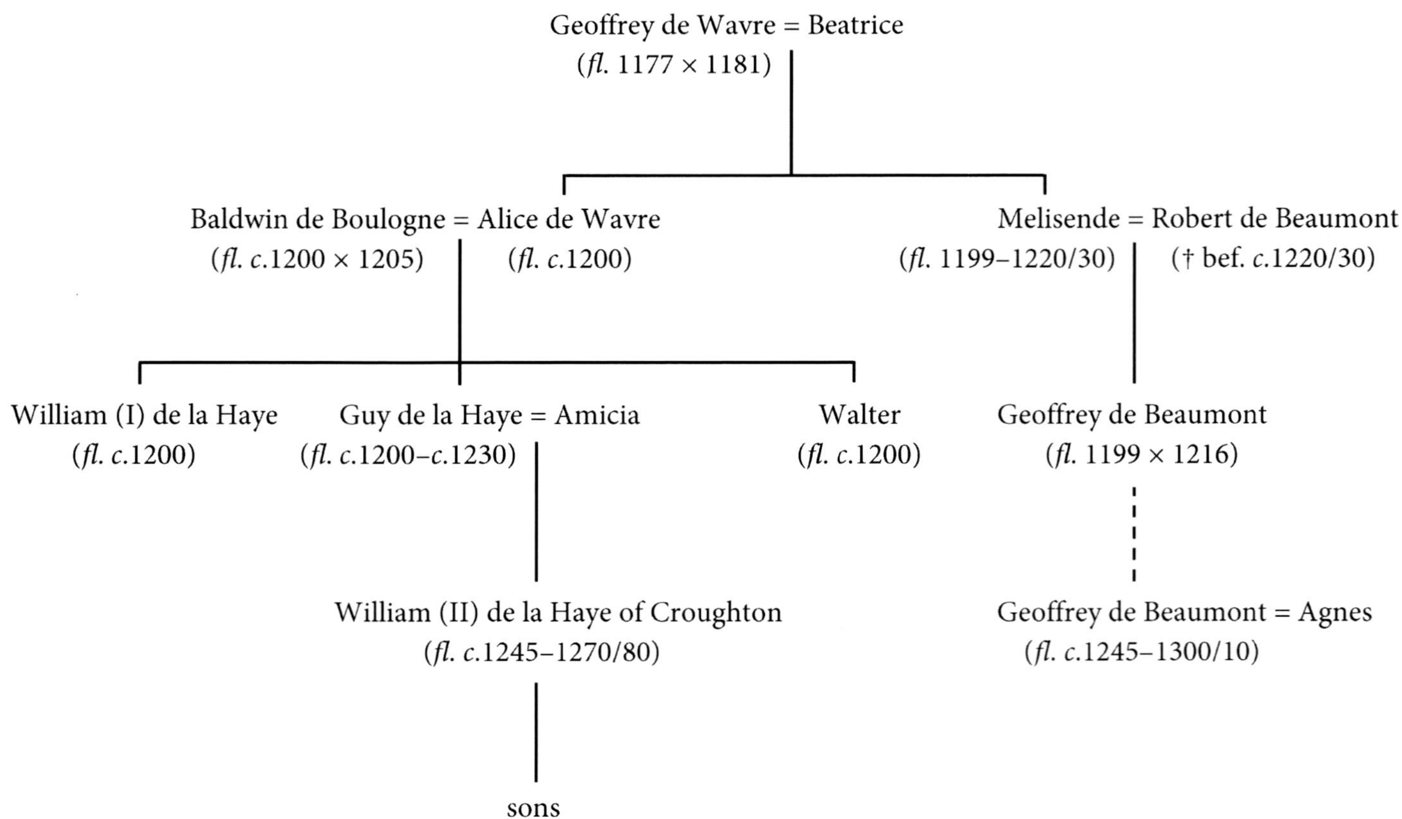


Genealogy 5. The descent of Geoffrey de Wavre.

# PART I

# STUDY

# INTRODUCTION

This book is the first to study, edit, and translate the important but hitherto little-known roll cartulary of the medieval 'wayfarer' hospital of SS James and John, Aynho (Northamptonshire), today held in the archives of Magdalen College, Oxford (EP/137/1). Made in the latter half of the thirteenth century, about a century after the hospital's foundation, the Aynho Cartulary contains the texts of some fifty-six acts, around half of which are still extant as originals. Despite being one of the earliest, largest, and best-preserved of its type in Britain and Ireland, this intriguing artefact has received virtually no scholarly attention to date, due in large part to its rediscovery only as recently as 1979. Roll cartularies (or cartulary rolls) in general have been relatively little studied by comparison with their more frequently encountered book-shaped cousins, and scholars are only just beginning to appreciate their true value and significance for our understanding of medieval documentary culture. At Aynho, this unusual choice of format appears to have been motivated by a combination of economic, logistical, pragmatic, and aesthetic factors that have deep roots in the hospital's history during the first hundred or so years of its existence, in the development of its property landscape and its patronage networks, and also in the scribal milieux and local documentary culture of which it was a part. Combining a contextual and historical exploration with a focussed examination of the cartulary's contents and a forensic scribal and material analysis, the present book offers its readers a holistic approach to – and a model for – studying these rare and still often underappreciated types of documents, one that sheds light on both the Aynho Cartulary itself and the wider culture and society that produced it.

## AYNHO HOSPITAL AND THE MAGDALEN COLLEGE ARCHIVES

Before outlining and contextualising our book's aim and methodological approach, it seems prudent to begin with a brief overview of the Aynho Cartulary's journey to the Magdalen College Archives. Founded in 1458 by William Waynflete, bishop of Winchester (1447–86), the college of St Mary

Magdalen in the University of Oxford, as it is officially known, is home to one of the largest collections of medieval deeds in the United Kingdom outside those kept in its national repositories. Numbering some 13,000 items, with the earliest dating from the first decades of the twelfth century, its size and chronological scope are the result of Waynflete's energetic efforts to ensure his new foundation had an adequate endowment. One major feature of Magdalen's early years was the annexation to it of decayed religious institutions, among them priories and hospitals.[1] Having fallen into a state of dilapidation, Aynho Hospital was of particular interest to Waynflete due to its proximity both to Oxford and to existing Magdalen estates. Conversely, it was likely of little value to its aristocratic patron, William Fitz Alan, earl of Arundel (1417–87), from whom Waynflete purchased the hospital in October 1483. Its archive, which included the Aynho Cartulary that is the focus of the present book, was subsequently transferred to Magdalen, with the majority of these records being stored in the college's purpose-built, late fifteenth-century muniment room, where they remain to this day (**Fig. I.1**). At some point in time, and for reasons unknown, the hospital's roll cartulary was separated from its collection of single-sheet charters,[2] such that it does not feature in the first comprehensive list of Magdalen's deeds, compiled *c.*1610,[3] nor in William Dunn Macray's (1826–1916) monumental (but unpublished) calendar of them, which he produced between 1864 and 1878.[4] It was eventually rediscovered only in 1979 by Christopher Woolgar, who was then employed by the college to list its late medieval and early modern estate records, among a bundle of papers relating to

1 For the founding of Magdalen and Waynflete's role in it, see V. Davis, *William Waynflete, Bishop and Educationalist* (Woodbridge, 1993), pp. 60–73.

2 Other cartularies that came into Magdalen's possession were similarly separated from their related archive of single-sheet deeds, being originally stored in the college's library. As this decision suggests, however, these are all codex in format, whereas the deed collection in the Muniment Tower is home to both flat and rolled items.

3 MCA, CP/3/31.

4 W.D. Macray, ['A Descriptive Calendar of the Muniments of St Mary Magdalen College, Oxford'], 48 vols, unpublished manuscript (1864–78). Save a handful of volumes, Macray's untitled manuscript calendar was typed and bound (but never published) in the 1920s. It is still an indispensable finding aid. Each volume is currently being retro-converted and uploaded as part of a multi-year project to Magdalen's online archives catalogue (<https://archive-cat.magd.ox.ac.uk/>). Macray outlined its contents in W.D. Macray, 'The Manuscripts of St Mary Magdalene College, Oxford', *Appendix to The Fourth Report of the Historical Manuscripts Commission* (London, 1874), pp. 458–65, and in W.D. Macray, 'St Mary Magdalen College', *Appendix to The Eighth Report of the Historical Manuscripts Commission* (London, 1881), pp. 262–69.

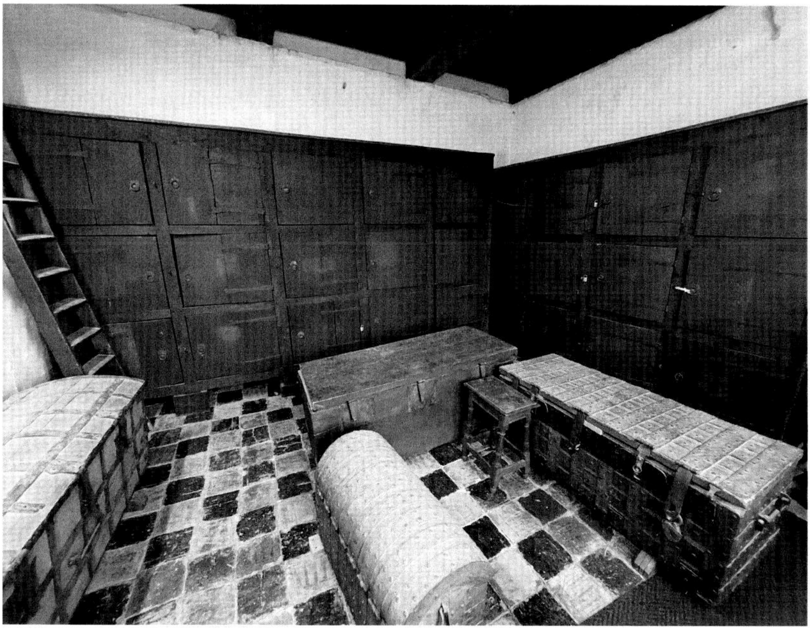

Fig. I.1. The Muniment Room of Magdalen College, Oxford.

Northamptonshire. Although a notice of his discovery was printed in 1981,[5] Woolgar's listing, like Macray's deeds calendar, is indispensable but unpublished,[6] such that the roll cartulary's existence has all but gone unnoticed save by a small handful of specialists.

## AIM OF THIS BOOK

This book positions itself at the crossroads of – and aims to create a conversation between – three prolific fields of research, each of which has seen increased scholarly activity during recent years, although rarely in conjunction with each other. The first of these (medieval cartulary studies) is represented by a steadily growing body of scholarship both inside and outside the anglophone academy, most notably in France and Germany, which has generated multiple book-length publications with helpful assessments of the *état présent* at different points during the twentieth and twenty-first

5 C.M. Woolgar, 'Two Cartularies at Magdalen College, Oxford', *Journal of the Society of Archivists*, 6 (1981), 498–9.

6 C.M. Woolgar, 'A Catalogue of the Estate Archives of St Mary Magdalen College, Oxford', 10 vols, unpublished typescript (1981).

centuries. Among the most recent is Joanna Tucker's monograph from 2020, which offers readers a concise yet detailed discussion of the field's development, as well as of its current state internationally.[7] There is little point in repeating this exercise or in rehearsing the findings of Tucker's comprehensive appraisal here, though we should at least note a few cartulary studies and/or editions that have appeared since, the findings of which have opened up new perspectives and lines of enquiry.[8] One is Yvonne Seale's and Heather Wacha's *editio princeps* (2023) of the thirteenth-century

7 J. Tucker, *Reading and Shaping Medieval Cartularies: Multi-Scribe Manuscripts and their Patterns of Growth* (Woodbridge, 2020), pp. 4–33; J. Tucker, 'Understanding Scotland's Medieval Cartularies', *Innes Review*, 70 (2019), 135–70. Previously P. Chastang, 'Cartulaires, cartularisation et scripturalité médiévale: La structuration d'un nouveau champ de recherche', *Cahiers de civilisation médiévale*, 49 (2006), 21–31; P. Chastang, 'Des archives au codex: Les cartulaires comme collections (XIe–XIVe siècle)', in B. Grévin and A. Mairey (eds), *Le Moyen Âge dans le texte: Cinq ans d'histoire textuelle au Laboratoire de médiévistique occidentale de Paris* (Paris, 2016), pp. 25–44; O. Guyotjeannin et al. (eds), *Les Cartulaires: Actes de la table ronde organisée par l'École nationale des chartes et le G.D.R. 121 du C.N.R.S* (Paris, 1993); A.J. Kosto and A. Winroth (eds), *Charters, Cartularies and Archives: The Preservation and Transmission of Documents in the Medieval West* (Toronto, ON, 2002); V. Lamazou-Duplan and E. Ramirez Vaquero (eds), *Les cartulaires médiévaux: Écrire et conserver la mémoire du pouvoir, le pouvoir de la mémoire* (Pau, 2013); A. Büttner et al. (eds), *Kopialbuch der Zisterzienserabtei Schönau (Generallandesarchiv Karlsruhe 67/1302)* (Heidelberg, 2020); H. Flachenecker et al. (eds), *Urkundenbücher, Chroniken, Amtsbücher: Alte und neue Editionsmethoden* (Torún, 2019); M. Mersiowsky, 'Urkunden, Kopiare, Zinsbücher: Die Esslinger Bettelordensklöster und ihre pragmatische Schriftlichkeit im Spätmittelalter', in M. Mersiowsky et al. (eds), *Schreiben–Verwalten–Aufbewahren: Neue Forschungen zur Schriftlichkeit im spätmittelalterlichen Esslingen* (Ostfildern, 2018), pp. 251–328; M. Gussone and M.B. Rössner-Richarz, 'Kopiare als Arbeitsinstrumente', in M. Gussone et al. (eds), *Adelige Lebenswelten im Rheinland: Kommentierte Quellen der Frühen Neuzeit* (Cologne, 2009), pp. 96–100; G. Vogeler, 'Digitale Urkundenbücher: Eine Bestandsaufnahme', *Archiv für Diplomatik*, 56 (2010), 363–92; S. Molitor, 'Das Traditionsbuch: Zur Forschungsgeschichte einer Quellengattung und zu einem Beispiel aus Südwestdeutschland', *Archiv für Diplomatik*, 36 (1990), 61–92. Most recently L. Agúndez San Miguel and F. Tinti, 'Introduction: New Perspectives after Thirty Years of Cartulary Studies', *Studia Historica. Historia Medieval*, 42 (2024), 3–8; J. Tucker, 'Recognising Cartulary Studies Thirty Years after *Les Cartulaires*', *Studia Historica. Historia Medieval*, 42 (2024), 9–24.

8 For example, B. Tabuteau (ed.), *Le Cartulaire de la léproserie d'Évreux* (Compiègne, 2021); L. Viaut (ed.), *Le cartulaire de l'abbaye du Palais Notre-Dame (XIIe et XIIIe siècles): Édition critique* (Pessac, 2021); C.B. Bouchard (ed.), *The Cartulary-Chronicle of St-Pierre of Bèze* (Toronto, ON, 2020); published just before but not referenced in Tucker's book is the useful collection of essays in R. Furtado and M. Moscone (eds), *From Charters to Codex: Studies on Cartularies and Archival Memory in the Middle Ages* (Turnhout, 2019).

cartulary of Prémontré Abbey, which champions material and book-historical analysis as a productive (if not altogether new) methodological approach to medieval cartulary studies, one that encourages 'a more inclusive understanding of the cartulary['s] history, its makers, its place of origin, its historical context, and its survival'.[9] This approach, wherein cartularies are viewed 'not only as the product of specific institutions but also as the representation of a constructed process that discloses the voices, actions, and agendas of various makers',[10] also underpins the present work. We use the Aynho Cartulary's material composition and uncommon format as a lens through which to study and bring into focus the wider socio-political and scribal milieux that produced it, thereby showcasing the cartulary itself and the charters that survive alongside it as a gateway to the society and documentary culture of thirteenth-century England.

This brings us to the second field of research addressed in this book: the study of medieval rolls and, more specifically, roll cartularies. Less common and, until very recently, less frequently studied by scholars than their codex-shaped counterparts, medieval roll cartularies or cartulary rolls (*cartulaires-rouleaux*) have been 'put on the map' by pioneering initiatives such as the ROTULUS project (2019–22) at the University of Lorraine, which has gathered and made openly accessible almost two hundred examples produced and preserved across France (https://rotuli.univ-lorraine.fr/), and the two Digital Humanities projects 'Rolls and Scrolls after the Codex' and 'English Manuscript Rolls, 1200–1600: A Collaborative Digitization Project' (both 2016) at the Beinecke Rare Book and Manuscript Library at Yale University, whose databases are yet to appear online or in published form.[11] Despite the regular and persistent use of rolls as instruments of governance, administration, and bureaucracy on both sides of the Channel from the twelfth and thirteenth centuries,[12] the study of roll cartularies

9 Y. Seale and H. Wacha (eds), *The Cartulary of Prémontré* (Toronto, ON, 2023), pp. 7–10, at pp. 7–8. A similar approach also characterises Tucker's study, which is referenced repeatedly by Seale and Wacha. As noted by Constance Bouchard in her review of Tucker's book, however, claiming that such an approach 'will break ground by combining codicology, pal[a]eography, and textual analysis' is at odds with the fact that 'those of us who work closely with cartulary manuscripts have long been doing so'; C.B. Bouchard, 'Review of J. Tucker, *Reading and Shaping Medieval Cartularies*', *TMR* (2021), <https://scholarworks.iu.edu/journals/index.php/tmr/article/view/32128/35956>.

10 *Cartulary of Prémontré*, ed. Seale and Wacha, p. 10.

11 On these two projects and their past activities (including collaborative workshops), see <https://digitalrollsandfragments.com/ms-rolls-projects/>.

12 J. Peltzer, 'The Roll in England and France in the Late Middle Ages: Introductory Remarks', in J. Peltzer et al. (eds), *The Roll in England and France in the Late Middle Ages: Form and Content* (Berlin, 2020), pp. 1–19; P. Robinson, 'The Format of Books:

in medieval England/Britain and our modern knowledge of them was/is a relatively modest affair. The revised edition (2010) of Godfrey Davis's standard reference work *Medieval Cartularies of Great Britain and Ireland* lists about twenty extant examples, the vast majority (*c*.70%) of which date between the fourteenth and early sixteenth centuries. Almost all are from monastic houses (mostly Benedictines or Cistercians), their dependent priories, and medieval England's great monastic cathedral priories (e.g., Ely, Exeter, York), with just a handful of secular examples.[13] The only roll cartularies produced by/for English hospitals other than Aynho date from the fourteenth and fifteenth centuries, which makes the Aynho Cartulary the earliest of its kind (see Chapter 4). Somewhat paradoxically, roll cartularies, while much fewer in number (less than 10% of Davis's corpus) than codex-types, might well have stood a better chance of survival. As has been noted repeatedly, the various important function(s) of cartularies for the daily life, administration, and liturgical/commemorative routine of religious communities would suggest that many (if not most) of them probably had their home not in the library, a facility that might barely have existed (if at all) in smaller institutions (especially hospitals), but rather in domestic archives, deed chests, or (fortified) muniment rooms (**Fig. I.1**), where they were kept together with the most valuable charters and privileges.[14] This

Books, Booklets and Rolls', in N.J. Morgan and R.M. Thomson (eds), *The Cambridge History of the Book in Britain. Vol. 2: 1100–1400* (Cambridge, 2008), pp. 41–54.

13 For their details and identifications, see Chapter 4. Perhaps the best-known British roll cartularies are those of Margam Abbey, which in recent years have received renewed attention thanks primarily to the work of Élodie Papin: É. Papin, 'Les cartulaires de l'abbaye de Margam: Le processus de cartularisation et l'administration des biens monastiques au pays de Galles au XIIIe siècle', *Médiévales*, 76 (2019), 11–24; É. Papin, 'Les cartulaires-rouleaux de l'abbaye de Margam: Matérialité et fonctions des rouleaux cisterciens au pays de Galles au XIIIe siècle', in J. Peltzer et al. (eds), *The Roll in England and France in the Late Middle Ages: Form and Content* (Berlin, 2020), pp. 197–215. On the *état présent* of medieval monastic cartulary studies, cf. Robert F. Berkhofer III, 'Interpreting Monastic Cartularies in Northwest Europe, 900–1200: Thirty Years of Scholarship', *Studia Historica. Historia Medieval*, 42 (2024), 25–46.

14 *Cartularies*, pp. xvii–xviii; Tucker, *Reading and Shaping*, pp. 16–25; *Cartulary of Prémontré*, ed. Seale and Wacha, p. 86 n. 110. Of the several hundred hospitals founded in medieval England, only just over fifty have left evidence of a domestic library or book collection; N. Ramsay and J.M. Willoughby (eds), *Hospitals, Towns, and the Professions* [= *CBMLC* XIV] (London, 2009), with discussion of hospital libraries and the book types typically kept therein (pp. xxxii–xxxvii). As Ramsay and Willoughby note, '[o]nly the better-endowed hospitals would have a cartulary, but each warden or master must have had some record-book with memoranda about its property' (ibid., p. xxxv). On archival storage solutions in the twelfth and thirteenth centuries, see now also R. Olney, *English Archives: An Historical Survey* (Liverpool, 2023), pp. 32–3, 38–40, and 81–7.

is especially true of rolls, which are recorded regularly – and occasionally depicted[15] – as being stored securely in the archives, charter houses (*domus cartarum*), and designated document chests of religious houses (and of their leaders) to help protect them from accidental damage, unauthorised access, and theft. This protection was sometimes so effective that they survived the dissolution or destruction of their medieval institutions intact, whereas the books stored in the library were looted, dispersed, or destroyed.[16]

The third major field of research to which this book pertains, and the one that has witnessed most activity in recent years, is the study of medieval hospitals and, by extension, medieval cultures of charity. Again, it would be superfluous to provide a comprehensive overview of the developments that have shaped this field since the publication more than a century ago of Rotha Clay's ground-breaking *The Mediæval Hospitals of England* (1909), as readers can conveniently be referred to multiple authoritative and widely accessible reviews of the *status quo* published at various points over the last forty years, several of them even in this very decade. These notably include, in chronological order, the important contributions by Miri Rubin (1987, 1989, 1991),[17] Nicholas Orme and Margaret Webster (1995),[18] Sheila Sweetinburgh (2004),[19] and, recently, Sethina Watson (2004, 2020) and Adam Davis (2021),[20] as well as Carol Fry's good (if unpublished) recapitulation of the historiography of medieval English hospitals up to 2020.[21] Their arguments and approaches are considered in Chapter 2 in the specific context

15 BL, MS Cotton Claudius E IV, fol. 124r, with photographic reproduction in B. Pohl, *Abbatial Authority and the Writing of History in the Middle Ages* (Oxford, 2023), p. 295.

16 Pohl, *Abbatial Authority*, pp. 304–13. Also cf. the discussion in Chapter 4.

17 M. Rubin, *Charity and Community in Medieval Cambridge* (Cambridge, 1987); M. Rubin, 'Development and Change in English Hospitals, 1000–1500', in L. Granshaw and R. Porter (eds), *The Hospital in History* (London, 1989), pp. 41–59; M. Rubin, 'Imagining Medieval Hospitals: Considerations on the Cultural Meaning of Institutional Change', in J. Barry and C. Jones (eds), *Medicine and Charity Before the Welfare State* (London, 1991), pp. 14–25.

18 N. Orme and M. Webster, *The English Hospital, c.1070–1570* (New Haven, CT, 1995).

19 S. Sweetinburgh, *The Role of the Hospital in Medieval England: Gift-Giving and the Spiritual Economy* (Dublin, 2004).

20 S. Watson, '*Fundatio*, *ordinatio*, and *statuta*: The Statues and Constitutional Documents of English Hospitals to 1300', unpublished PhD dissertation, University of Oxford, 2004; S. Watson, *On Hospitals: Welfare, Law, and Christianity in Western Europe, 400–1320* (Oxford, 2020); A.J. Davis, *The Medieval Economy of Salvation: Charity, Commerce, and the Rise of the Hospital*, rev. pb. edn (Ithaca, NY, 2021).

21 C. Fry, '"Hospitality, Chantries, and Other Works of Piety": A Select Study of the Functions and Longevity of Hospitals in Small Towns and Villages in Medieval England, *c*.1150-*c*.1450', unpublished PhD dissertation, University of Oxford, 2020, pp. 3–17.

of the medieval spiritual economy of charitable donation, gift-giving, and exchange. The role of the gift (in its various guises) in medieval society is a subject that has received a fair amount of attention, with some recent publications focusing specifically on England during the high/later Middle Ages and in the early modern period.[22] As others have noted, expectations of reciprocity and reward on the part of the giver(s) were crucial for the endowment of medieval hospitals, many of which – particularly small 'wayfarer' foundations like Aynho, which was built to welcome pilgrims and the sick-poor – could not rely on major gifts and prestigious sponsorship from royal or comital patrons, but were instead dependent on the concerted and continuous support of individuals and families from among the aspiring ranks of medieval society, as well as on voluntary (and sometimes actively solicited) acts of common charity by virtually anyone able to give something to them.[23] Their dynamic and distinctive position at the local intersections of socio-economic, socio-political, spiritual, and – thanks to rare sources such as the Aynho Cartulary – documentary activity places hospitals such as Aynho among the chief witnesses of everyday life and community building in medieval England and wider Europe.

By making an original contribution to not one but three fields of study, the present book deliberately situates the Aynho Cartulary at a lively interdisciplinary and methodological juncture to reconstruct the process of its production and, viewed through this lens, explore the history of the various individuals and families whose lives and interactions it records. These include not only members of the local aristocracy and landholding classes, but also groups who are often marginalised in medieval diplomatic records (and modern studies thereof), such as professional scribes, local clerks and witnesses, women, and the sick, poor, and impaired,[24] all of whom were

22 L. Kjær, *The Medieval Gift and the Classical Tradition: Ideals and the Performance of Generosity in Medieval England, 1100–1300* (Cambridge, 2019); N. Perkins, *The Gift of Narrative in Medieval England* (Manchester, 2021); see also the recent contributions to L. Kjær and G. Strenga (eds), *Gift-Giving and Materiality in Europe, 1300–1600: Gifts as Objects* (London, 2022). On the early modern period, see I. Krausman Ben-Amos, *The Culture of Giving: Informal Support and Gift-Exchange in Early Modern England* (Cambridge, 2008); F. Heal, 'Good Gifts, the Household and the Politics of Exchange in Early Modern England', *Past and Present*, 199 (2008), 41–70.

23 Cf. the discussions by Sweetinburgh, *Role of the Hospital*, pp. 35–47; Orme and Webster, *English Hospital*, pp. 84–106; Davis, *Economy of Salvation*, pp. 115–63.

24 In line with wider scholarly practice, we are using the terms 'impaired' and 'impairment' to refer indistinctly to various physical and/or mental conditions that put individuals in need of the kind of care provided by medieval hospitals; cf. I. Metzler, *Disability in Medieval Europe: Thinking about Physical Impairment during the High Middle Ages, c.1100–1400* (London, 2006).

important agents at Aynho Hospital and had their activities – and their voices – recorded in its cartulary, often uniquely so. Close study and edition of the cartulary allows for these voices to be heard in concert for the first time and to be placed in conversation with groups that more regularly constitute the subject of scholarly enquiry. What is more, the cartulary itself can be placed in close dialogue with the hospital's archive of original deeds, also conserved at Magdalen College, thereby allowing us to capture with unusual definition the social, political, and economic profiles of (and relationships between) the people attached to this relatively obscure rural hospital, from the high and mighty down to the meek and lowly – a true 'microcosm' of medieval English society in a locality that, while 'off the beaten track' today, was at the centre of (and embedded within) various important networks in the later twelfth and thirteenth centuries.

## STRUCTURE OF THIS BOOK

To help reveal this microcosm, the book has been organised into two parts. Part I comprises a comprehensive study of Aynho Hospital and its cartulary (Chapters 1–4), framed by an Introduction and Conclusion.

Chapter 1 sets out the general historical context by situating Aynho and its hospital within the wider religious, social, and political landscape of medieval Northamptonshire and England in the first century after the hospital's foundation (*c.*1170–*c.*1280). It identifies and introduces key figures associated with both the institution and Aynho's ecclesiastical life more generally, including the founding family and their dynastic relations, regular benefactors, and prominent individuals like the celebrated English chronicler, Ralph de Diceto. We demonstrate that the hospital's foundation, traditionally dated to *c.*1180 (and sometimes much later), in reality took place in 1170/1, thus placing it at the very forefront (if not ahead) of the 'second wave' of hospital foundations in medieval England. We further situate the hospital's establishment and early history within the wider movements of medieval charity and hospitality, specifically as they played out in small towns and villages, before beginning to explore the *raison(s) d'être* for the creation of its roll cartulary.

Chapter 2 then continues and expands these considerations by establishing Aynho Hospital more firmly within the socio-political and socio-economic network(s) of which it was a part and from which it benefited both spiritually and materially. It identifies further patrons and property donors, traces the familial and feudal connections between them, and investigates their participation in the medieval spiritual economy. Going beyond the remit of prosopography, this chapter also examines the patchwork of local landscapes and markets in which the hospital was situated and which it managed and manipulated in turn, with particular attention being paid to the modes of landholding, investment, and estate building that defined and sustained rural institutions and communities such as Aynho.

Chapter 3 contextualises Aynho Hospital and its cartulary within the wider documentary culture(s) of thirteenth-century Northamptonshire and neighbouring Oxfordshire. Using the hospital's extant original charters, as well as those issued in relation to other hospitals in nearby Brackley and Oxford, we examine the work of those scribes known to have written Aynho charters, something that has hitherto escaped scholarly investigation but is essential for understanding the Aynho Cartulary. We show how a forensic survey of Brackley and Oxford deeds allows for otherwise anonymous scribes responsible for producing Aynho acts to be identified and, in some instances, even named for the first time. Taken together, this situates the work of the main Aynho cartularist, who himself worked anonymously, within these wider scribal milieux, and it examines the sort of documentary resources that a rural hospital like Aynho could muster in-house or call upon from outside.

Chapter 4 shifts the focus away from Aynho Hospital as an institution towards the Aynho Cartulary as a material and literary artefact. It introduces readers to the physical object by exploring in detail the cartulary's format, design, material composition, and scribal preparation. Using both internal and external evidence, we establish a new date for the cartulary's original creation, showing that it was likely produced *c.*1260 (certainly pre-1270) during the mastership of Peter of Windsor, rather than *c.*1280 as previously assumed. This situates it among the earliest roll cartularies to survive from medieval England and makes it the only one known to have been produced by a hospital anywhere in Britain and Ireland before the fourteenth century. Chapter 4 also provides the first full palaeographical (handwriting) and codicological (materiality) analysis of the Aynho Cartulary with identifications of six different scribes who contributed to it over the period *c.*1260–*c.*1270 × 1280, some of whose penmanship can also be identified in the corpus of the hospital's extant original charters. The reasons why the cartulary was created in the uncommon format of a parchment roll, rather than as a codex as was customary in the period under consideration, are explored from both pragmatic and economic points of view. The advantages this format might have offered to the cartulary's intended users at Aynho are discussed and the human and material resources involved in its production considered in detail.

These studies in Part I are rounded off with a Conclusion that draws together their respective findings and offers concrete suggestions for future work in the fields of study to which it pertains.

Part II of this book consists of a full photographic facsimile that reproduces the cartulary's seven membranes (recto and verso) as high-definition colour plates commissioned especially for this book, thereby enabling readers to appreciate the Aynho Cartulary's intriguing materiality and helping them to visualise the various palaeographical and codicological arguments in the book's preceding part. This is accompanied by a full critical edition and English translation of the cartulary's contents, which is designed both to facilitate and inspire future research and university-level teaching. An Appendix provides critical editions and summary descriptions of extant Aynho charters *not* copied in the Aynho Cartulary, which are used and cited as primary evidence throughout this book, followed by a bibliography and indices of people, places, and subjects.

As at least one scholar has noted, the sheer number of independently founded hospitals in medieval England, a great many of which were located in rural settings, would have made them institutions much more familiar and accessible to the average person than their better-known – and hence more frequently studied – monastic counterparts.[25] The fact that hospitals such as Aynho's have not hitherto received the scholarly attention they deserve risks rendering one-dimensional the multifaceted landscapes in which they operated. By placing Aynho Hospital and its thirteenth-century cartulary at the centre of our analyses, this book looks not only to bring some overdue perspective to the lively charitable and documentary worlds in which this hospital was situated, and to which it contributed, but also to amplify and contextualise the different and diverse voices, activities, and aspirations of the remarkably wide cross-section of individuals and families preserved in its records. In doing so, we showcase the Aynho Cartulary as an instructive source for scholars and students interested in the history of hospitals, the spiritual economy, and the documentary cultures of England and Europe in the central and later Middle Ages.

25 S. Watson, 'The Origins of the English Hospital', *Transactions of the Royal Historical Society*, 16 (2006), 75–94, at p. 76.

# 1

# FOUNDATION AND EARLY HISTORY OF AYNHO HOSPITAL (*c.*1170–*c.*1280)

This chapter establishes Aynho Hospital within its various historical contexts during the first century or so of its existence. It identifies the key figures associated with the hospital, including the founding family (the lords of Warkworth, later known as the house of Clavering) and some of its regular benefactors, as well as those individuals associated with the ecclesiastical life of Aynho more generally, among them the celebrated chronicler, Ralph de Diceto (*c.*1120–*c.*1202). It shows how the hospital's foundation, traditionally dated to *c.*1180 (and sometimes much later), in fact took place a decade earlier in 1170/1, thereby placing it at the forefront (and perhaps even slightly ahead) of what might be called the 'second wave' of hospital founding in medieval England. It also situates the hospital's establishment within the wider movement of hospitality in the Middle Ages, specifically as it played out in small towns and villages, a subject hitherto little studied. This chapter concludes by examining the circumstances at Aynho Hospital towards the second half of the thirteenth century, thereby exploring and contextualising the historical conditions surrounding the creation of its cartulary, the production process of which will be studied in detail in Chapter 4.

## THE SETTLEMENT OF AYNHO

The Northamptonshire village of Aynho (/ˈeɪnhoʊ/) lies to the east of the Cherwell valley on the edge of gentle uplands, approximately 10 km south-east of Banbury near the border with Oxfordshire. Its current proximity to the M40 motorway makes it a convenient place to live for any of its residents wishing to commute to major cities like Birmingham or London, but, like many such villages in England, it is also somewhere that is today more often driven past at great speed than visited with any specific intent. In this respect, it is a far cry from its medieval predecessor. Located in the ancient

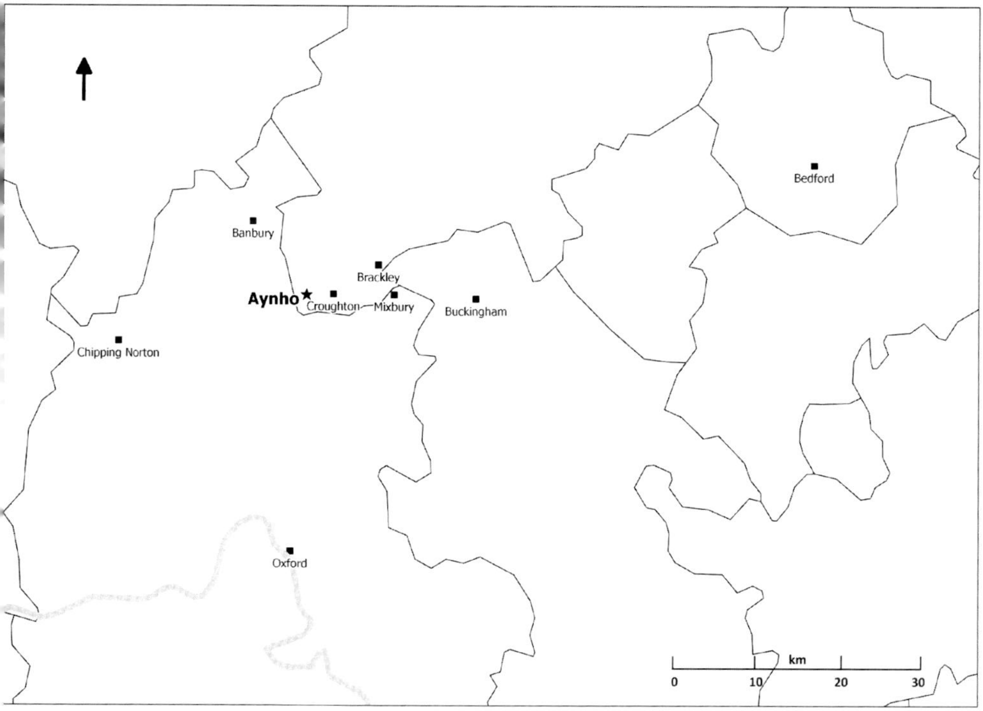


Fig. 1.1. Aynho and its surroundings.

diocese of Lincoln in what was King's Sutton Hundred, the vill of Aynho sat on the ancient ridgeway linking Buckingham to Chipping Norton in the west and Banbury in the north. It is some 27 km north of Oxford and 9 km southwest of Brackley (**Fig. 1.1**), land to the south of which was, by the late twelfth century, one of only five approved sites for tourneying, thereby making Aynho a place through which knights and their large retinues routinely passed.[1] Its proximity to the Cherwell also made Aynho an important point for crossing the river, traffic across which was controlled, from at least as early as 1226, by a bridge to which travellers were encouraged to give alms.[2] Although there is evidence of prehistoric settlement in

[1] A decree of Richard I (1189–99) stipulated that tournaments could be held between Brackley and Mixbury, which is just 9 km due east of Aynho on the road between Chipping Norton and Buckingham. For Richard's decree, see J. Barker, *The Tournament in England, 1100–1400* (Woodbridge, 1986), pp. 11, 53.

[2] *Rot. Welles*, vol. 2, p. 220. Later known as Nell Bridge: P. Goodfellow, 'Medieval Bridges in Northamptonshire', *Northamptonshire Past and Present*, 7 (1986), 143–58.

the surrounding area,[3] Aynho's origins in the documentary records can be traced back no earlier than the mid-eleventh century, with the first written mention of its existence coming from Domesday Book. There it is recorded as having belonged (before the Conquest) to Esgar the Staller, a known royal official and a leading citizen of London,[4] with its combined holdings in 1086 being valued at £8 and its population given as forty households.[5] Under William the Conqueror (1066–87), Esgar's extensive estates passed, in general, to Geoffrey (I) de Mandeville (†*c.*1100), who granted the tithe of the manor of Aynho to his monastic foundation at Hurley, Berkshire,[6] and through whose descendants the manor would eventually be granted to Alice of Essex and her husband, Roger Fitz Richard, founder of Aynho Hospital (see below).

Little today remains of Aynho's medieval parish church, dedicated to St Michael, of which there is no written record before the twelfth century. Its advowson belonged to the priory (later abbey) of Walden, to which the church had been granted *c.*1140 by the priory's founder, Geoffrey (II) de Mandeville, earl of Essex (†1144).[7] Walden's other possessions included the nearby church of Kingham, Oxfordshire, in which Ralph de Diceto, archdeacon of Middlesex and subsequent chronicler of the times, was instituted as parson by Robert Cheney, bishop of Lincoln (1148–66), around 1160.[8] It was likely at this same time (and certainly before 12 December 1164) that Ralph was also instituted as rector in the church of Aynho. He did not reside there, however, but instead installed as his perpetual vicar Turbert, son of Turbert, who discharged all the obligations of the cure and paid to Ralph two gold pieces a year.[9] Turbert, whose name is also rendered as Turbern

3 *An Inventory of the Historical Monuments in the County of Northampton* (6 vols, London, 1975–), vol. 4, p. 12.

4 A. Williams, 'Asgar the Staller (d. after 1066)', in *ODNB*, vol. 2, pp. 596–7.

5 *Domesday*, vol. 12: *Northamptonshire*, ed. F. Thorn and C. Thorn, 45.1.

6 Geoffrey's foundation charter for Hurley states that he granted to the priory the third part of the tithe of all his grain (*annona*) in all the manors that were at that time in his demesne ('… in omnibus maneriis que in dominio meo tempore erant […] tertiam partem decimae totius annone mee'): Dugdale, *Monasticon*, vol. 3, p. 433. That this included the tithe of Aynho appears confirmed by a charter of Richard of Ely, bishop of London (1189–98), although its form is suspect: *EEA*, vol. 26, no. 19, pp. 20-1.

7 L. Watkiss and D. Greenway (eds and trans.), *The Book of the Foundation of Walden Monastery* (Oxford, 1999), Appendix 2, no. 2, pp. 172–4. The priory's ownership was confirmed in 1156 × 1162 by Henry II: Vincent (ed.), *Henry II*, vol. 5, no. 2753, pp. 161–2.

8 *EEA*, vol. 1, no. 277, pp. 171–2.

9 The details of Ralph's installation are recorded in an act of Hugh of Avalon, bishop of Lincoln (1186–1200), concerning the presentation of his successor at Aynho. This

in Aynho documents, and who is therein described as 'parson' (*persona*) or 'rector' (*rector*),[10] was almost certainly the son of the Turbert/Turbern whose half a hide of land was granted to Aynho Hospital as part of its foundational endowment (see Chapter 2). Turbert/Turbern 'the younger' was still in post as perpetual vicar/parson in the early 1190s, since his position was confirmed at the petition of Ralph de *Verineto*, canon of Lincoln,[11] who had succeeded Ralph de Diceto as rector and was likely a relation of Warin de *Verineto*, a witness of five Aynho charters (nos. **36–9**, **41**). Shortly thereafter, Geoffrey Fitz Peter, earl of Essex (†1213), quit-claimed the church of Aynho to the abbot of Walden in return for the advowson during his and his son's lifetimes.[12] Half a century later, Isabella, widow of Roger Fitz John (†1249), great-grandson of Roger Fitz Richard, attempted to lay claim to the right of advowson, brandishing a somewhat suspicious looking charter supposedly kept in the archives of Langley Abbey, which had been founded by her late husband's grandfather.[13]

A century after the Domesday inquest, the manor of Aynho was valued at £30, and was home to four ploughs, 400 sheep, and thirteen pigs.[14] The nucleus of its church and central dwellings was surrounded by an open-field system, the distinctive organisation of which (at least in Northamptonshire terms) seems to have been determined in large part by the patchwork nature of the hospital's endowment (see Chapter 2). It was also via the hospital, which was located towards the vill's west end near a spring running down

act records how Ralph was installed at the presentation of William, prior of Walden, who was dead by 12 December 1164. The same act records the two gold pieces paid by Turbert to Ralph's successor, which is likely the amount Ralph also received: *EEA*, vol. 4, no. 204, p. 134.

10 See, nos. **3–4**, **39**, **41**, **46**, **A1**. Turbert/Turbern the parson is presumably also the same person as Turbert, chaplain, who appears in nos. **36–8**.

11 *EEA*, vol. 4, no. 204, p. 134. For Ralph as canon, see *Fasti*, vol. 3, p. 136.

12 Watkiss and Greenway (eds and trans), *Walden Monastery*, Appendix 2, no. 10.

13 BL, Harley MS 3697, fol. 49v (64v). The text of this charter, which is included in a broader account in the cartulary of Walden Abbey of the resolution of Isabella's claim, is essentially a garbled version of the act by which William de Mandeville granted the manor of Aynho to Roger Fitz Richard in 1170 (see below p. 22 n. 40), wherein Roger's name has been replaced by that of his son, William. The authors consulted the Walden manuscript at the British Library in September 2023, making a preliminary transcription of the act on folio 49v *in situ* (personal photography of the item not being allowed). Plans to consult this manuscript at greater length and to produce a critical edition of the act for inclusion in this book were thwarted by the Rhysida cyber-attack upon the British Library of 28 October 2023, which at the time of writing continues to prohibit all access to and reproduction of the document.

14 *Rot. de Dominabus*, p. 30.

to the Cherwell,[15] that Ayhno became connected with the nearby vill of Croughton, the chapel of which was donated to Aynho Hospital at the turn of the thirteenth century. Its parish church was under the patronage of the locally influential Neirenuit family,[16] who were also hospital benefactors (no. **28**).[17] From 1207, the brothers there had the right to hold a three-day fair each year around the feast of St James (see below), while by the early fourteenth century the right to hold both a fair and market had been granted to the lord of the manor, John (II) Fitz Robert (†1332), grandson, thrice removed, of Roger Fitz Richard.[18] By the 1480s, however, not only had Aynho manor passed from Clavering control to the earls of Arundel, but an endowment that in previous centuries had been sufficient for the hospital's charitable obligations was now no longer being put to such uses.[19] Moral, physical, and financial dilapidation nevertheless had a value of its own, especially to a man like William Waynflete, bishop of Winchester, who was then looking for properties with which to endow his new foundation at Oxford. Having acquired the hospital from the earl of Arundel, it was to Magdalen College's benefit that its landed possessions were transferred, along with its archive, in October 1483.[20]

## THE FOUNDING FAMILY

Aynho Hospital was founded by Roger Fitz Richard, second husband of Alice of Essex. Both figures have had much written about them over the last four centuries, although little of it is accurate. Roger was lord of Warkworth in Northumberland, the castle of which was granted to him by Henry II

15 Its precise location is unknown. The hospital is often said to have been on the site of 'College Farm' (e.g., Cooper, p. 31), now situate between Banbury Road and Station Road. However, archaeological investigations revealed no medieval remains in either the buildings or the wider area of the site: I.R. Scott, *College Farm, Aynho, Northamptonshire. Archaeological Evaluation Report* (Oxford, 1999). The antiquarian John Bridges (1666–1724), in describing the spring that issues to the west of the village 'near the spital', notes that it 'runs through the hospital down into the Cherwell': P. Whalley (ed.), *The History and Antiquities of Northamptonshire. Compiled from the Manuscript Collections of the Late Learned Antiquary John Bridges, Esq* (2 vols, Oxford, 1791), vol. 1, p. 134.

16 *EEA*, vol. 2, no. 117, p. 96.

17 For Miles Neirenuit, see Keats-Rohan (ed.), *Domesday Descendants*, pp. 1048–9.

18 *CChR*, 1300–26, p. 463.

19 The papal document authorising Aynho's appropriation to Magdalen College notes that 'hospitality had not for a long time been observed, and was not being observed': *CPL*, 1484–92, p. 183.

20 Davis, *William Waynflete*, pp. 146–7.

Plantagenet (1154–89) in 1157 × 1164,[21] and patriarch of the eventual house of Clavering, Essex. He certainly was not the son of Richard Fitz Eustace, constable of Chester (†1163), whose father, Eustace Fitz John (†1157), rose to prominence under Henry I (1100–1135),[22] a spurious assertion first made (as far as we are aware) by Henry Peacham (1578–*c.*1644), which has been repeated by generations of antiquarians (and sometimes scholars) thereafter.[23] Roger's grandchildren nevertheless had a connection to the Fitz Eustace line (the eventual house of Vescy), which traced its origins to Normandy and a certain Ranulf the moneyer,[24] since his daughter, Alice, married Richard Fitz Eustace's son, John Fitz Richard, constable of Chester (†1190), whose own grandchild, John, would be made Earl of Lincoln in 1232 (**Genealogy 2**). Aynho charters issued by his in-laws show John Fitz Richard among the witnesses, along with his sons Roger and Geoffrey (nos. **3**, **6–7**), the latter of whom would later be married to the daughter of Hubert de Rye at the direction of his uncle, Robert (I) Fitz Roger (see below).[25]

Roger Fitz Richard's actual origins are difficult to determine, save for the self-evident fact of his father's name. A note in a now-lost life of St Osyth by William de Vere, canon of the priory of St Osyth's, Essex, and later bishop of Hereford (1186–96), styles Roger as 'nepos comitis Hugonis Bigot',[26] which

[21] Vincent (ed.), *Henry II*, vol. 2, no. 997, pp. 221–2.

[22] For Eustace, see P. Dalton, 'Eustace Fitz John and the Politics of Twelfth-Century England: The Rise and Survival of a Twelfth-Century Royal Servant', *Speculum*, 71 (1996), 358–83.

[23] H. Peacham, *The Compleat Gentleman* (London, 1622), p. 190. For subsequent examples, see W. Dugdale, *The Baronage of England* (2 vols, London, 1675–6), vol. 1, p. 106; G. Ormerod, *The History of the County Palatine and City of Chester* (3 vols, London, 1819), vol. 1, p. 509; E. MacKenzie, *An Historical, Topographical, and Descriptive View of the County of Northumberland*, 2nd edn (2 vols, Newcastle upon Tyne, 1825), vol. 2, p. 29; Baker, vol. 1, p. 546; J. Burke, *A Genealogical and Heraldic History of the Commoners of Great Britain and Ireland* (4 vols, London, 1835–8), vol. 1, p. 238; C. Hartshorne, *Feudal and Military Antiquities of Northumberland and the Scottish Borders* (London, 1858), p. 189; J. Hodgson, *A History of Northumberland* (15 vols, Newcastle upon Tyne, 1899), vol. 5, p. 21; H. Colvin, *The White Canons in England* (Oxford, 1951), p. 150.

[24] Ranulf the moneyer held a mill at Bacilly in the parish of Vains (Manche, cant. Avranches), which had been sold to him by Suppo, abbot of Mont Saint-Michel (1033–42/8): M. Fauroux (ed.), *Recueil des actes des ducs de Normandie de 911 à 1066* (Caen, 1961), no. 148, pp. 330–3; D. Bates (ed.), *Regesta regum Anglo-Normannorum: The Acta of William I (1066–1087)* (Oxford, 1998), no. 214, p. 672–5.

[25] A fifteenth-century history of the Lacy family says only that John had sons called Roger and Eustace, along 'with many others' (*et plures alios*): Oxford, Bodleian Libraries, MS Dodsworth 157, fol. 2v (printed Dugdale, *Monasticon*, vol. 5, p. 534).

[26] L. Toulmin Smith (ed.), *The Itinerary of John Leland in or About the Years 1535–1543* (5 vols, London, 1906–10), vol. 5, p. 172.

can only be a reference to Hugh Bigod, 1st Earl of Norfolk (†1177). Since the note's author was Roger's brother-in-law, we can be reasonably confident that his description is an accurate one. That said, Hugh is not known to have had a brother called Richard, while none of his known sisters married a man by that name.[27] Both J.H. Round and C.T. Clay nevertheless thought that *nepos* should be understood here to mean 'nephew', with Clay arguing that Roger's mother was likely an unknown daughter of Hugh Bigod,[28] but the term might also be translated as 'cousin', 'kinsman', or 'grandson' (the last of which is not applicable in this instance).[29] As both Clay and Katharine Keats-Rohan have observed, William de Vere's genealogical notes in the life of St Osyth also qualify Roger as being the nephew of a certain Thomas, who is identified, again in a marginal note, as 'Thomas de Candelent'.[30] Frustratingly, his origins are as difficult to pin down as Roger Fitz Richard's, with Clay proposing 'Candelent' as a possible corruption of 'Cauntelo' (i.e., Canteloup, Normandy),[31] the anglicised form of which (Cantelupe/Cantilupe) was borne by a prominent gentry dynasty in twelfth-century East Anglia. Keats-Rohan suggests a connection with the manor of Candlet in Suffolk,[32] which was held, in 1086, by Northmann the sheriff from Roger Bigod to whom he was also bound in friendship forged through intercession for the dead.[33]

Whatever his precise relationship to the Bigods, Roger and his children certainly shared links with major aristocratic families embedded throughout both the secular and ecclesiastical hierarchies of the twelfth-century Anglo-Norman realm. The most important of these links, especially insofar as this book's subject is concerned, came as a result of Roger's marriage. Like her husband, Alice of Essex has been identified over the years with various people she was not, most frequently as either the wife or daughter of Henry of Essex (†aft. 1163), lord of Rayleigh and

27 For a family tree of the Bigods and their kin, see A. Wareham, 'The Motives and Politics of the Bigod Family, *c.*1066–1177', *ANS*, 17 (1995), 223–42, at p. 230.

28 J.H. Round, 'Who was Alice of Essex?', *Transactions of the Essex Archaeological Society*, n.s. 3 (1889), 243–51, at p. 247; C.T. Clay, 'The Ancestry of the Early Lords of Warkworth', *Archaeologia Aeliana*, 32 (1954), 65–71, at p. 68.

29 R. Latham, D. Howlett, and R. Ashdowne (eds), *Dictionary of Medieval Latin from British Sources* (London, 1975–2013), fasc. 7. N, p. 1906.

30 Toulmin Smith (ed.), *Itinerary of John Leland*, vol. 5, p. 172.

31 Clay, 'The Ancestry', p. 69.

32 Keats-Rohan (ed.), *Domesday People*, pp. 29, 306; Keats-Rohan (ed.), *Domesday Descendants*, p. 948.

33 A. Wareham, *Lords and Communities in Early Medieval East Anglia* (Woodbridge, 2005), p. 148.

second son of Robert Fitz Swein (†aft. 1130).[34] She was, in reality, the daughter of Aubrey (II) de Vere, royal chamberlain and justiciar (†May 1141), and his wife, Alice de Clare,[35] and therefore sister-in-law (through her first marriage) to Henry of Essex; sister to Aubrey de Vere, 1st Earl of Oxford (1141–94); sister-in-law (through her sister's marriage) to Geoffrey (II) de Mandeville, 1st Earl of Essex (†1144); and aunt to William de Mandeville, 3rd Earl of Essex (1166–89) (**Genealogy 3**).

Alice's first husband, Robert of Essex (†1132/40), eldest son of Robert Fitz Swein, died without issue. The date of her betrothal to Roger Fitz Richard is unknown, but it must have taken place not long after Robert's death, since Alice was born in 1105/6,[36] meaning that by 1140 she would have been approaching an age when childbearing became more difficult. She instead had three children with Roger Fitz Richard: two sons, Robert (the eventual heir) and William, as well as a daughter, Alice, all of whom appear in Aynho charters (and, in William's case, seemingly uniquely so).[37] Alice continued to be known as 'of Essex' following her second marriage, as at least one of the hospital's charters bears witness (no. **3**), most likely because her new husband's social status was considered inferior to that of her first. Her marriage portion of Clavering, in the fee of Henry of Essex,

34 For daughter, see R. Eyton, 'Robert Fitz Wimarch and his Descendants', *Transactions of the Shropshire Archaeological and Natural History Society*, 2 (1879), 1–34, at pp. 27–9; for wife, see Dugdale, *Baronage*, vol. 1, p. 463; Hartshorne, *Feudal Antiquities*, p. 191.

35 Alice's origins are largely unpicked in Round, 'Who was Alice?', pp. 243–51. However, Round believed Alice to have been the second wife of Robert Fitz Swein and thus stepmother to Henry: ibid., p. 246. Katharine Keats-Rohan has demonstrated convincingly that Robert cannot have married Alice and that she instead married his son by that name: Keats-Rohan (ed.), *Domesday Descendants*, pp. 450–1, 761.

36 Alice appears twice in the 1185/6 royal inquest of widows and wards then in the king's gift. Her age is given as 60 in one instance and as 80 in another: *Rot. de Dominabus*, pp. 29, 76. The earliest date at which her first husband was dead is 1132 and the latest 1140. Had Alice been born in 1125/6 and thus aged 60 in 1185/6, she would have been betrothed to Robert of Essex as a child either under the age of 10 or only just over it (assuming, of course, that Robert died shortly after the marriage). Such a young age is not impossible (the *Rotuli dominabus* records, for example, that Matilda de Bidune was a widow at 10: ibid., p. 49), but it seems more likely that Alice was born in 1105/6 and was therefore either 27 or 35 at the time of her first husband's death.

37 The *Foundation for Medieval Genealogy's* 'Medieval Lands' dataset lists four other children alongside Robert and Alice (it does not list William at all), namely Richard, Roger, Thomas, and Emma: <https://fmg.ac/Projects/MedLands/ENGLISHNOBILITYMEDIEVAL3D-K.htm#RogerFitzRicharddiedbefore1185>. However, there is no direct evidence linking any of these individuals to Roger Fitz Richard. Since their activities relate to Lancashire and Yorkshire, in which Roger Fitz Richard is not known to have had any interest, their origins are to be sought elsewhere.

nevertheless descended to her sons by Roger Fitz Richard.[38] It was also via her Essex connections that Alice received the manor of Aynho in free dower from Earl William (II) de Mandeville 'over and above those lands that were given her in dower by Roger Fitz Richard',[39] to whom the earl of Essex granted Aynho in 1170 in exchange for the manor Roger held from the earl at Long Compton, Warwickshire.[40] The date of Roger's death is unclear, but he was still alive during what is now known as the 'Great Revolt' against Henry II Plantagenet in 1173/4. The revolt must have proved a particularly awkward moment for Roger, given that his 'uncle' Hugh Bigod was among the rebels and his wife's nephew an ally of the king.[41] He was nevertheless one of the few northern barons to side with Henry, as was his daughter's brother-in-law, William de Vescy.[42] As a result, the castle of Warkworth, the defences of which Jordan Fantosme describes as 'feeble' (*fieble*), was sacked in 1174 by William the Lion, king of Scots (1165–1214).[43] Roger subsequently moved to defend Newcastle upon Tyne, where he held land from the king,[44] refusing to surrender the city.[45] Nothing is known of his fate after the rebellion, but he was certainly dead before 1185, when his widow, Alice, was registered as being in the king's gift with regard to her manors at Clavering and Aynho.[46] The date of her own death is also unknown, but it must have been shortly after 1185, as it was Henry II who granted her manor

38 A return appended to the 1166 *Cartae baronum* shows Clavering had been granted to Roger Fitz Richard at an undetermined date: H. Hall (ed.), *The Red Book of the Exchequer* (3 vols, London, 1986), vol. 1, p. 359.

39 This charter is known only by a seventeenth-century description of it, first noticed by J.H. Round (Round, 'Who was Alice?', p. 245), citing BL, MS Harley 259, fol. 67r. It is actually to be found in BL, MS Lansdowne 259, fol. 67r.

40 J.H. Round, 'A Charter of William, Earl of Essex (1170)', *EHR*, 6 (1891), 364–7. Roger's then or future son-in-law, John, constable of Chester, is among the witnesses of this act.

41 For a full account of the revolt, see M. Strickland, *Henry the Young King, 1155–1183* (New Haven, CT, 2016), pp. 151–205.

42 J. Green, 'Aristocratic Loyalties on the Northern Frontier of England, circa 1100–1174', in D. Williams (ed.), *England in the Twelfth Century: Proceedings of the 1988 Harlaxton Symposium* (Woodbridge, 1990), pp. 83–100, at p. 99.

43 R.C. Johnston (ed.), *Jordan Fantosme's Chronicle* (Oxford, 1981), p. 42; '… et ipse [rex Scottorum] cum reliqua parte et baronum suorum devastans, et cepit armis […] castellum de Werkeurda, quod Rogerus filius Ricardi custodivit': Roger of Howden, *Gesta regis Henrici secundi Benedicti abbatis: The Chronicle of the Reigns of Henry II and Richard I, A.D. 1169–1192*, ed. W. Stubbs (2 vols, London, 1867), vol. 1, p. 65.

44 The Pipe Rolls of Henry II record Roger in receipt of an annual allowance of £20 for *terra data* in Newcastle: *PR* 2–4 Henry II, pp. 177–8; 5 Henry II, p. 13; 6 Henry II, p. 56.

45 Johnston (ed.), *Fantosme's Chronicle*, p. 42.

46 *Rot. de Dominabus*, pp. 29–30, 76–7.

of Clavering to her son, Robert.[47] Alice was buried in the Lady Chapel of Walden Abbey, to which she had apparently retired in widowhood at the instigation of her nephew, William de Mandeville.[48]

Of Roger's and Alice's children, all three were alive when their father founded Aynho Hospital. As has already been noted, their younger son, William Fitz Roger, is known only from the hospital's charters, but it is possible that he is the William Fitz Roger named by Roger of Howden as being among the adherents of Henry the Young King (1155–83).[49] Kate Norgate identified this William as the William Fitz Roger recorded as holding land in Hampshire in the 1158 Pipe Roll, although seemingly on grounds no more substantial than that the two men shared the same name.[50] We, admittedly, have little more to go on. It is interesting to note, however, that a William Fitz Roger can be found among the witnesses of a charter of the Young King issued at Alençon around September 1180 for Waltham Abbey, Essex, located some 30 km (as the crow flies) from Clavering.[51] Had our William indeed joined the young Henry in rebellion, then he would have also found himself in opposition to his own father, who stayed loyal to Henry II throughout.[52] Of course, participation in revolt does not necessarily imply action without familial consent, as the splitting of loyalties at a time of internecine conflict was a long-established tactic among the nobility, guaranteeing a family's fortunes no matter the outcome. But it may yet explain William's subsequent absence from the historical record. Having hitched his star to the Young King, William Fitz Roger may have found himself in the wake of 1173/4 estranged from both the royal court and his father, wandering northern France with Henry's household as the disaffected and defeated royal prince made his way around the tournament circuit.[53]

That said, the charters of Aynho Hospital also allow us to paint a somewhat different – and, on balance, rather more likely – picture, one in which William Fitz Roger was not necessarily an erstwhile opponent of the Crown

47 Vincent (ed.), *Henry II*, vol. 2, no. 1001, pp. 223–4.

48 Watkiss and Greenway (eds and trans), *Walden Monastery*, p. 76.

49 Roger of Howden, *Gesta regis Henrici*, vol. 1, p. 46.

50 K. Norgate, *England under the Angevin Kings* (2 vols, London, 1887), vol. 2, p. 139 n. 2.

51 J. Conway Davies (ed.), *The Cartae Antiquae, Rolls 11–20* (London, 1960), no. 359, pp. 42–4. For its date, see R.J. Smith, 'Henry II's Heir: The *Acta* and Seal of Henry the Young King, 1170–83', *EHR*, 116 (2001), 297–326, at p. 326 (no. 32).

52 On the young Henry's exploitation of tensions between fathers and sons, see Strickland, *Young King*, pp. 141–50. See also, D. Power, *The Norman Frontier in the Twelfth and Early Thirteenth Centuries* (Cambridge, 2004), pp. 400–1.

53 For Henry after the Great Revolt, see Strickland, *Young King*, pp. 206–38.

but simply a second son who, like all too many of his contemporaries, died prematurely. Interpreted in this context, these charters offer insights into emerging patterns of inheritance in later twelfth-century England, and, more specifically, into the role played by Earl William de Mandeville in the administration of his estates, which, in the wake of his death in 1189, became the subject of a protracted dispute.[54] As noted above, the manor of Aynho was given to Alice of Essex in free dower by her nephew, who then granted it to Roger Fitz Richard to administer on her behalf (just as Roger would have continued to do with the lands he himself gave Alice in dower from his own estates).[55] Although inheritance practices at this time were still in a state of flux, it was customary for second sons to inherit the marriage portion of their mothers' estates, with major feudal lords like William de Mandeville explicitly acknowledging the rights of some younger sons in this respect.[56] That the earl might similarly have acknowledged William Fitz Roger as heir to his mother's dower lands at Aynho is suggested by the latter's acts in the Aynho Cartulary. The first is known only by the cartulary copy (no. **5**), the original being lost, but its reference to William de Mandeville's brother and predecessor, Earl Geoffrey, suggests that it was issued shortly after the hospital's foundation. Its content, whereby William Fitz Roger confirms his father's grant without adding anything to it, is typical of the sort of consent sought from someone with a future vested interest (i.e., an heir). By 1185, Roger Fitz Richard was dead, with his widow, Alice, recorded as holding her Aynho manor from William de Mandeville, and both her sons as being still alive.[57] However, William Fitz Roger's second act in the cartulary (no. **6**), whereby he both confirms the hospital's foundation *and* contributes to it (or at least claims to be doing the latter),[58] suggests that, by this point, it was he who had been entrusted by the earl with Aynho's administration in the same way as his father had before him. The instrument by which this transaction took place is no longer extant,[59] but the cartulary does

54 For discussion, see R.V. Turner, 'The Mandeville Inheritance, 1189–1236: Its Legal, Political and Social Context', *Haskins Society Journal*, 1 (1989), 147–72.

55 On women and their landed property, see J. Ward, *Women of the English Nobility and Gentry, 1066–1500* (Manchester, 2013), pp. 85–121.

56 See, for example, William's acknowledgement of Geoffrey de Say, younger son of Beatrice de Mandeville, as the heir apparent to his mother's marriage portion: J.C. Holt, *Colonial England 1066–1215* (London, 1997), pp. 313–14.

57 'Arenho quod est manerium ejus, quod etiam tenet de comite Willelmo', *Rot. de Dominabus*, pp. 29–30. The same source also shows that William Fitz Roger was still living, as it records (in the present tense) that Alice 'has two sons, knights' ('habet ii. filios milites').

58 See Chapter 2.

59 It is possible that the memory of just such a lost act is conserved in the garbled charter produced by Isabella, widow of Roger Fitz John, in support of her claim

contain an act in which William de Mandeville confirms the donations made to Aynho Hospital not just by Roger and his wife, but also specifically by William (no. **10**). William's older brother, Robert, on the other hand, is conspicuously absent from this act, and while he himself would later issue a charter similar to no. **6** both confirming the hospital's foundational grant *and* making his own contribution to it (no. **7**), this can be clearly dated to the early 1190s, when Robert was in full enjoyment of the manor. In the period that separates these acts, Alice herself had retired to Walden Abbey, whose foundation chronicle records an episode that suggests her younger son and heir, William, had predeceased her, thus making Robert the sole remaining male heir to both his mother's and father's estates.[60]

Alice's daughter, also called Alice, married John Fitz Richard, constable of Chester, taking her story away from Warkworth, Clavering, and Aynho. Her husband departed for the Holy Land in March 1190 as part of the Third Crusade, probably in the stead of his lord, Ranulf III, earl of Chester (1181–1232), but died shortly thereafter at the siege of Acre or while convalescing at Tyre in 1190.[61] Alice herself was still alive in 1185,[62] but it is not known whether she predeceased her husband or he her. Her eldest brother, Robert, inherited the manor of Clavering and the castle of Warkworth from their father during the final years of Henry II's reign,[63] at which time we must assume that the manor of Aynho also passed to him (and at least, it would

concerning the advowson of Aynho's church (see above p. 17 n. 13), for while this act is almost certainly a forgery, it seems difficult to explain why it should have been forged in William's name unless there was some (distant) recollection of him as administrator of the manor.

60 The *Walden Foundation Book* records how Alice held land she had received from her first husband, Robert, and, 'having retained possession of this land until her own death, [she] left it to her son and heir Robert whom she had had by her second husband Roger' (*terram iam dictam usque ad mortem propriam retinens, filio suo et heredi Roberto quem de alio viro nomine Rogero susceperat dimisit)*: Watkiss and Greenway (eds and trans), *Walden Monastery*, p. 76. Given how William Fitz Roger seems to have been recognised in relation to Aynho, which had come to Alice through her second marriage to Roger Fitz Richard, it is plausible that he might similarly have been heir to the land she had through her previous marriage – unless, of course, William had died by then.

61 S. Bennett, *Elite Participation in the Third Crusade* (Martlesham, 2021), pp. 104, 143, 320. A fifteenth-century history of the Lacy family printed by Dugdale incorrectly gives his date of death as 11 October 1183, which is the one encountered most frequently in the historiography: Dugdale, *Monasticon*, vol. 5, p. 534. However, the original manuscript of this history actually gives his date of death as 'idus octobris anno Domini M. C. LXX. III°': Oxford, Bodleian Libraries, MS Dodsworth 157, fol. 2v.

62 Her existence and marriage to John is recorded in *Rot. de Dominabus*, p. 29.

63 For Clavering, see above, p. 22 n. 38. For Warkworth, see *Rot. Chart.*, p. 187b.

seem, before the Mandeville estates became embroiled in the inheritance dispute following Earl William's death). It was during the reigns of King Richard I the Lionheart (1189–99) and King John (1199–1216), however, that the family's interests began to expand beyond its traditional holdings in Northumberland, Northamptonshire, and Essex. In the first instance, at some point before Michaelmas 1190, Robert Fitz Roger married Margaret (†1231), widow of Hugh de Cressy (†1188/9) and daughter and heir of William de Chesney (*Caisneto*) (†1174), who had himself been hereditary High Sheriff of Norfolk and Suffolk and was founding patron of the abbey of Sibton, Suffolk.[64] Through his marriage, Robert Fitz Roger received seisin of his wife's significant estates in East Anglia and subsequently served, like his late father-in-law before him, as sheriff of Norfolk and Suffolk (1190–94; 1197–1200).[65] Robert also became a monastic patron, again in imitation of his father-in-law, founding the Premonstratensian abbey of Langley (Norfolk) in 1195.[66]

Outside East Anglia, Robert was able to expand his estates both into new parts of England and within his family's traditional heartlands. Thus, in 1194 (and again, in 1198), Richard the Lionheart confirmed to Robert the manor of Iver in Buckinghamshire, which in the time of Henry II had been held by Gilbert de Vere, Robert's maternal uncle,[67] and which Robert himself now held of the king for the service of one knight's fee.[68] In 1199, after the accession of John, Robert paid 100 marks to decide the marriage of his stepson, Roger de Cressy (†1246).[69] He also gave 300 marks to secure all the lands he had received under kings Henry and Richard, and an equivalent sum to have the youngest daughter of Hubert de Rye in marriage for his nephew, Geoffrey, son of his sister, Alice, and John Fitz Richard, late constable of Chester.[70] Though not all of these endeavours

64 On the de Chesney family, see S. Yarrow, *Saints and Their Communities: Miracle Stories in Twelfth-Century England* (Oxford, 2006), pp. 145–6; J. Green, *English Sheriffs to 1154* (London, 1990), p. 61.

65 On Robert as sheriff and on the lands acquired through his marriage, see J.H. Round, 'The Early Sheriffs of Norfolk', *EHR*, 35 (1920), 481–96, at pp. 492–5.

66 The foundation was confirmed by Richard the Lionheart on 1 September 1197 (*CChR*, 1300–26, pp. 480–1) and again by King John on 7 July 1199 (Dugdale, *Monasticon*, vol. 6, part 2, p. 930).

67 *BF*, vol. 1, p. 116.

68 L. Landon (ed.), *The Cartae Antiquae, Rolls 1–10* (London, 1939), no. 549, pp. 155–6; TNA, PRO C52/29, Cartae Antiquae Roll 29, m. 2, no. 7.

69 *PR* 1 John, p. 273; H.G. Richardson (ed.), *The Memoranda Roll for the Michaelmas Term of the First Year of the Reign of King John, 1199–1200* (London, 1943), p. 79.

70 *Rot. Fin.*, p. 14. Geoffrey is not mentioned by name in the oblation and fine rolls, but we know he married Hubert's daughter, Isabella, since Roger de Cressy, Robert Fitz Roger's stepson, married Isabella, who is described as Geoffrey's former wife,

bore fruit, it was under King John that Robert's fortunes expanded greatly. In Northumberland, where he served as sheriff for the greater part of the king's reign (1200–12) and was a generous benefactor of Durham Cathedral Priory,[71] the *Book of Fees* shows that by 1212 Robert, in addition to Warkworth, held lands at Whalton, Rothbury, Newburn, and Corbridge.[72] It is possible that the considerable amount of money spent by Robert in 1199 had been underwritten by credit, for on 9 September 1208 three merchants of Bologna were licensed to spend 820 marks on buying and exporting Stamford cloth. This sum derived from the repayment of a loan made to Robert Fitz Roger, which makes him the earliest known English layman to receive such an Italian advance. Whatever the case may be, Robert was also trading under his own initiative, having been licenced in April 1206 to export corn from Tynemouth.[73] He died on 22 November 1214,[74] and was buried in his monastic foundation at Langley.[75]

The one thing so far missing from this potted narrative of Robert's life is, of course, Aynho and its hospital. Robert issued three charters in favour of his father's foundation, two of which certainly date from the beginning of his majority (nos. **7**–**8**), as is also likely the case with the third (no. **9**). At first glance, one might be forgiven for thinking that these three acts reflect Robert's disinterest in Aynho, given their limited number, the relatively small scale of the donations, and their concentration in the earlier part of his lordship. On 10 June 1207, however, the king himself granted to the hospital the right to hold a fair (*feria*) for three days before, during, and after the feast of St James (25 July), a significant concession that was perhaps made with Robert's encouragement or in reward for his loyal service to the Crown.[76] Of course, by the beginning of the thirteenth century, the manor and hospital of Aynho formed just one part of Robert's increasingly expanding network of estates. What is more, as John Holt noted in his seminal study of the northern lords under John, those barons like Robert

without royal permission: *PR* 9 John, p. 178. As punishment, Roger's lands were escheated not to Robert Fitz Roger but to Robert of Burgate: S.D. Church, *The Household Knights of King John* (Cambridge, 1999), p. 54.

71 Robert made various grants to the monks from his estates at Warkworth and Follingsby: Durham University Archives, 1.1.Spec.50, 2.4.Spec.8, 4.3.Sacr.3.

72 *BF*, vol. 1, pp. 200–1.

73 For both the loan and the licence to trade, see M. Prestwich, *The Place of War in English History, 1066–1214* (Woodbridge, 2004), pp. 57–8.

74 Colvin, *White Monks*, p. 152.

75 J. Weever, *Antient Funeral Monuments, of Great-Britain, Ireland, and the Islands Adjacent* (London, 1767), p. 548, who cites a lost copy of the abbey's annals.

76 *Rot. Chart.*, p. 167b. For the markets and fairs of Northamptonshire more generally, see P. Goodfellow, 'Medieval Markets in Northamptonshire', *Northamptonshire Past and Present*, 7 (1987–8), 305–23.

with estates divided between the north and south frequently found their attentions – not to mention their loyalties – similarly divided.[77] In a period of expanding fortunes and political turmoil, it is therefore little wonder that the relatively small operation at Aynho might have captured only a similarly small but not insignificant part of its lord's benevolence.

Robert, who remained a trusted and important member of the royal household until the end,[78] did not live to see the dramatic denouement of John's reign. By contrast, his son and heir, John (I) Fitz Robert, would come to play a central role in it. Best known today as one of the Twenty-Five barons chosen to act as surety for Magna Carta, the seeds of John's rebellion against his namesake were likely sown early on. His widowed mother had proffered £1,000 for seisin of her husband's estates, an exceptionally large sum, only for the king to insist on holding Norwich castle for himself.[79] John Fitz Robert eventually had the castle in his custody,[80] as well as the shrievalty of Norfolk and Suffolk, in which role the king commanded the son of his openly rebellious half-brother, Roger de Cressy, be handed over to him,[81] but he was never elevated to the same level of royal trust as his father had been. John's precise role in the eventual rebellion in the North is difficult to determine, but it has been suggested that he may have been second in command to Eustace de Vescy (†1216), his distant relative.[82] The immediate consequences of his actions are much easier to establish, since, by 25 June 1215, the king, angry and bruised, had commanded that the shrievalty of Norfolk and Suffolk be handed over to John Marshal.[83] Some six months later, John paid a visit to Iver in Buckinghamshire, the manor of which belonged to John Fitz Robert, as part of a progression around rebel baron estates that was likely designed with intimidation and reprisals in mind.[84] Three months after that, he gave John's manor of Aynho over to Thomas de Saint-Valery.[85]

77 J.C. Holt, *The Northerners: A Study in the Reign of King John* (Oxford, 1992), pp. 62–3.

78 For Robert's lasting place within John's inner circle, and his wider place within this circle, see Holt, *The Northerners*, pp. 217–50.

79 *PR* 16 John, p. 175.

80 Round, 'Early Sheriffs', p. 495.

81 T. Stapelton (ed.) *Magni rotuli Scaccarii Normanniae sub regibus Angliae* (2 vols, London, 1840–4), vol. 2, p. cxix.

82 S. Painter, *The Reign of King John* (Baltimore, 1949), p. 355.

83 *Rot. Litt. Pat.*, p. 144.

84 *Rot. Litt. Claus.*, vol. 1, p. 242a. On John's motivations for visiting Iver in December 1215, see 'King John's Diary & Itinerary: John tours the lands of rebels' at <https://magnacartaresearch.org/read/ itinerary/John_tours_the_lands_of_rebels>.

85 *Rot. Litt. Claus.*, vol. 1, p. 254a (act dated 17 Mar 1216).

The minority and early years of Henry III's (1216–72) reign proved comparatively less turbulent for John Fitz Robert, even if he continued under the new regime to feel the consequences of his rebellion.[86] Now loyal to the Crown,[87] which was not something that could be said of his half-brother, Roger de Cressy,[88] he spent the next decades slowly doing under Henry what his father had done under John, expanding his estates and influence (although not, it should be noted, with the young king himself, whose household was tightly controlled until 1221 by Peter des Roches).[89] The most significant development at this time concerned John's marriage to Ada, daughter of Hugh de Balliol (†1229). Ada brought with her not only a further estate at Stokesley, Yorkshire, but important connections that would eventually extend the family's interests beyond England's borders.[90] These were to be capitalised upon most significantly via the couple's own children, two of whom married into the line of the earls of Dunbar (**Genealogy 1**). By the mid-1220s, John himself seems to have moved somewhat closer to the royal orbit. He was present with Henry on 18 August 1224, along with a notable gathering of former rebels, shortly after the siege of Bedford Castle,[91] in the build up to which John had perhaps granted what is his only known act for the hospital at Aynho (no. **14**).[92] By April 1225, and presumably as reward for his perceived loyalty, the king had not only given John custody of the county of Northumberland, but also specific privileges concerning its ports, coastline, and forests,[93] as well as the right to hold a fair for two days around the feast of Thomas Becket (29 December) in his

[86] On 8 November 1217, the king granted the farm of John's manor of Corbridge to Philip de Ulecot, his seneschal: *CPR*, 1216–25, p. 124.

[87] He is recorded as being so on 25 July 1217: *Rot. Litt. Claus.*, vol. 1, p. 316b.

[88] Roger was among those captured fighting at Lincoln against Nicholaa de la Haye and royalist forces in May 1217: Round, 'Early Sheriffs', p. 495.

[89] For the early entourage of Henry III, see D. Carpenter, *Henry III: The Rise to Power and Personal Rule, 1207–1258* (New Haven, CT, 2021), pp. 20–2.

[90] According to an inquest held in the reign of Edward I, John received the manor of Stokesley from Ada's father 'in maritagium': W. Illingworth (ed.), *Placita de quo warranto temporibus Edw. I. II. & III. In curia receptæ scaccarij Westm. asservata* (London, 1818), p. 194a.

[91] *CPR*, 1216–25, p. 495.

[92] Prior to besieging Bedford, the king was at Northampton, where he had summoned his magnates for counsel and whence royal forces were directed on Bedford: D. Carpenter, *The Minority of Henry III* (Berkeley, CA, 1990), pp. 359–62. Given the proximity of Aynho to these events (just 36 km, as the crow flies, from Northampton and 56 km from Bedford), and the fact that John was with the king in August, it is possible that he visited his Northamptonshire estates at this time.

[93] *Rot. Litt. Claus.*, vol. 1, pp. 618b, 643b (acts of 29 Aug 1224); *CPR*, 1216–25, pp. 496 (act of 12 Nov 1224), 522 (act of 27 Apr 1225).

manor of Stokesley.[94] On 20 July 1226, Henry issued a writ to replevy the land in Aynho given in alms to the hospital by a certain Hugh of Compton (*Cu[m]pton'*) until it could be determined whether it had been given as surety for a debt owed to the Jews.[95] Four years later, and after a number of abortive attempts to cross to France, Henry III finally set sail with his army from Portsmouth on 1 May 1230 to lay claim to his inheritance there.[96] John Fitz Robert was with the royal host, since he is listed among those magnates given letters of protection eleven days earlier,[97] while Henry, having been subsequently bogged down at Nantes, granted him further such letters on 24 June 1230 'for as long as [John] might be in service of the lord king in parts overseas' (*quamdiu fuerit in servicio domini regis in partibus transmarinis*).[98] On the fringes of the royal court, and without family lands to recover in France, John can hardly have found the expedition an appealing prospect.[99] By October, the king was back at Portsmouth, the whole enterprise having proved an abject failure. John Fitz Robert largely disappears from royal records in the expedition's aftermath, and, when he does noticeably resurface in 1237/8, it is to be constrained on no fewer than four separate occasions to hand over land in Northumberland and Cumbria to Alexander II, king of Scots (1214–49).[100]

John Fitz Robert died in late 1240 or early 1241. His passing is recorded by Matthew Paris, who not only described John as 'a noble man and one of the foremost barons of northern England' (*vir nobilis et unus de precipuis baronibus in plaga Anglie boreali*), but also preserved for us a drawing of his shield.[101] John's sons were still not of age, but his widow, Ada, was able to

94 *Rot. Litt. Claus.*, vol. 1, p. 618b (act of 29 Aug 1224).

95 *Rot. Litt. Claus.*, vol. 2, p. 130a. The writ, addressed to the sheriff of Northamptonshire, ends by saying that it is specifically 'for John son of Robert' (*pro Iohanne filio Roberti*).

96 For the background to this expedition, which was first mooted in 1227, see Carpenter, *Henry III*, pp. 77–85.

97 *CPR*, 1225–32, pp. 357–62, at p. 362.

98 *CPR*, 1225–32, p. 380.

99 Even for those magnates with significant estates lost in France, the expedition's aim of recovering them seemed to present more of a can of worms than a golden opportunity: Carpenter, *Henry III*, pp. 95–6.

100 *CPR*, 1232–47, pp. 197, 199, 213, 215 (acts of 28 Sep 1237, 27 Oct 1237, 16 Mar 1238 and 7 Apr 1238). For the context in which this land was to be given to Alexander, see M.A. Pollock, *Scotland, England and France after the Loss of Normandy, 1204–1296: 'Auld Amitie'* (Woodbridge, 2015), pp. 127–8.

101 Paris places his death in 1240: H.R. Luard (ed.), *Matthæi Parisiensis, monachi Sancti Albani, Chronica majora* (7 vols, London, 1872–83), vol. 4, p. 80. John was certainly dead by 14 February 1241, when a die he held in Canterbury of the archbishop of Canterbury was granted to Edward, son of Odo of Westminster: *CPR*, 1232–47,

purchase their guardianship for 2,000 marks, receiving in addition all the lands John held through their marriage as well as the manors of Newburn, Whalton, and Iver.[102] It was seemingly at her initiative that a double marriage alliance was forged with the family of Patrick II, earl of Dunbar (1232–49), first through her daughter, Cecilia, who married the earl's eldest son, the future Patrick III (1249–89), and secondly through her eldest son, Roger, who was betrothed to the earl's daughter, Isabella, to whom Aynho was given in dower.[103] Whatever hopes Ada may have had for her husband's heir were abruptly ended a few years later, however, when Roger Fitz John, then still an adolescent (*etate adolescens*), was trampled to death in May 1249 at a tournament at Argences, Normandy. His mother offered 1,200 marks for the guardianship of Roger's infant son, Robert (II) Fitz Roger, aged only eighteen months,[104] but the king instead handed him over, along with the castle of Warkworth and many other of his lands, to his own half-brother, William de Valence, 1st Earl of Pembroke (†1296).[105]

His father dead, and his mother having married a second time,[106] Robert Fitz Roger then lost his paternal grandmother in 1251.[107] His mother, however, was able to dispute Valence's title to Corbridge, where it has been argued she raised her young son.[108] It would seem that Robert's maternal grandmother, Euphemia, countess of Dunbar (†1267), who had been widowed in the same year as her daughter, was also living at Corbridge and there played a significant role in her grandson's upbringing, for Robert would later grant 40s of rent to Aynho Hospital on condition that its

p. 245. See also C. Roberts (ed.), *Excerpta è rotulis finium in Turri londinensi asservatis, Henrico Tertio rege, A.D. 1216–1272* (2 vols, London, 1835-6), vol. 1, p. 337. The drawing of John's shield can be found in Cambridge, Corpus Christi College, MS 16II, fol. 140r.

102 Roberts (ed.), *Excerpta è rotulis*, vol. 1, p. 342; *CCR*, 1237–42, pp. 279, 298.

103 The connection between the two families was first identified by A. MacEwen, 'A Clarification of the Dunbar Pedigree', *The Genealogist*, 9 (1988), 229–41, at pp. 231–4, who nevertheless considered the evidence he gathered to be 'circumstantial' (p. 231). The connection between Patrick II's daughter and Roger Fitz John is confirmed by an Aynho document (see below), of which MacEwen was unaware. Isabella was granted seisin of the manor of Aynho on 9 August 1249 after her husband's death: *CCR*, 1247–51, p. 190.

104 His age is given in a writ issued after the inquisition *post mortem*, dated 22 June 1249, meaning Roger was born in early 1248: *CIPM*, vol. 1, p. 41.

105 Luard (ed.), *Chronica majora*, vol. 5, p. 92; F. Madden (ed.), *Matthæi Parisiensis, monachi Sancti Albani, Historia anglorum* (3 vols, London 1866–9), vol. 3, p. 67.

106 Isabella's second husband was Simon Baard of Northumberland: MacEwen, 'Clarification', p. 233.

107 Roberts (ed.), *Excerpta è rotulis*, vol. 2, p. 115.

108 H.H.E. Craster, *A History of Northumberland* (15 vols, Newcastle upon Tyne, 1914), vol. 10, p. 68.

brothers maintained a suitable chaplain, to be chosen by Robert and his heirs, who would celebrate the divine office for his grandmother's soul (no. **A10**). This act, which has all but escaped scholarly notice, not only suggests an especially close bond between Robert and Euphemia but also provides a key piece of evidence linking Robert's father to a daughter of the Dunbar line.[109] That Robert chose Aynho as the place to institute this chaplain – rather than somewhere like Blythburgh Priory, of which he was a benefactor, the manor having passed to him in 1263,[110] or his great-grandfather's foundation at Langley, where some of his ancestors were buried – also illustrates the continuing importance of Aynho Hospital within the nexus of Clavering estates. Robert also clearly felt some affection for his paternal grandmother's family, since he referred to Ada's brother, Hugh de Balliol (†1292), as 'his very dear uncle' (*son tres cher oncle*),[111] and was an early benefactor of her other brother's new foundation at Oxford.[112] But, as this suggests, if Aynho and the family's foundational estates were not insignificant, Robert's activities, which played out largely in the reign of Edward I (1272–1307), frequently took him far from Northamptonshire and beyond

[109] The original charter, the text of which is not copied in the Aynho Cartulary, is damaged at the point containing this clause, such that most of Euphemia's name has been obscured. William Macray, who calendared the Aynho deeds at Magdalen College (see Introduction), drew attention to the charter's existence, although without a reference number and with only the first letter of Euphemia's name: *Fourth Report of the Royal Commission on Historical Manuscripts. Part I. Report and Appendix* (London, 1874), p. 460. She is misidentified as 'Elizabeth' in VCH, *Northampton*, vol. 7, p. 150. The first two letters ('Eu–') are, in fact, still visible. Andrew MacEwen, who was the first to make the connection between Roger Fitz Robert and Isabella of Dunbar, was unaware of the Aynho act at the time of his 1988 article (see above, n. 103), although later communicated Macray's notice to Douglas Richardson: D. Richardson, *Magna Carta Ancestry: A Study in Colonial and Medieval Families*, 2nd edn (Salt Lake City, UT, 2011), p. 489 n. 269. Euphemia is also correctly identified in Fry, 'Hospitality', p. 78, although without any further commentary.

[110] C. Harper-Bill (ed.), *Blythburgh Priory Cartulary* (2 vols, Woodbridge, 1980–1), vol. 1, no. 41, p. 46. The manor passed to Robert following the death of Stephen de Cressy, grandson of Robert's great-grandmother, Margaret, without issue.

[111] Oxford, Bodleian Libraries, MS Dodsworth 49, fol. 45v. Calendared in A.M. Oliver (ed.), *Northumberland and Durham Deeds: From the Dodsworth MSS. in Bodley's Library, Oxford* (Newcastle upon Tyne, 1929), p. 283. For the identification of this Hugh as Ada's brother, rather than her nephew through her brother, John, see A. Beam, *The Balliol Dynasty 1210–1364* (Edinburgh, 2008), p. xix.

[112] J. Bain, G. Simpson, and J. Galbraith (eds), *Calendar of Documents Relating to Scotland preserved in Her Majesty's Public Record Office, London* (5 vols, Edinburgh, 1881-6), vol. 2, no. 326, p. 89.

the chronological scope of this book,[113] such that there is neither room nor need to chronicle them in detail here. He died in debt at some point before 1310,[114] and was succeeded by his son, John (II) Fitz Robert, to whose wife, Hawise, he had given £100 in dower from his manor at Aynho.[115]

## FOUNDING AYNHO HOSPITAL

Having set Aynho Hospital within the wider contexts of the vill itself and its founding family, we now turn to look at its establishment, both from a chronological and motivational perspective. In terms of chronology, while we are fortunate to have the hospital's 'founding charter' (no. **4**), this, like many others issued in relation to England's medieval hospitals, contains no precise dating clause. Previous scholarship has therefore traditionally placed Aynho Hospital's foundation around 1180, with some even impossibly pushing its foundation into the first decade of the thirteenth century.[116] The *terminus a quo* for any such foundation is, of course, the grant of the manor of Aynho to Roger Fitz Richard by the earl of Essex in 1170. Moreover, the hospital must have been in existence before 1185, when Alice of Essex is recorded as being a widow. We would otherwise have to content ourselves with a rather broad date range of 1170 × 1185, were it not for the survival of Roger Fitz Richard's founding charter in the original. Its witness list, which is omitted by the cartulary scribe, would appear at first glance to be of little help in narrowing the date any further, but the hitherto unnoticed mention therein of a certain Stephen, brother of the earl of Richmond, allows us to date the charter with unusual precision.[117] Stephen was a little-known

113 We find him, by way of example, being dispatched to the Scottish marches in May 1299: *CPR*, 1292–1301, p. 413. His seal is one of those attached to an act formalising the alliance between Edward I and the count of Flanders in 1296: Paris, Archives nationales, J 543, no. 6.

114 He died owing £149 for his manor of Corbridge: *CFR*, 1307–19, p. 61.

115 *CCR*, 1272–79, pp. 487–8.

116 For the date of *c.*1180, which is no doubt based on the date assigned by William Dunn Macray to the founding charter in his unpublished calendar of Aynho's deeds, see Woolgar, 'Two Cartularies', p. 498; Fry, 'Hospitality', p. 36. Knowles and Hadcock give the foundation as '–1200' (D. Knowles and R. Hadcock, *Medieval Religious Houses: England and Wales* (London, 1953), p. 252) and as '–1189?' and '*t.* Henry II' in the revised edition of their work (D. Knowles and R. Hadcock, *Medieval Religious Houses: England and Wales*, rev. edn (London, 1971), pp. 313, 341). The *Victoria County History* claims Aynho was founded 'towards the close of the twelfth century': VCH, *Northampton*, vol. 2, p. 150. Clay gives the wildly incorrect date of 1208: Clay, *Mediæval Hospitals*, p. 309.

117 His presence has not been noticed in part because the charter text has never been edited and published before, and in part because the word 'Richemund' has

bastard son of Alan the Black, earl of Richmond (†1146).[118] He appears elsewhere in a handful of charters issued by his relatives, but always as either 'filius comitis' or 'avunculus comitisse' (that is, uncle of Constance, duchess of Brittany and countess of Richmond).[119] His qualification in the Aynho act in relation to his brother Conan IV, duke of Brittany and earl of Richmond, is therefore not only unusual, but also suggests that Conan, who died on 20 February 1171,[120] was still very much alive at the time the act was issued. As such, it seems safe to conclude that Aynho Hospital was founded before February 1171, with the balance of probability suggesting it was established in 1170. As for explaining Stephen's presence among the witnesses of Roger's act, it is possible that he was a local landowner, having been granted the property in nearby Croughton which was once held by his great-uncle, Brian Fitz Count, illegitimate son of Duke Alan IV of Brittany (1084–1112).[121] Or he may at that point have been in the retinue of Roger's son-in-law, John, constable of Chester, since he witnessed one of his acts (also as the brother of Earl Conan) alongside a number of other individuals who were also witnesses to Roger Fitz Richard's act for Aynho.[122]

Our ability to date Roger's charter more precisely is important not just within the specific context of Aynho Hospital itself, but also for our understanding of the wider movement of hospitality in twelfth-century England. The period before *c.*1180 is one for which much remains unknown with regard to the founding of England's hospitals, in part because of the haphazard way in which they appear in the historical record.[123] To be able to fix Aynho's foundation precisely is therefore important in terms of establishing something concrete in relation to this otherwise nebulous period, one during which the murder of Thomas Becket on 29 December 1170 had a material impact on England's charitable landscape and the needs that

been partially obliterated due to damage to the parchment. Macray's unpublished calendar of the Aynho acts does not attempt to transcribe the missing word.

118 C.T. Clay (ed.), *Early Yorkshire Charters* (10 vols, York, 1935–65), vol. 5, p. 352.

119 J. Everard (ed.), *The Charters of Duchess Constance of Brittany and her Family, 1171–1221* (Woodbridge, 1999), nos. C3, C5, C19, pp. 45–7, 54–5.

120 The date of Conan's death is recorded in the '*Chronicon Kemperlegiense*', ed. É. Baluze, *Miscellanea nova ordine digesta*, ed. J.D. Mansi (4 vols, Lucca, 1761–4), vol. 1, p. 266.

121 Brian's holdings at Croughton are recorded by a twelfth-century survey of Northamptonshire, sometimes referred to as its 'Hydarium': Keats-Rohan (ed.), *Domesday People*, p. 100.

122 *Early Ches. Charts.*, no. 6, p. 14. For further discussion, see no. **4**.

123 Watson, 'The Origins', p. 77.

wayfarer hospitals like that at Aynho subsequently fulfilled.[124] Of course, individual motives might also underpin the founding of a hospital (or the benefaction thereof), which are discussed in more detail in Chapter 2. Let us simply note here that Aynho is but a short distance from Brackley, where Robert de Beaumont, earl of Leicester (1104–68), had established a hospital for pilgrims and the sick-poor just a few years earlier in 1166 × 1167/68.[125] Although not of the same aristocratic class, Roger Fitz Richard may very well have felt the need to imitate Robert's foundation, which the earl had entrusted to his clerk, Salomon, who became the hospital's first master.[126] Alternatively, while Aynho's founding charter is issued in Roger's name, it is possible that his wife, Alice, played a formative part in the venture. As Sethina Watson has shown, aristocratic women often played a crucial role in the foundation of medieval hospitals, one which the hospital's own deeds have a tendency to silence.[127] The manor of Aynho had been granted to Alice in dower by her nephew, William de Mandeville, and, while he subsequently granted it to Roger Fitz Richard in 1170, it was to Alice that the

124 In her seminal work on England's hospitals, Clay summarised key periods in the development of various charitable foundations, identifying the period 1170–1270 as one in which wayfarer hospitals, which had previously been confined to monasteries, sprung up across southern England to accommodate the pilgrim traffic heading to Becket's shrine at Canterbury: Clay, *Mediæval Hospitals*, pp. 4–6. It is difficult, however, to establish a direct link between the location of England's rural hospitals and pilgrimage: M. Satchell, 'Towards a Landscape History of the Rural Hospital in England', in J. Henderson, P. Horden, and A. Pastore (eds), *The Impact of Hospitals 300–2000* (Oxford, 2007), pp. 237–56, at p. 243.

125 The date of Robert's foundation is often given as *c.*1150 (Knowles and Hadcock, *Religious Houses*, pp. 315, 345; S. Watson, 'A Mother's Past and her Children's Futures: Female Inheritance, Family and Dynastic Hospitals in the Thirteenth Century', in C. Leyser and L. Smith (eds), *Motherhood, Religion, and Society in Medieval Europe, 400–1400: Essays Presented to Henrietta Leyser* (London, 2016), pp. 213–49, at p. 243) or 1148 × 1151 (Watson, '*Fundatio*', pp. 79 n. 6, 86, 306; Watson, 'The Origins', p. 79; Fry, 'Hospitality', p. 46). The hospital's foundation charter, however, contains among its witnesses a certain Geoffrey the monk, brother of the abbot of Lyre ('Gaufrido monacho, fratre abbatis de Lira'): MCA, Brackley 39. This is Geoffrey, future abbot of Lyre (1177–1206), who was made *procurator generalis* of the monks of Lyre in England during the abbacy of his brother, Osbern (1166–77): V. Gazeau, *Normannia monastica* (2 vols, Caen, 2007), vol. 2, p. 189; *EEA*, vol. 18, no. 79, p. 56. The charter cannot, therefore, have been issued before 1166, and must have been issued before the earl's death in 1168. The act is also witnessed by Richard, abbot of Leicester (1143/4–1167/8), such that the *terminus ad quem* may be 1167.

126 MCA, Brackley 5, Brackley 39 and Brackley B184.

127 Watson, 'Mother's Past', pp. 213–49.

manor reverted upon her husband's death.[128] Aynho Hospital was therefore built on Alice's (and her family's) lands, rather than those at the heart of her husband's patrimony in Northumberland, a move that suggests that either Alice played an active role in encouraging the hospital's foundation or that her husband tacitly recognised the importance to his new venture of his wife's lands and the more important network of connections within which they were embedded. Whatever the case may be, both her apparent heir, William Fitz Roger, and her nephew, William de Mandeville, recognised her as having made a material contribution to the hospital, referring to Alice in their acts as a donor (nos. **6**, **10**).

Once founded, the identity of the individual to whom the stewardship of Aynho Hospital was initially entrusted is not anywhere explicitly stated, although the first act in the cartulary, issued by Innocent III (1198–1216) on 25 October 1202 (no. **1**), is addressed 'to T., the proctor' (*T. procuratori*). This is likely Turbert/Turbern, son of Turbert/Turben, parson/rector of Aynho (see above),[129] who, in an act not transcribed in the cartulary, makes it known that, as rector, he has no right in the custody and governance of Aynho Hospital, save only at the request of the lord of the manor, declaring that he and his successors in the rectory may not hereafter claim for themselves any right over it (no. **A1**). Like the aforementioned Salomon at Brackley, Turbert also appears to have held the title of chaplain (*capellanus*; nos. **36–7**).[130] His immediate successor at the hospital was a certain Jordan. Presumably the chaplain by that name mentioned in Aynho documents (nos. **36–7, 41**), he is referred to as the hospital's 'prior and proctor' (*prior et procurator*; no. **2**) and 'master' (*magister*; nos. **12–13, 17**),[131] the latter being the title also applied to those who succeeded him. Almost nothing is known about these individuals. At least two, Adam of Stuchbury (*Stutesber'*) and

[128] According to the 1185 survey of widows in the king's fief, Alice held 'her manor of Aynho of Earl William' ('Arenho quod est manerium ejus, quod etiam tenet de comite Willelmo'): *Rot. de Dominabus*, pp. 29–30. As pointed out by Liesbeth van Houts, '[t]he extent of the husband's control over the dowry and dower is a […] historiographical problem with […] a distinct northern and southern European aspect to it […] As for the north[,] there is scholarly consensus that dower assigned at the church's door on the occasion of the wedding was controlled by the husband and only after his death, when legally transferred, became the widow's property'; E.M.C. van Houts, *Married Life in the Middle Ages, 900–1300* (Oxford, 2019), p. 12, with reference to J. Green, *The Aristocracy of Norman England* (Cambridge, 1997), pp. 364–82.

[129] William Macray thought this the case: W. Macray, *Notes from the Muniments of St Mary Magdalen College, Oxford, from the Twelfth to the Seventeenth Century* (Oxford, 1882), p. 4.

[130] For Salomon as chaplain, see MCA, Brackley 5.

[131] See also, MCA, Whitfield 106.

Geoffrey of Croughton (*Crouleton*'), were locals,[132] but others were clearly recruited from Clavering lands further afield (**Table 1.1**). Peter of Maldon (*Maldone*), a canon of Blythburgh originally from Essex, was presented by Roger de Cressy, who then held the manor of Aynho in farm from his half-brother John (I) Fitz Robert.[133] Likewise, William of Occold (*Acolt/Hokkehalte/Okholt*), who was presented by Robert (II) Fitz Roger on 12 May 1282, hailed from the Suffolk place of that name, while the roll of Richard of Gravesend, bishop of Lincoln (1258–79), gives Master Peter's toponymic as Windsor (*Wyndesover*'),[134] just 8 km (as the crow flies) from the Clavering estate at Iver.

Similar patterns can be traced in relation to some of those individuals outside the founding family who made material contributions to the hospital. In certain cases, therefore, it is clear that the expansion of Clavering influence beyond Northumberland and Northamptonshire brought with it new benefactors to Anyho, such as Robert of Sheering (*Schiringe/Schyringe/Scyring*') and Paulinus of Marlow (*Merlawe*), whose toponymic surnames suggest they came from (or at least traced their family origins to) places in the vicinity of Clavering estates in Essex and Buckinghamshire.[135] In other instances in which we cannot demonstrate a direct feudo-vassalic link between the Claverings and other Aynho Hospital benefactors, analysis of the manorial landscape and the prosopographical connections that underpinned it shows how the hospital's founding family would have been given ample opportunity to rub shoulders with – and perhaps even directly encourage – some of those individuals who ended up giving to it.

Such is the case with members of the Turville family, who appear regularly in the hospital's charters. The earliest to do so are Robert de Turville and his son, Simon (e.g., nos. **15–17, 22**). This Robert is presumably the same Robert de Turville who in the twelfth century granted land in

132 Adam was local in the sense that he was chaplain at Stuchbury prior to his appointment as master. His institution as chaplain shows that his toponymic was 'of Barby' (*de Bereweby/de Beregheby*), which means he likely hailed from the vill by that name located approximately 6 km southeast of Rugby: *Rot. Welles*, vol. 2, pp. 142, 231.

133 *Rot. Welles*, vol. 2, p. 171, where the editor mistakenly identifies 'Bliburge' as Blythe Bridge in Staffordshire.

134 *Rot. Gravesend*, p. 113.

135 Sheering (Essex) is approximately 18 km (as the crow flies) from Clavering, and Marlow (Bucks) about 10 km from the Clavering estate at Iver. For evidence that individuals might move between Clavering estates, taking their toponymic surnames with them, see a 1286 inquisition concerning Richard le King, of Walden [Uttlesford and Freshwell Hundred, Essex], and Walter of Aynho (*Eynho*), of Essex: TNA, C 241/18/114. See also, W.H. Ward, *A History of the Manor and Parish of Iver* (London, 1933), p. 46, which seems to suggest that Hubert of Aynho, a regular witness of Aynho Hospital charters, became a tenant of the manor of Iver.

Table 1.1. The Masters of Aynho Hospital (*c.*1190–1294).

| Datable mentions | Master | Source(s) |
|---|---|---|
| 1194 × 1202 | Turbert/Turbern | no. **A1** |
| 25 Oct 1202 | | no. **1** |
| after 25 Oct 1202 × 1210 | Jordan | no. **22** |
| *c.*1210 | | no. **17** |
| Nov 1214 × 1232 | | nos. **12–13** |
| 27 Nov 1215 | | no. **2** |
| *c.*1228 | | MCA, Whitfield 106 |
| 1232 (presented by Roger de Cressy) | Peter of Maldon | *Rot. Welles*, vol. 2, p. 171 |
| 1235 (presented by Roger de Cressy) | Adam of Stuchbury | Hoskin (ed.), *Grosseteste*, no. 608 |
| 1244 (presented by Ada de Balliol through Thomas de *Barwe*, clerk, her proctor) | Stephen | Hoskin (ed.), *Grosseteste*, no. 799 |
| *c.*1245 × 1250 | | no. **30** |
| *c.*1260 | Peter of Windsor | no. **A8** |
| 19 Sep 1269 (presented by Simon Bayard and Isabella, his wife) | John of Gra(nt)ham | *Rot. Gravesend*, p. 113 |
| *c.*1270 | | no. **A12** |
| 1270 × 1280 | | nos. **52, A13, A17, A18** |
| 12 May 1282 (presented by Robert [II] Fitz Roger) | William of Occold | *Rolls of Sutton*, vol. 2, p. 17 |
| *c.*1285 | | no. **A21** |
| 18 Mar 1288 | | MCA, Aynho 11 |
| *c.*1290 | | MCA, Aynho 16 |
| 16 Feb 1294 (presented by Robert [II] Fitz Roger) | Geoffrey of Croughton | *Rolls of Sutton*, vol. 2, p. 108 |

Adstone, Northamptonshire, to the monks of Canons Ashby.[136] He was therefore a relative (perhaps a cousin?) of Geoffrey de Turville, whom a twelfth-century Northamptonshire survey shows held land at Adstone,[137] and who was the patriarch of a family with various holdings in the Honour of Leicester.[138] This included the manor of Helmdon, some 13 km to the northeast of Aynho.[139] Outside Northamptonshire, there were Turville estates in Buckinghamshire at Weston Turville, Penn, and Taplow, all of which came into the family's possession (or are recorded as being in it) at the same time as Robert Fitz Roger received the nearby manor of Iver.[140] By 1222, Petronilla, daughter or sister of William de Turville junior (†bef. 1217), had been married to a certain Simon of Croughton,[141] a union that would have brought the family even closer to the Clavering orbit, given the connections between this vill and Aynho Hospital. This Simon, who is recorded in the *Book of Fees* as holding land in Croughton from the earl of Leicester as 'Simon de Turville',[142] was likely the grandson of the aforementioned Robert, whose grant to Canons Ashby he confirmed.[143] He was

136 TNA, E 326/309; BL, MS Egerton 3033, fol. 31r.

137 'In Atteneston Galfridus de Turuill iii paruas uirg'': Keats-Rohan (ed.), *Domesday People*, p. 102.

138 For useful but by no means complete (or always accurate) pedigrees of the Turville family, see G.H. Fowler and M.W. Hughes, 'A Calendar of the Pipe Rolls of the Reign of Richard I for Buckinghamshire and Bedfordshire, 1189–1199', *Publications of the Bedfordshire Historical Record Society*, 7 (1923), 204–7; J.R. Delafield, *Delafield, the Family History* (2 vols, New York, 1945), vol. 2, pp. 638–41.

139 'In Helmenden' Willelmus de Torewell' iiii. hid' de feodo Comitis Leycestrie': Keats-Rohan (ed.), *Domesday People*, p. 101.

140 William de Turville and Isabel, his wife, are the first to be mentioned in connection with Penn in 1197–1200: J. Hunter (ed.), *Fines, sive pedes finium ... A.D. 1195–A.D. 1214* (2 vols, London, 1835–44), vol. 1, pp. 158, 180, 193, 226; F. Palgrave (ed.), *Rotuli Curiæ Regis: Rolls and Records of the Court held before the King's Justiciars or Justices* (2 vols, London, 1835), vol. 1, p. 357. Penn is around 17 km (as the crow flies) from Iver. In 1197, William and Isabel subinfeudated Taplow to the Prior of Merton: D. Stenton (ed.), *The Chancellor's Roll for the Eighth Year of the Reign of King Richard I Michaelmas 1196* (London, 1930), p. 163. Taplow is around 12 km from Iver.

141 F.W. Maitland (ed.), *Bracton's Note Book: A Collection of Cases decided in the King's Courts during the Reign of Henry III* (3 vols, London, 1887), vol. 2, p. 165.

142 *BF*, vol. 2, p. 940. He appears elsewhere in the *Book of Fees* as Simon de Turville in relation to other Turville estates (ibid., vol. 1, p. 507; vol. 2, pp. 876, 895). He is sometimes referred to in the modern literature as 'Simon de Turville of Croughton' (P. Coss, 'Identity and Gentry c. 1200-c. 1340', *Thirteenth-Century England*, 6 (1997), pp. 49–60, at p. 53 n. 26), but never appears as such in the sources cited (e.g., *CRR*, 1230–2, nos. 1769, 2318).

143 For Simon's confirmation, in which he styles himself as Simon, son of Simon de Turville, see above, n. 136. For the suggestion that Simon was Robert's grandson, see Delafield, *Family History*, vol. 2, p. 641 n. 1.

succeeded by his son and heir, William de Turville (†bef. 1296/7), at some point before 1278.[144] As tenants of the Leicester fee, we therefore might reasonably expect to find William and his heirs acting as benefactors to the hospital at Brackley, even if its patronage had since passed to the earls of Winchester. Instead, it was to Aynho that William turned, granting a messuage and half a virgate of land in Croughton, and even going so far as to state that he would defend his donation against any wrongful action by the earl of Leicester (nos. **57–8**),[145] who, as we shall see, was perhaps then in open rebellion against the Crown.

The precise role (if any) played by the Claverings in facilitating this donation is, of course, unknown, but the fact of its existence is likely the result of a combination of proximity and personal connections. The same is also likely true of the important donations made by the descendants of Geoffrey de Wavre, who granted and repeatedly confirmed the chapel at Croughton to Aynho Hospital (nos. **41–5**). It has proven difficult to identify Geoffrey himself with certainty, but we do know that he held his demesne lands in Croughton from William de Mandeville, nephew of Roger Fitz Richard's wife (no. **40**). The Latin form of Geoffrey's toponymic (*Wavere*), which is also rendered as *Waffre*/*Wafre*/*Wavre* in the cartulary, can be found as an element in various English place names, but he cannot be linked to any of the places in question.[146] Instead, it is likely Geoffrey traced his origins to the Low Countries, whence we find a Geoffrey de Wavre (*Wavere*) – perhaps a relative or descendant? – being installed under King John as lord of Dennington, Suffolk, which he held in fee from Henry I, duke of Brabant (1190–1235), in whose duchy the city of Wavre lay.[147] The idea that Geoffrey shared similar links is supported by the marriage of his daughter, Alice, to a certain Baldwin de Boulogne (*Bolonia*/*Bolunia*/*Buluinia*),[148] whose toponymic speaks to connections with the counts of that name, in whose former

[144] VCH, *Buckingham*, vol. 2, p. 366.

[145] William's son, Nicholas, confirmed this donation in turn on 1 August 1306: MCA, Aynho 54.

[146] The toponym '*Wavere*' is often rendered as 'Over' in modern English place names, such Brownsover, Churchover and Cesters Over (all Warwickshire): *EPNS*, vol. 13, pp. 100, 103–4, 113. It is also used in the Middle Ages for Woore (Shropshire): *EPNS*, vol. 82/83, p. 325.

[147] For Geoffrey and Dennington, see R. Mortimer (ed.), *Leiston Abbey Cartulary and Butley Priory Charters* (Ipswich, 1979), no. 18, p. 68. Despite the similarities in their first name, these must have been two different people, since Geoffrey de Wavre first appears in the historical record in May 1177 × Sep 1181 (no. **40**), while his Suffolk namesake was still alive in 1230. The authors are extremely grateful to Liesbeth van Houts for her guidance as to their initial findings on this point.

[148] The rubricator of the Aynho Cartulary appears to style Baldwin as 'of Byfield' on one occasion (no. **36**), although we should probably here understand '*Carta Baldowini*

honour of Eye the manor of Dennington lay. Or it may signal a connection with the Anglo-Flemish community that had become established in England since the days of the Conquest,[149] a prominent member of which is also recorded as holding lands in Northamptonshire from the Mandeville fee.[150] Earl William himself had close links with the Low Countries. He had been sent by his father to be raised by Philip I, count of Flanders (1168–91), with whom he remained friends, and subsequently acted as a key conduit between England and Flanders.[151] What is more, the Aynho Cartulary contains a copy of an act for land in Croughton issued in the name of a certain Geoffrey de *Lonhoud* (no. **18**). His unusual toponymic cannot be found elsewhere in English sources outside acts for Brackley Hospital, of which he was also a benefactor,[152] but it does appear in continental records relating to the village of Loenhout (*Loenhoudt*/*Lonhout*/*Lonout*), again located in the duchy of Brabant,[153] which therefore suggests that it was to here that Geoffrey traced his origins.

What brought these men to England cannot be known. As Eljas Oksanen has noted, however, Northamptonshire was one of the centres of Flemish landholding from the eleventh century onwards, with its networks of relationships serving both to attract and then bind together would-be

---

*de* Bifeld' to mean 'Baldwin's charter *concerning* Byfield', since he appears in all other instances as 'Baldwin de Boulogne'.

149 For Flemish contacts with and migration to England between 1066 and 1216, see E. Oksanen, *Flanders and the Anglo-Norman World, 1066–1216* (Cambridge, 2012), pp. 178–213; more recently S. Levelt and A. Putter, *North-Sea Crossings: The Literary Heritage of Anglo-Dutch Relations 1066–1688* (Oxford, 2021).

150 'In Eston' [Aston le Walls] et Apeltreya [Appletree] Willelmus de Bolonia vii. hid. de feodo Comitis de Mandeuille': Keats-Rohan (ed.), *Domesday People*, p. 101. This is William de Boulogne († bef. 1130), son of Geoffrey, illegitimate son of Count Eustace II (1049–87).

151 Bennett, *Elite Participation*, p. 140.

152 MCA, Astwick and Evenley 86A, 91A, 95A, 101A, 102A, 108A, and 129A, in which his toponymic is rendered as *Londhold*, *Luneholte*, *Lonhoud*, *Lonhout*, and *Lunhot*. An act issued after his death refers to him as 'Geoffrey de Loenhout, knight' ('Godefridi de Lunhout', militem'): MCA, Aswtick and Evenley 64A.

153 H.P.H. Camps et al. (eds), *Oorkondenboek van Noord-Brabant tot 1312* (4 vols in 2, 's-Gravenhage, 1979–2000), vol. 2.1, nos. 1028–29, 1143, 1149–51, pp. 328–30, 546–7, 555–9. Admittedly, these mentions are from the mid-thirteenth century onwards, but one of the points of Jean de Sturler's seminal study of Anglo-Brabantine relations is that Flemish and Brabantine individuals are to be found more readily in English sources of the twelfth and early thirteenth centuries than those of the Low Countries, where record keeping was only just beginning at this time: J. de Sturler, *Les relations politiques et les échanges commerciaux entre le duché de Brabant et l'Angleterre au moyen âge* (Paris, 1936), p. 13.

immigrants from the Low Countries.[154] What held true for migrants from Flanders was likely also the case for their neighbours in Brabant, whose aristocratic leaders played a crucial role in fostering diplomatic and economic relations with England from the reign of Henry I (1100–35) onwards.[155] Moreover, the movements of those at the top of medieval lay society usually brought those below them in their wake, no more so than in the hiring of paid soldiers, the most readily identifiable of which at this period are Flemings and Brabanters.[156] Geoffrey de Wavre first appears in the historical record shortly after the Great Rebellion of 1173/4, during which Henry II is known to have shipped over such mercenary troops.[157] Alternatively, he and Geoffrey de Loenhout may have found themselves recruited at a knightly tournament on the continent, a world in which Flemish and Brabantine soldiers had a conspicuous presence.[158] Whatever the case may be, what the acts of the Aynho Cartulary may preserve for us is the legacy of just such service in a royal or comital retinue. At the very least, they seem to capture a snapshot of an enclave of Anglo-Brabantine settlers (or their descendants) installed at Croughton, just a stone's throw from the Brackley-Mixbury tournament circuit, where their patriarch (Geoffrey de Wavre) held his lands from a figure (William de Mandeville) with close links to the region from which they had come. Whatever their origins, it was such feudo-vassalic links that almost certainly underpinned subsequent de Wavre generosity to Aynho Hospital, especially since the family also held and gave land to it at Byfield (nos. **36–39**), the church of which belonged to the Norman abbey of Saint-Évroult by a gift of the earls of Chester,[159] to whom the hospital's founding family were connected through Robert (I) Fitz Roger's brother-in-law, John Fitz Richard, constable of Chester.

## CONCLUSION

Whatever connections existed between these individuals and the Claverings, the analysis of the hospital's charters presented here reveals that the endowment of even a modest rural foundation like Aynho relied on a

154 Oksanen, *Flanders*, pp. 192–208.

155 N. Ruffini-Ronzani, 'The Counts of Louvain and the Anglo-Norman World' (*c*.1100–*c*.1215), *ANS*, 42 (2020), 135–54.

156 Oksanen, *Flanders*, p. 138.

157 *PR* 20 Henry II, p. 135.

158 Oksanen, *Flanders*, pp. 133–42.

159 G. Barraclough (ed.), *The Charters of the Anglo-Norman Earls of Chester, c. 1071–1237* (Chester, 1988), no. 1, pp. 1–2; no. 11, pp. 20–1. A twelfth-century survey shows eight hides were also held there by the earls of Leicester: Keats-Rohan (ed.), *Domesday People*, p. 101.

subtle and yet significant patchwork of relationships and obligations that stretched well beyond its immediate vicinity. To be able to trace these with some degree of accuracy is significant, not least in the light of Max Satchell's recent observation that, while the ratio of rural to urban hospitals was actually greater in the twelfth and thirteenth centuries, making them an institution more familiar to most than larger (and generally better studied) religious institutions,[160] over half of all rural hospitals have lost their charters.[161] Ironically, Aynho is not among those houses studied by Satchell, who remains one of the few people to look at England's medieval rural hospitals in any detail before 1300, even though it falls within his definition of such an institution (i.e., not named after an urban centre and located more than 4.8 km from the nearest one). Nevertheless, Aynho Hospital certainly had many of the hallmarks identified by Satchell, chief among them that it was at the centre of a local community (at least in terms of its material impact upon the landscape, if not necessarily its precise location), close to a supply of water (the spring running down to the Cherwell), and near a site of passing alms traffic (in the form of the bridge over that same river). Its proximity to the frequently used tournament site between Brackley and Mixbury, which, in October 1249, attracted no less a figure than the king's half-brother and Robert (II) Fitz Roger's guardian, William de Valence,[162] would almost certainly have made it a routine destination for knights and their large retinues.[163] This is vividly illustrated by Robert Fitz Roger's act for Aynho Hospital in memory of his grandmother (see above). Its witness list includes the famous Anglo-Norman knight and poet, Walter of Bibbesworth (†*c.*1270), whom Robert probably knew through William de Valence,[164] as

160 As Sethina Watson notes, the sheer number of hospitals in England would have made it an institution 'more widely and intimately known' to the typical person: Watson, 'The Origins', p. 76.

161 Satchell, 'Rural Hospital', p. 238.

162 For Valence and his tourneying circuit in 1248 and 1249, see Luard (ed.), *Chronica majora*, vol. 5, pp. 17–18, 54–5, 83.

163 The size of a medieval tournament can be estimated via a heraldic roll for a tournament held at Dunstable in 1309, which gives some 235 shields, with each of these knights bringing a sizeable retinue with them: A. Tomkinson, 'Retinues at the Tournament of Dunstable, 1309', *EHR*, 74 (1959), 70–89, at pp. 78–9. A mid-thirteenth-century document shows Edmund de Lacy, constable of Chester (*c.*1230–58), travelling to a 1249 tournament with a retinue of 20 knights: M. Carlin and D. Crouch (eds and trans.), *Lost Letters of Medieval Life. English Society, 1200–1250* (Philadelphia, PA, 2013), p. 207.

164 We can be confident that the 'domino Waltero de Bybeswrd" who appears first in the list of witnesses for Robert's act is the Walter of Bibbesworth best known for his *Tretiz*, a rhyming vocabulary of French written at some point between the years 1230 and 1270. According to a prologue transmitted in some manuscripts, this was

well as two knights attached to the Clavering nexus of estates, all of whom may very well have been present with Robert as he passed through Aynho on his way to or from a Brackley-Mixbury tournament.[165] At the time this charter was issued, Aynho Hospital was nearing its one hundredth year of existence. It was under the stewardship of Peter of Windsor,[166] whose toponymic speaks to connections well beyond Northamptonshire, and it had amassed a small but not unimportant network of properties within the county itself at Aynho, Croughton, Brackley, and Byfield. Its ever growing – and perhaps increasingly difficult to navigate – archive of charters would have reflected this slow but steady expansion, as would the hospital's small 'library', which we know at the very least contained its book of obits (*martilogium*; no. **33**). Like its larger counterparts in Oxford and Brackley, Aynho's hospital also had its own seal (no. **A8**). It owed such circumstances to the continued, multi-generational support of its founding family, as well as to an engaged network of local and regional benefactors. It is to these individuals and their motivations that we shall now turn in Chapter 2.

---

written at the request of Dyonise de Munchensi, wife of Warin de Munchensi (†20 July 1255). Dyonise was stepmother to Joan de Munchensi (†1307), who at some point before 13 August 1247 married William de Valence, the king's half-brother and Robert (II) Fitz Roger's eventual guardian: A. Dalby (ed. and trans.), *The Treatise of Walter of Bibbesworth* (Totnes, 2012), p. 5. Walter was also a landholder in Essex at Saling, Latton, and Waltham, not too far from Clavering.

165 These are Hugh Gubiun and John de Mohaut (or Montalt). A Hugh *Gubyum*/*Gubyun* can be found serving members of the Balliol family (M. Drexler, 'Dervorguilla of Galloway', *Transactions of the Dumfriesshire and Galloway Natural History and Antiquarian Society*, 79 (2005), 101–46, at p. 129) and was among those knights who accompanied Robert Fitz Roger to the Scottish march in May 1299 (*CPR*, 1292–1301, p. 413). He also appears as witness to a quit-claim of the burgesses of Corbridge: Craster, *Northumberland*, vol. 10, p. 70 n. 1. John de Mohaut (*Muhault*) is perhaps the 'king's knight' who in the 1270s played an important role in the Welsh wars, and whose family held the hereditary stewardship of Chester: N. Denholm-Young, *Collected Papers on Mediaeval Subjects* (Oxford, 1946), p. 80 and n. 3. Whatever the case may be, a John le Muhaut, knight, also appears in act of Robert's son, John, issued for Aynho Hospital around 1290: MCA, Aynho 16.

166 Peter of Windsor's installation as Master is not recorded in the institution rolls of Robert Grosseteste, bishop of Lincoln (1235–53), while his death is recorded in those of Richard of Gravesend (1258–79). As such, it seems he must have been installed as Master during the reign of Henry of Lexington (1254–58), for whom only one roll (for Huntingdonshire) survives.

# 2

# PROPERTY, NETWORKS, AND BENEFACTORS

The previous chapter set out the foundation and early history of Aynho Hospital during the first hundred or so years of its existence (*c.*1170–*c.*1280), allowing us to introduce various key figures associated with the institution and to contextualise its domestic history within cultures of charity and hospitality in later twelfth- and thirteenth-century England. Building on this crucial framework, the present chapter establishes the hospital more firmly within the socio-political and socio-economic networks of patronage and property of which it was a part, and from which it benefited both spiritually and materially. Using the primary evidence of the Aynho Cartulary alongside original documents not copied in it, we can identify the hospital's major patrons and benefactors, trace their connections (familial, political, feudal, etc.), and investigate their participation in what is known as the medieval spiritual economy. Going beyond this prosopographical analysis, this chapter also examines in detail the patchwork of local landscapes and markets in which the hospital was situated, and which it managed and manipulated, paying specific attention to modes of rural landholding, investment, and property accumulation that defined and sustained communities such as Aynho in the central Middle Ages.

## ESTATE BUILDING

Like many medieval religious institutions, Aynho Hospital occupied a position at the crossroads of spiritual and temporal life, a juncture where secular and ecclesiastical spheres of influence converged, and where social, political, and economic interests entered into direct conversation (and sometimes competition) with one another. To assert and sustain itself within this increasingly crowded and competitive – and, from the later twelfth and thirteenth centuries, commercialised – environment, the hospital had to learn to manage and manipulate the local landscape by drawing on its socio-political and socio-economic networks. Much of what was needed to run a small institution such as Aynho and to feed, wash, and clothe its inhabitants on a day-to-day basis would have been provided through common acts of charity. Impromptu donations (food, clothing, money, etc.) by individuals who passed the hospital or engaged with its inhabitants in public spaces (towns, markets, on the road, etc.) would have been a regular occurrence. Many would have given to the brothers out of their own volition and initiative in keeping with what has been labelled 'a broader pan-European religious culture of charity',[1] which also included other kinds of institutions such as dedicated leprosaria.[2] Others might have needed a little more encouragement and some gentle (or perhaps not so gentle) 'nudging' to part with whatever they could spare in resources and/or alms. One of the two papal privileges copied at the opening of the Aynho Cartulary (no. **2**), neither of which has ever been edited, therefore 'beseech[es], admonish[es], and encourage[s]' all good Christians living within the province of Canterbury to do just that by declaring that 'whenever the same prior and the [afore]mentioned brothers [of Aynho] or their envoys (*nuntii*) come to you requesting alms (*elemosinam*), you should listen to them kindly, giving to them liberally from the goods bestowed on you by God'.[3] This, Pope Innocent III explains, shall be done in fulfilment of God's own command, set down in Scripture (2 Corinthians 5:10 and 9:6), since 'it is proper that we prepare for the day of harvest (*diem messionis*) with works of the utmost mercy, and to sow on Earth, with a view to eternity (*eter[n]-orum intuitu*), that which, with God repaying [it] with multiplied fruit, we ought to reap in heaven', being forever mindful that 'he who sows sparingly reaps sparingly'.

1 Davis, *Economy of Salvation*, p. 4.

2 Satchell, 'Towards a Landscape'; M. Satchell, 'The Emergence of Leper-houses in Medieval England, 1100-1250', unpublished PhD dissertation, University of Oxford, 1998; S. Watson, 'Responding to Leprosy in the Twelfth and Thirteenth Centuries', in A. Medcalf et al. (eds), *Leprosy: A Short History* (Hyderabad, 2016), pp. 29–38; C. Rawcliffe, 'Learning to Love the Leper: Aspects of Institutional Charity in Anglo-Norman England', *ANS*, 23 (2001), 231–50; C. Rawcliffe, 'Isolating the Medieval Leper: Ideas—and Misconceptions—about Segregation in the Middle Ages', in P. Horden (ed.), *Freedom of Movement in the Middle Ages* (Donington, 2007), pp. 229–48; ead., *Leprosy in Medieval England* (Woodbridge, 2006).

3 Innocent's bulls for Aynho are mentioned briefly in J.E. Sayers, *Papal Government and England During the Pontificate of Honorius III (1216–1227)* (Cambridge, 1984), p. 114, and in N. Vincent, 'Some Pardoners' Tales: The Earliest English Indulgences', *Transactions of the Royal Historical Society*, 12 (2002), 23–58, at p. 53. On the use of *nuntii* to solicit gifts, cf. Sayers, *Papal Government*, p. 114, as well as Davis, *Economy of Salvation*, p. 9, who notes that '[w]hile some potential donors might have been reluctant to give away a portion of their wealth to the poor, preachers sought to reassure them that they were making the wisest kind of investment by earning credit with God and funding "a heavenly treasure"'.

Innocent's use of the term 'dies messionis' is ambiguous – possibly deliberately so – since it can refer to both the actual harvest and the day of reckoning (i.e., Last Judgement),[4] thus encouraging gifts of food and produce when they were in abundance at the same time as emphasising these gifts' spiritual value and their givers' eternal reward.

Swaying hesitant or reluctant donors may well have required a more concrete – and perhaps more compelling – incentive, however, which explains why Innocent III's privilege also offers forty days of penance 'to all those conferring any benefits to the same prior or the aforementioned brothers [of Aynho] or their envoys, and especially to all who, from the vigil of St James until the octave day, should visit the church built there in his honour'. As the document makes clear, these regular donations are a necessity because, without them, the hospital would not have sufficient resources to minster liberally to its inhabitants (*cum ad hoc proprie non suppetant facultates*), thus underscoring the institution's crucial dependence on *continuous* gift-giving to enable and help sustain even its most basic yet vital operations. The high frequency and spontaneous nature of these gifts, whether given voluntarily or prompted by (pro)active 'fundraising' in the local community and solicitation on the part of the hospital's agents, explains why they tend to be unrecorded, and why their donors, though known and acknowledged for their charity at the time, remain anonymous today. While frustrating to the modern historian seeking to quantify a medieval hospital's elementary means of material provision (and its ultimate survival), such ephemerality presumably would have troubled neither the beneficiaries nor the benefactors of these gifts in the Middle Ages. For them, charity of any quantity was guaranteed to be duly registered in their favour by the highest judge and ultimate accountant: God Himself.

This is not to say, however, that donations made to medieval hospitals were never recorded for posterity by the giving and receiving parties. While day-to-day acts of charity like those described above typically elude us, those involving what can be considered 'major gifts', which contributed to a hospital's estate, were usually put in writing, sometimes on multiple occasions. The extant charters, confirmations, and cartularies from hospitals in medieval England (and wider Europe) are instructive testimony of this documentary practice,[5] and Aynho forms no exception here. What is

4 Cf. *Word-List*, p. 297; *Lexicon*, vol. 1, p. 880.

5 Cartularies (in the form of codices) survive from many medieval English hospitals, both independent houses and ones attached to monasteries, including Abingdon, Anglesey, Beck, Bolton, Brackley, Bristol, Burton Lazars, Bury St Edmunds, Cambridge, Canterbury, Castleton, Chichester, Clerkenwell, Clitheroe, Cockersand, Conishead, Creake, Doncaster, Dover, Durham, Edisford, Elsham, Exeter, Great Yarmouth, Harbledown, Heytesbury, Holborn, Ickburgh, Ilford, King's Lynn,

exceptional about it, though, making it an ideal case study of estate building and property management on a local level, is that over half of the acts of donation and confirmation copied in the Aynho Cartulary also survive as originals. There is also a sizeable corpus of originals not copied in the cartulary, which likewise give important information about both the hospital's initial estate and the means by which it was expanded over time (**Tables 2.2–2.3**). The remainder of this section utilises this unusually comprehensive and complementary documentation to trace the gradual accumulation of the hospital's property through major charitable gifts by members of the local community and, in some cases, even donors from further afield. Occasional *lacunae* notwithstanding, this discussion will operate chronologically according to the dates (or, where exact dates cannot be established, date ranges) of these donations, rather than following the order in which

Kirkby in Kendal, Ledbury, London, Lowcross, Maiden Bradley, Newcastle upon Tyne, Norwich, Ospringe, Oxford, Pontefract, Preston, Royston, St Mary-de-Pre, Salisbury, Sandwich, Southampton, Southwark, Sprotbrough, Tandridge, Thanington, Winchester, Worcester, Wymondley, and York; cf. the relevant entries in *Cartularies*. Some of the above have had their contents edited: C. Wordsworth (ed.), *The Fifteenth-Century Cartulary of St. Nicholas' Hospital: With Other Records* (Salisbury, 1902); H.E. Salter (ed.), *A Cartulary of the Hospital of St John the Baptist* (3 vols, Oxford, 1914–17); C.D. Ross (ed.), *Cartulary of St Mark's Hospital, Bristol* (Bristol, 1959); N.J.M. Kerling (ed.), *Cartulary of St Bartholomew's Hospital, Founded 1123: A Calendar* (London, 1973); C. Rawcliffe, 'The Cartulary of St Mary's Hospital, Great Yarmouth', in C. Rawcliffe et al. (eds), *Poverty and Wealth: Sheep, Taxation and Charity in Late Medieval Norfolk* (Norwich, 2007), pp. 157–230; M.G. Underwood (ed.), *The Cartulary of the Hospital of St John the Evangelist, Cambridge* (Cambridge, 2008); D.X. Carpenter (ed.), *The Cartulary of St Leonard's Hospital, York* (2 vols, Woodbridge, 2015). On the written sources for medieval English hospitals, cf. also S. Watson, 'The Sources for English Hospitals 1100 to 1400', in M. Scheutz et al. (eds), *Quellen zur europäischen Spitalgeschichte in Mittelalter und Früher Neuzeit / Sources for the History of Hospitals in Medieval and Early Modern Europe* (Vienna: Böhlau, 2010), pp. 65–104; Watson, 'Origins', pp. 81–7. On hospitals' archives, see C. Rawcliffe, 'Passports to Paradise: How English Medieval Hospitals and Almshouses Kept Their Archives', *Archives*, 27 (2002), 2–22. Hospital cartularies from across the Channel include the recently edited cartulary of Saint-Nicolas d'Évreux (Évreux, Archives départementales de l'Eure, H-dépôt Évreux G7) from the mid-thirteenth century and the illuminated fifteenth-century cartulary of Saint-Jacques de Tournai (Tournai, Bibliothèque de la Ville, Cod. 4A); Tabuteau (ed.), *Cartulaire d'Évreux*; B. Tabuteau and F. Epaud, 'Le prieuré-léproserie de Saint-Nicolas d'Évreux: Dossier historique et patrimonial', *Bulletin des Amis des Monuments et Sites de l'Eure*, 138 (2011), 11–50; D. Vanwijnsberghe, 'Cartulaire de l'hôpital Saint-Jacques de Tournai [Tournai, Bibliothèque de la Ville, Cod. 4A (conservé n° 27)]', in M. Smeyers and J. Vander Stock (eds), *Manuscrits à peintures en Flandre, 1475–1550* (Ghent, 1997): pp. 186–87 (= no. 30); D. Vanwijnsberghe, 'Cartulaire de l'hôpital Saint-Jacques de Tournai: Description commentée des images', *Art de l'enluminure*, 73 (2020), 31–61.

they are copied in the cartulary. Our natural starting point must be the donations by the hospital's founder and original patrons, Roger Fitz Richard and Alice of Essex,[6] as well as those by their sons.

The earliest major gift recorded in the Aynho Cartulary (no. **4**), as well as in a corresponding original (Aynho 71), is the hospital's 'foundational endowment' by Roger, made 1170 × 20 February 1171, of one hide (*c.*120 acres) of land in the vill of Aynho.[7] As we saw in Chapter 1, the history through which Roger's family came to possess and administer this land is only partially recorded, but we can be certain that the manor of Aynho – recorded in Domesday Book as comprising just over three hides (*c.*384 acres) of land (*terrae*), of which just over one (*c.*144 acres) were in demesne (i.e., so-called 'lord's land'), plus eight hides (*c.*960 acres) of ploughland (*carucata*), twenty acres of meadow, and a mill, with a combined annual value of £8 – was re-allocated post-Conquest to a new Norman tenant-in-chief, Geoffrey (I) de Mandeville (†*c.*1100). The manor then passed from Geoffrey, via two intermediate generations (i.e., William (I) and Geoffrey (II), 1st Earl of Essex), to his great-grandson, William (II) de Mandeville, 3rd Earl of Essex and Chief Justiciar of England (†1189), who gave it in dower to his aunt, Alice, to be administered by her husband as per the earl's grant of 1170.[8] Why William de Mandeville chose to 'top up' Alice's dower 'over and above' what she had received in dower from her husband is unknown, but it may well suggest that he considered Roger's provision insufficient. Still, by granting Roger the right to administer this dower on Alice's behalf as if Roger had given it to her himself, the earl allowed Roger to save face and keep his reputation as a landholder and husband intact. According to Roger's foundation charter, the hide of land he gifted (perhaps with Alice's encouragement or at least consent) to his new hospital at Aynho had formerly been held between a certain Turbern (half a hide), who was probably the father of the Aynho parson by the same name, and Svein (half a hide), who, as a later cartulary act (no. **10**) reveals, was Turbern's brother.

6 On Roger and his family's ancestry, see Chapter 1.

7 The cartulary's preceding act (no. **3**) records the grant of one virgate (around thirty acres) of land and a messuage, likewise located in the vill of Aynho, by Roger Fitz Richard to his servant (*servienti meo*), Azurus. It is not clear whether – and, if so, in what capacity – this Azurus and/or the land granted to him (which had previously been held by one Robert le Brankere) were connected to the foundation of Aynho Hospital, which is why they are excluded from the present discussion.

8 *Domesday*, vol. 12: *Northamptonshire*, ed. F. Thorn and C. Thorn, 45.1; also cf. the online entry in Open Domesday: <https://opendomesday.org/place/SP5133/aynho/>. On the early post-Conquest succession of the manor of Aynho, cf. Cooper, pp. 13–19. The summary account of Aynho's manorial history by Baker, vol. 1, pp. 543–5 continues to provide a useful overview. On William (II) de Mandeville's grant to Roger and Alice, see Chapter 1.

Henceforth, this same land was to be enjoyed entirely by the hospital 'in pure and perpetual alms, for sheltering poor brothers seeking to be received there for the love of God' (*in puram et perpetuam elemosinam, ad hospitandum pauperes fratres qui hospitium ibi pro amore Dei petierint*). Such *in elemosinam* gifts had become increasingly common practice in the twelfth and thirteenth centuries, especially in grants to monastic houses, where they gradually replaced the more traditional *pro anima* benefactions as the new preferred means of 'redemptive almsgiving', to borrow Adam Davis's fitting expression.[9] We return to this in the next section of this chapter.

A single hide of arable land was not a huge endowment, even for a newly founded hospital such as Aynho. Under Roger's sons and (eventual) successors, further property was added to the hospital's estate, with his firstborn, Robert (I) Fitz Roger, sheriff of Norfolk and Suffolk (1190–4; 1197–1200), appearing as the main donor of this generation. Having confirmed his father's original bequest, Robert gave the hospital a messuage (no. **7**) and half a virgate (⅛ hide = around fifteen acres) of land (no. **8**) in the vill of Aynho alongside a meadow known as *Refam* and a pasture called *Stenirul* (no. **9**).[10] As we saw in Chapter 1, the younger son, William Fitz Roger, had previously confirmed his father's donation without adding to it (no. **5**). However, the cartulary's subsequent act (no. **6**), which also survives in the original (Aynho 31), is peculiar. In it, William Fitz Roger once more confirms the foundational grant, specifically the half hide of land formerly held by Turbern (*dimidiam hidam terre que fuit Turberni, quam pater meus et mater mea dederunt eidem hospitali*), but this time he himself claims to be increasing it with the half hide previously held by Svein (*in incrementum donationis eorum ego do eidem hospitali dimidiam hidam que fuit Sueini*), as if to imply that this portion of the grant was actually his own to give, rather than his father's. One possible explanation could be that Svein had held one hide of land total, half of which was granted by Roger and the other half by William. But if this were so, then it would seem very strange indeed for William to confirm in the 1180s only Turbern's half hide without mentioning the existing half hide of Svein, which we know his father had given to the hospital as early as 1170/1 (no. **4**). As Aynho manor's apparent

9 Davis, *Economy of Salvation*, pp. 131–9.

10 *Refam* is one of the ancient forms of those place names with the modern form Reepham. For examples from Lincolnshire and Norfolk, see *EPNS*, vol. 85, p. 76; A.D. Mills, *A Dictionary of British Place Names* (Oxford, 2003), p. 388. Derived from Old English, it means 'the village, homestead of the reeve'. Since no such place name appears on modern maps of Aynho and its environs in the location where *Refam* is marked on those from earlier centuries, its old forms (*Refam*/*Rifam*) are used throughout this book.

heir (see Chapter 1), it would surely have been in William's interest to mention and confirm the existing endowment in full before adding to it.

The much more likely explanation, therefore, is that William overplayed his own contribution to the hospital's nascent estate by trying to 'pass off' part of the original grant as his own, thereby fashioning himself, somewhat disingenuously, as a benefactor in his own right. Neither Robert Fitz Roger's subsequent bequests nor the respective confirmations of Roger's grant by William (II) de Mandeville (no. **10**) and Hugh of Avalon, bishop of Lincoln (1186–1200) (no. **11**) show William in the capacity of an independent donor.[11] Why, then, would William have made such a spurious claim? Perhaps the most plausible explanation is that he tried to protect his own inheritance against possible infringement by future rivals, first and foremost his elder brother. William certainly issued no. **6** while his mother Alice was still alive, and possibly after the death of his father Roger, in which case he would already have been tasked with administering Aynho as part of Alice's dower but had not yet come into its full inheritance. If this was the case, and later twelfth-century inheritance custom notwithstanding, then there might well have been a risk – real or perceived – of Robert contesting William's right in the future by claiming Aynho for himself after their mother's death. Indeed, as Ralph Turner put it very aptly with regard to the inheritance disputes among the heirs of William of Mandeville (from whom Alice had, after all, received Aynho in dower), 'although the common law was drawing up careful rules of seniority for heirs and heiresses, the descent of the Mandeville lands [...] illustrates the improbability of strict linear succession'.[12] Such 'sibling rivalry' over part of the hospital's endowment derived from Alice's dower might have been exacerbated further by the considerable commemorative capital and social prestige attached to these gifts in the context of the medieval spiritual economy, in which pious donations, 'whether to monasteries or hospitals, were understood as reciprocal and dynamic exchanges, whereby the donor reaped valuable and calculable assets in the form of spiritual benefits'.[13] And, if William Fitz Roger had indeed been involved in the Great Revolt against Henry II in 1173/4,

11 It is significant, in this regard, that William de Mandeville's confirmation (no. **10**) speaks of Roger, Alice, and William collectively as having made a single (i.e., joint) donation to the hospital ('donationem quam Rogerus filius Ricardi et Aelicia uxor sua et Willelmus filius eorum donaverunt hospitali'), rather than separate or independent ones (in which case one may expect to see the plural *donationes* instead of the singular *donatio* in the earl's act; cf. no. **25**, for example).

12 Turner, 'Mandeville Inheritance', p. 147. On inheritance rights in a rural context, cf. M. Müller, *Childhood, Orphans and Underage Heirs in Medieval Rural England: Growing Up in the Village* (London, 2019), pp. 79–117.

13 Davis, *Economy of Salvation*, p. 133.

then this involvement might have increased even further his desire to be recognised and recorded as a benefactor alongside his brother Robert. Either way, by claiming the role of active donor for himself during the mid-1180s, exaggerated though it might have been, William made a statement as to his wish to step out of his elder brother's shadow – a role into which he could have grown more fully still had he not predeceased (so it seems) both his brother and mother.[14]

As a family unit, Roger, Alice, and their son(s) together endowed the newly founded hospital with about 135 to 195 acres of land, plus a meadow, a pasture, and one (perhaps two) messuage(s), all in/near the vill of Aynho, which, as we saw above, the family had possessed since 1170. The foundational grant of land was perhaps even as much as 225 acres, if the donation to Azurus, detailed without contextualisation in the so-called 'founder's charter' (*carta fundatoris*; no. **3**), relates to the hospital's foundation, which seems impossible to ascertain in the absence of corroborating evidence.[15] Expressed in modern terms, this amounted to between fifty-four (min.) and ninety-one (max.) hectares, an area the size of between seventy-five and 126 football (soccer) fields, which could be used in various ways to generate revenues and income for the fledgling hospital. According to David Hall's extensive survey of Northamptonshire's open fields and their development over the centuries, the township of Aynho comprised, at the point of its maximum recorded expansion between the sixteenth and eighteenth centuries, about 1,262 ½ acres, not much more (and perhaps slightly less) than it did at the time of the aforementioned Domesday survey of 1086.[16] A township can usefully be defined with Hall as 'a basic land-unit characterized by one complete, self-contained field system',[17] usually consisting of a single block of land, which on occasion could be supplemented with

14 See the discussion in Chapter 1.

15 It is perfectly possible, for example, that Roger's grant of one virgate of land in Aynho to his servant Azurus had nothing at all to do with the original foundation of Aynho Hospital, and that its inclusion in the Aynho Cartulary is owed entirely to a desire on the part of the hospital's subsequent managers to gather all documents relating to this location conveniently in one place.

16 Hall, *Northamptonshire*, Appendix. The numerical data for Aynho in Hall's summary table of Northamptonshire's open fields (ibid., pp. 157–64, at p. 157) only starts in the first quarter of the sixteenth century (1521), listing the township as comprising 2 fields (increasing to 3 and 4 in the seventeenth and eighteenth centuries, respectively), with half an acre each and a grand total of 50 ½ yardlands (*c.*1,262 ½ acres) in 1545; also cf. the entry for Aynho in the open-field gazetteer in ibid., pp. 184–85. Some earlier historic data specific to Aynho that reaches back to the mid-fifteenth century (before 1463) is analysed in D. Hall, 'Aynho Fields, Open and Enclosed', *Northamptonshire Past and Present*, 59 (2006), 7–22.

17 Hall, *England*, p. 7.

meadows, woodlands, and pastures so as to be turned into a more versatile – and thus more valuable – multi-purpose landscape. Such an arrangement, while relatively rare in thirteenth-century England, was created for and by Aynho Hospital. This was no happy accident, but the result of a carefully planned and systematically executed endowment strategy on the part of the hospital's major benefactors.

There is clear evidence of this mid-to-long-term endowment strategy in both Roger Fitz Richard's foundational bequest and the subsequent grants and confirmations by his family. When granting the hospital its first hide of land, Roger had been explicit that this donation included all associated woodland, open land, meadows, pastures, roads, paths, and mills (*in bosco, in plano, in pratis, in pasturis, in viis, in semitis, in molendinis*, [etc.]; no. **4**). This formula was then repeated (*sans* mills) by his son, Robert, when appending another half virgate of land to his father's endowment (*in bosco et in plano, in pascuis et in pratis, in viis et semitis, et in omnibus que ad eandem dimidiam virgatam pertinent*; no. **8**), who added, during a separate donation, the pasture of ten oxen and four draught horses and the oxen in Robert's other pastures (*pasturam decem bovum et quatuor affrorum, cum bobus meis in dominica mea pastura et in aliis meis pasturis omnibus ubi boves mei dominici se pascentur*; no. **9**). William Fitz Roger's confirmation of his father's original grant specifically states that the land thus bequeathed could be expected to generate sufficient revenues for the hospital to provide whatever was necessary to the poor seeking its hospitality (*ut de exitu illius terre habeant necessario pauperes hospitari querentes propter Deum*), explicitly forbidding the transfer or use of these lands and revenues for any other purpose (*ut nichil in alios usus transferatur, nisi tamen in usus pauperorum*; no. **5**). The likely intention – certainly the result – of Roger's concerted efforts, and those of his direct heir(s), was the creation of a sustainable estate that provided the(ir) hospital with a stable source of income and varied resources of a kind that could not be generated from sporadic acts of charity and random gifts.

In the years and decades that followed, this estate was consolidated and expanded further by others who followed the founding family's example and endowed the hospital with properties. The exact chronology of these donations is difficult – and sometimes impossible – to establish, given that almost all of them have no dates of issue (and usually no witness list, if known solely from the cartulary), meaning they can only be dated (if at all) relative to certain other acts by which they are preceded or succeeded. Any attempt to arrive at a definitive timeline is also frustrated by the fact that the cartulary's contents are not always arranged in strict chronological order. Such caveats notwithstanding, and due in no small measure to the sizeable corpus of original acts relating to Aynho Hospital that survive alongside the cartulary, we can get some sense of how and by whose donations the hospital's estate developed between the late twelfth and the late thirteenth/early fourteenth century. Most bequests made during the hospital's second 'wave' of endowment (*c.*1190 × 1220) by benefactors of the same generations as Roger's children and grandchildren were grants of land. Among the earliest was another virgate of land (around thirty acres) in the vill of Aynho, with a messuage, which were bequeathed by a certain Ralph the clerk and his wife Matilda (nos. **12–13**) and confirmed by John (I) Fitz Robert (†1240), Robert (I) Fitz Roger's son (no. **14**). This would remain the hospital's last property acquisition in Aynho for some time. The only subsequent acts that concern property in Aynho granted to/by the hospital not mentioned explicitly in previous donations are from the second half of the thirteenth century, only one of which is included in the cartulary. The first of these, dated *c.*1260, records a grant by the hospital's then master, Peter of Windsor, to a certain Roger of Leyton, cook, of a messuage formerly held in Aynho by Richard Sewat, which was located next to the house held of the hospital by John Payn (no. **A8**). The second grant (*c.*1250 × 1270) – this time to the hospital – was made in two instalments by William (II) de la Haye (nos. **32**, **A7**), consisting of 1 ½ acres in his 'outlying meadow' (*pratum forinsecum*) in the meadow of Croughton next to the Cherwell, which an eighteenth-century map (**Fig. 2.1**) shows was adjacent to the hospital's field in Aynho called *Refam*. The final grant – again to the hospital – was made *c.*1290 by yet another descendant of the founding family, John (II) Fitz Robert (aka Clavering; †1332), son of Robert (II) Fitz Roger, who gave a walled fishpond (*unum vivarium muratum*) in Aynho, located between a courtyard (*curia*) already belonging to the hospital and the donor's own arable land (*terra arabilis*).[18]

As far as we know, John II's grant of *c.*1290 marked the end of the hospital's estate expansion in Aynho itself in the period under consideration. Judging from the available documentary evidence, it seems that every time the hospital acquired land or other property in Aynho between its foundation in 1170/1 and the end of the thirteenth century, it did so either directly from Roger Fitz Richard and his descendants or, as the case of John (I) Fitz Robert suggests, by their permission and agency. And yet, Aynho was not the only – and, arguably, not even the primary – location in which the hospital came to acquire property for its growing estate. Beginning with the second wave of endowment and gathering momentum during the third (*c.*1220–70) and fourth (*c.*1270–1300), the nearby vill of Croughton took centre stage and, before long, overtook Aynho as the main source of property for the hospital's estate. Like Aynho, Croughton is recorded in

[18] MCA, Aynho 16.

Domesday Book, where it is said to have had eighteen households in 1086 (less than half the number of Aynho with its forty households) split between three post-Conquest tenants-in-chief.[19] Two were close companions of the Conqueror: Geoffrey de Montbray, bishop of Coutances (1049–93), and Robert, count of Mortain (1049–90) and 1st Earl of Cornwall (1068–90), the king-duke's half-brother. The third tenant-in-chief was none other than Geoffrey (I) de Mandeville, grandfather of Roger Fitz Richard's wife, Alice. According to Domesday, Geoffrey de Mandeville held just over three hides (*c.*396 acres) of ploughland in Croughton (more than double what his episcopal namesake and Robert of Mortain held between them), as well as a mill, with a combined annual value of £1 13s.

It was not the founding family who gave Aynho's newly established hospital its first property in Croughton, however. In fact, the earliest grants in this locality are recorded not in the hospital's cartulary, but in its extant original charters. Judging from their evidence, the first – and indeed the most important – property acquired in Croughton was the chapel of St Michael, which was given and/or confirmed to the hospital on multiple occasions, and by various related individuals, within just a few years of each other. At the beginning stands a grant by Alice de Wavre to a certain Osmund the clerk (*Osmundus clericus*), made *c.*1200 (no. **A2**) and confirmed by Alice's relatives (nos. **A3–A4**). Exactly how this grant relates to Aynho Hospital is unclear, though the same could be said of no. **3**, the contents of which only became hospital property via subsequent grants. As for the chapel in Croughton, this was transferred into the hospital's ownership by Alice and her husband, Baldwin de Boulogne (nos. **41–2**), at some point before October 1202, when it was confirmed thus by Innocent III (no. **1**). Subsequent confirmations of the same chapel as being in the hospital's possession were issued by Alice's and Baldwin's sons, William (no. **43**) and Guy (no. **44**) de la Haye, by Hugh (II) of Wells, bishop of Lincoln (1209–35), and his dean (nos. **47–8**), and by Walter Chamberlain and his wife, Roeis (no. **46**),[20] as well as by Robert de Beaumont and his wife, Melisende (no. **45**), who further granted the hospital half a virgate of land in Croughton (nos. **20–1**) – a grant that was confirmed first by their son, Geoffrey de Beaumont (no. **24**), and then by one Richard son of Osbert (no. **25**) – plus a messuage situated between the same land and the chapel (nos. **22–3**). That these were all complementary rather than competing grants is shown by the fact that the wives of Robert (Melisende) and Baldwin (Alice) were both

[19] *Domesday*, vol. 12, ed. Thorn and Thorn, 4.29, 18.64, 45.2–3; <https://opendomesday.org/place/ SP5433/croughton/>.

[20] On these grants and their chronology, cf. the discussion by Fry, 'Hospitality', pp. 72–4.

daughters of Geoffrey de Wavre (**Genealogy 5**), who, as we have shown in Chapter 1, had close links to the Low Countries, specifically Brabant. Another donor with direct connections to Brabant, Geoffrey de Loenhout, confirmed the donation of yet another virgate of land (with a croft) in Croughton to Aynho Hospital (no. **18**), which had once been held from him by Ralph Blunt, and by Roger de Bray (whose granddaughter, Mabel, was Geoffrey de Loenhout's wife) after him, and which was then donated to Aynho Hospital by the same Walter Chamberlain who also played a part in the bequest of St Michael's chapel (nos. **15–17**, **19**) to the hospital. Given these close mutual relationships, the gift to the hospital of Croughton's chapel and some adjacent properties almost certainly formed yet another case of a 'family venture', similar to what we saw above among Roger Fitz Richard's descendants. We return to the chapel's significance for both the hospital and its benefactors in the next section of this chapter.

The parallels between these families and their respective endowments for Aynho Hospital can be traced further during subsequent decades. Like Roger Fitz Richard's and Alice of Essex's children and grandchildren, the first- and second-generation descendants of Baldwin de Boulogne and Alice de Wavre followed in their parents' footsteps by donating additional (and related) property to the hospital. One of their sons, William (I) de la Haye, seems merely to have confirmed his parents' grants without adding to them, rather like William Fitz Roger (see above). The other, Guy de la Haye – who, as we saw, confirmed the parental grant of the chapel (no. **44**) and Walter Chamberlain's grant of the land he held from Geoffrey de Wavre (no. **19**), as well as another of his parents' gifts to the hospital of one virgate of land in the vill of Byfield (nos. **36–9**) – acted as a benefactor in his own right on at least two separate occasions, once by giving the hospital two acres of land in Croughton *c.*1220 (no. **29**), and again by adding, at an unspecified date, two houses in the same vill, which were confirmed *c.*1260 × 1270 by his son, William (II) de la Haye (no. **31**). This William (Baldwin's and Alice's grandson) would, in turn, advance to become the hospital's most prolific benefactor not only of his own generation, but of his entire lineage to date. Three of the cartulary's acts (nos. **30**, **32–3**), plus an original deed not copied therein (no. **A7**), provide testimony of his serial endowments of property in both Croughton and Aynho during the period *c.*1245 × 1270, together comprising one part of land (presumably one virgate) with a house (*domus*), one acre of arable land (i.e., half an acre in the northern and half an acre in the southern field), and 1 ½ acres of meadowland. William's close contemporary (perhaps his cousin), Richard de Beaumont, added another four acres of land in Croughton to the hospital's estate *c.*1270 × 1280 (no. **A16**), which some years later were released by Alice le Beaumont (Richard's mother?) after the death of her husband (Richard's father?), one Robert

Sergeant (no. **A20**), plus one further acre, also in Croughton, donated *c.*1270 × 1280 (no. **A13**). Subsequent generations of both the Beaumonts and the de la Hayes also gave property in this location to Aynho Hospital, with John de la Haye donating one acre of arable land *c.*1270 (no. **A11**) and one Geoffrey de Beaumont (who is not to be confused with the son of Robert and Melisende by the same name) and his wife, Agnes, a generous five acres *c.*1300 × 1310 (Aynho 5).

There are other individuals and families besides those discussed above that gave property located in and around Croughton to Aynho Hospital in the period under consideration here. Most notably, these include Thomas Newman, son of Robert Newman, who, from 1259 to *c.*1280, donated (or sold) a total of eight acres and one rood of land with a tenement (nos. **56**, **A12, A15, A17–A18, A21**); Robert of Sheering, who gave six acres of land in the same period (nos. **50, 55, A14**); Paulinus of Marlow, who a generation earlier had gifted three acres plus an unspecified number of lands and tenements (no. **51** and, issued by later generations but mentioning Paulinus' grants, Aynho 60–61, 67); William de Turville, who, across the second half of the thirteenth century, donated a total of 1 ½ virgates and three messuages (nos. **57–8** and, a subsequent charter mentioning William's donation, Aynho 54); and a few others who appear but once in the corpus and, for reasons of space, can be excluded from further enumeration. What the numbers presented here show beyond doubt, however, is that over the course of the thirteenth century – specifically during the third and fourth waves of endowment – Croughton soon rivalled and ultimately replaced Aynho itself as the hospital's primary estate location and major revenue stream. This development and shifting priority must prompt us to revisit our previous observation that the Aynho Cartulary's contents do not follow a consistent internal chronology but were instead copied (seemingly) out of sequence. Upon closer inspection, however, it transpires that the cartulary's overarching principle of organisation is less chronology than it is location – a principle encountered with some frequency in medieval cartularies and known as 'topographical organisation'[21] – with acts that relate to Aynho itself (nos. **4–14**) copied first after the two papal privileges and the 'founder's charter', and acts that relate to Croughton (nos. **15–34**, **41–58**) thereafter. Other – albeit comparatively minor – locations are Byfield (nos. **36–9**) and,

[21] For example, in the monastic cartulary of Kirkstead: K. Dutton, 'The Cartulary of the Cistercian Abbey of Kirkstead, Lincolnshire: The Landscape Realities and Documentary Defences of an Abbey Site in the Thirteenth and Fourteenth Centuries', *Journal of Medieval Monastic Studies*, 12 (2023), 77–121, at pp. 84 and 91–2; K. Dutton, 'The Cistercian Abbey of Kirkstead, Lincolnshire: Rethinking a Twelfth-Century Foundation and its Thirteenth-Century Cartulary', *ANS*, 46 (2023), 161–83, at pp. 166–8.

documented solely by original acts, Brackley (nos. **A5**, **A19** and Aynho 11). Both these vills are recorded in Domesday Book, the latter being home to its own hospital,[22] though neither came anywhere close to Croughton and Aynho in their respective contribution to and significance for the hospital's estate building.

Once we look below the level of vills and manors like Aynho, Byfield, Brackley, and Croughton to individual plots of open and enclosed land such as fields, furlongs, meadows, pastures, and crofts, then locating the property acquired by Aynho Hospital during the twelfth and thirteenth centuries with any degree of precision becomes extremely difficult and mostly impossible. This is due, to some extent, to the 'patchwork' character of the hospital's estate, which, instead of being planned and plotted out systematically by a single donor, developed gradually as a product of multiple endowment campaigns by different individuals and families, often over several generations, each of whom gave from their respective landholdings without much consideration of how this would fit within the hospital's existing property landscape. Add to this the irregular typology and nomenclature of Aynho's medieval fields (see below), as well as the transformative changes brought about by their early modern enclosure(s) (1619–1792), and it is not difficult to see why hardly any of them can be pinpointed accurately (or at all) on extant maps of the later seventeenth and early eighteenth centuries,[23] let alone on Ordnance Survey maps (including the preparatory Ordnance Surveyors' Drawings (OSDs) produced *c.*1789–1840).[24] A notable exception is *Refam*, a meadow which is named twice in the cartulary (nos. **1**, **9**), and which also appears on an eighteenth-century estate plan made for Magdalen College (**Fig. 2.1**).[25] Unfortunately, this is not the case with the other locations in the Aynho Cartulary and/or Aynho charters, none of

22 *Domesday*, vol. 12, ed. Thorn and Thorn, 21.1–2, 22.1, 23.12; <https://opendomesday.org/place/ SP5153/byfield/> and <https://opendomesday.org/place/SP5837/brackley/>. See also the respective gazetteer entries in Hall, *Northamptonshire*, pp. 205 (Brackley), 226–8 (Byfield).

23 Take for example Edward Grantham's map of Aynho's upper fields and meadows in/before 1721, which he based on an earlier map of *c.*1681: Northampton, Northamptonshire Archives, CA/9/1/4; *olim* 6268.

24 Grantham's 1721 map and another map made in 1696 (Northampton, Northamptonshire Archives, Map/5077; *olim* 4612) together form the basis of the annotated maps in Hall, 'Aynho Fields', pp. 8, 10, 13, 19 (= Figs. 1–4), none of which, however, shows place names recorded in the Aynho Cartulary and/or charters. Though Aynho features on the margins of three Ordnance Surveyors' Drawings – Bicester (OSD 223), Barford St. John (OSD 224), and Banbury (OSD 225), all produced *c.*1811–5 and freely available via the British Library/Wikidata, <https://w.wiki/3B9Z> – these drawings do not give the medieval names of the surrounding fields, woodlands, etc.

25 MCA, MP/1/54(i). It appears here as *Rifam*.

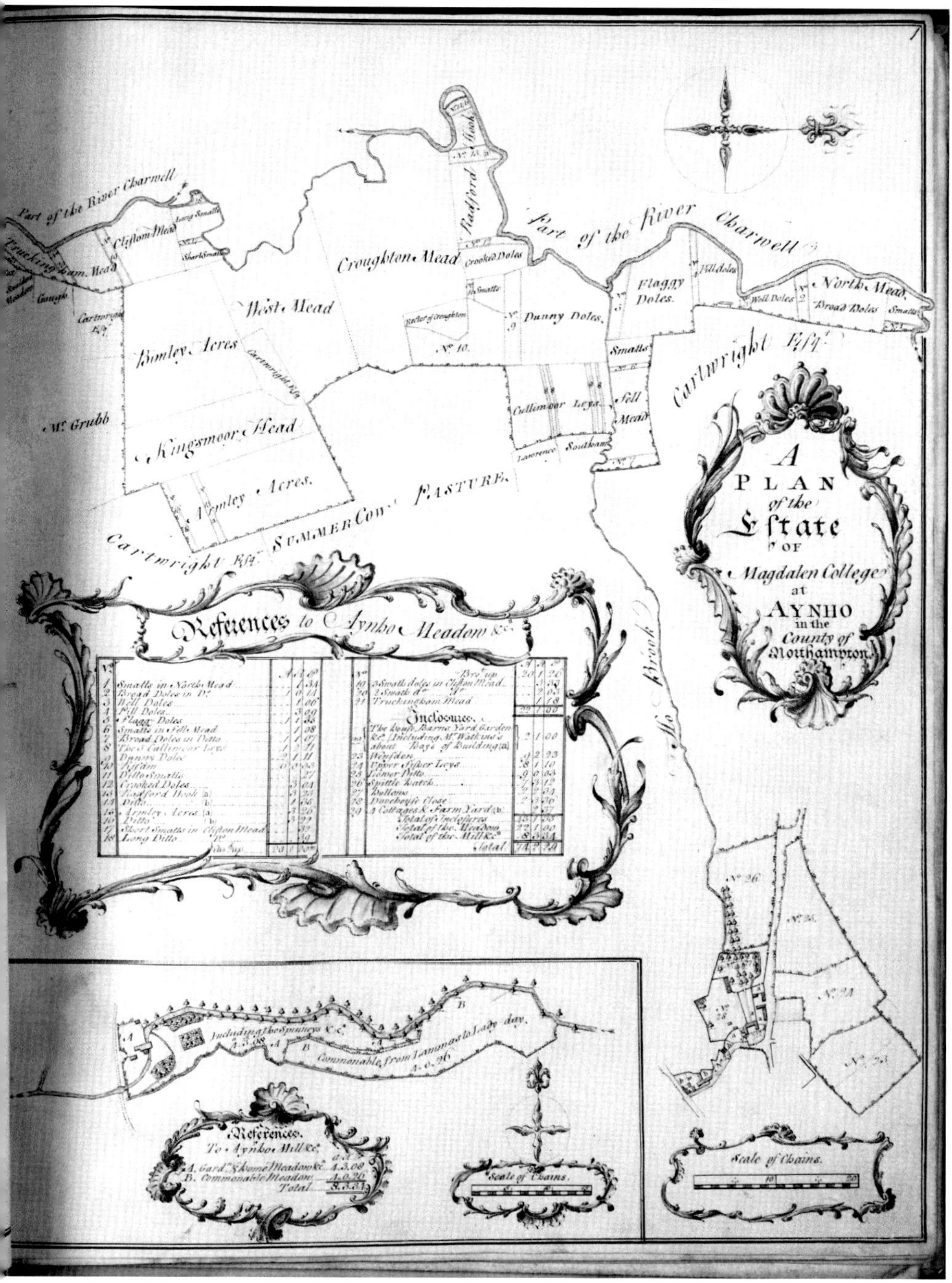


Fig. 2.1. MCA, MP/1/54(i).

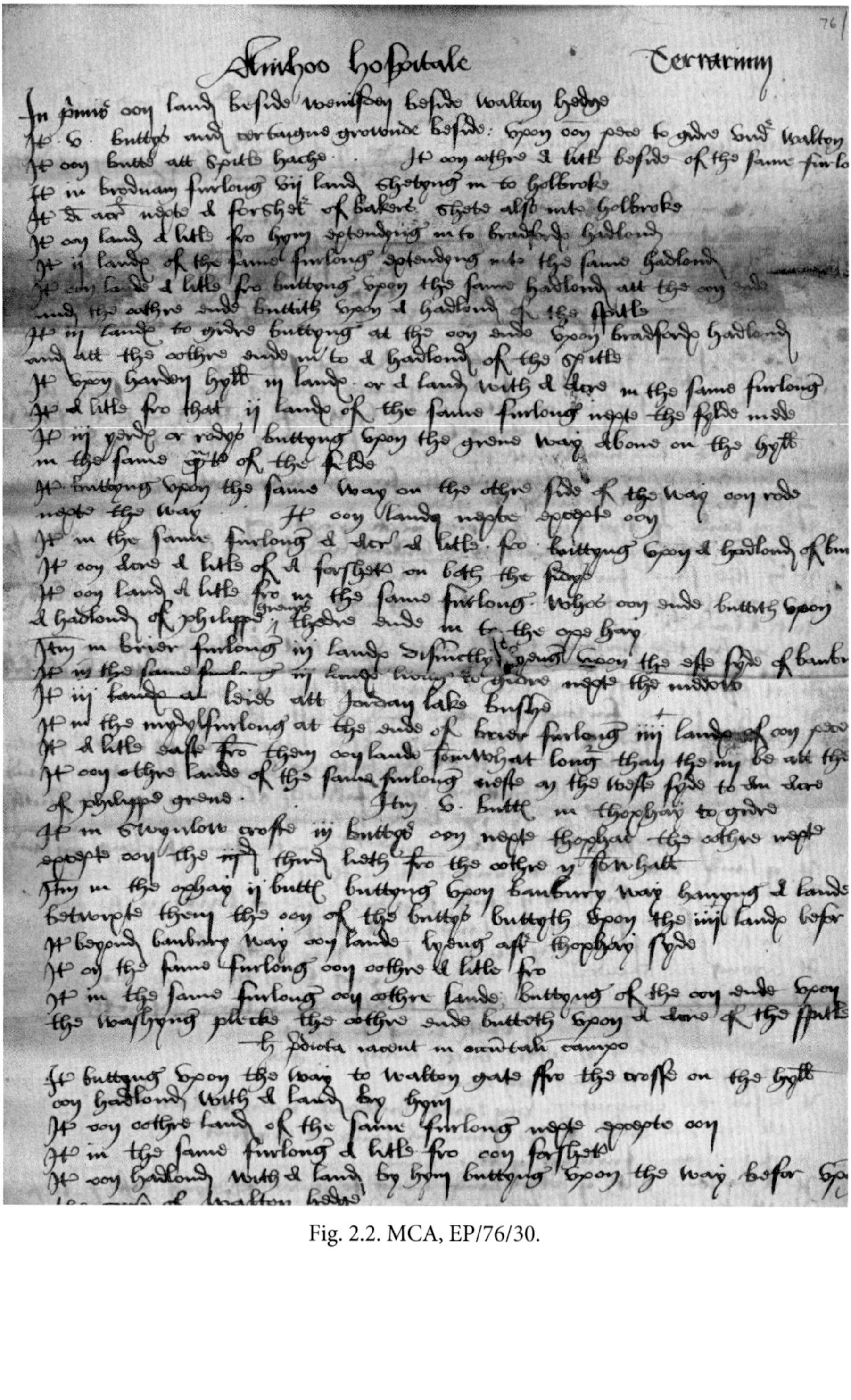

Fig. 2.2. MCA, EP/76/30.

which – with the possible exception of *Smethenhulle* – features in its earliest terrier (*Ainhoo hospitale terrarium*) produced before 1463 (**Fig. 2.2**),[26] suggesting that the thirteenth-century system (or, at the very least, its designations) had disappeared by the mid-fifteenth century, if not earlier.[27] **Table 2.1** below gives the names both of places granted to the hospital and of places mentioned in the cartulary/charters as located near or adjacent to – and serving as reference points for – granted property. References to the corresponding *lemmata* in the English Place-Name Society's Northamptonshire survey (*EPNS*, vol. 10) are also provided where available. Major locations discussed earlier in this chapter (Aynho, Croughton, etc.) and mapped in Chapter 1 (**Fig. 1.1**) have been excluded.

Table 2.1. Place names in the Aynho Cartulary and charters.

| Place name | Recorded in | See also |
|---|---|---|
| *Affegore* | Aynho 5 | |
| *Alnettesaker/Alnettes Aker* | nos. **A16**, **A20** | |
| *Astermere* | no. **A13** | |
| *Bereford* | no. **35** | |
| *Charewell'* (= river) | no. **A7** | *EPNS*, vol. 10, 2, 18 |
| *Chereslawe* | no. **A14** | |
| *Coliersforlong* | no. **A15** | |
| *Eastbernel'* | nos. **49–50** | |
| *Fhurteneakeres* | nos. **49–50** | |
| *Foxholeforlong* | nos. **A16**, **A20** | |
| *Godboldesmilne* | no. **A10** | |
| *Grundhole* | no. **29** | *EPNS*, vol. 10, 278 |
| *Helkesden/Elkesdene* | no. **A13**, Aynho 5 | |
| *Hethermersforlong* | Aynho 5 | |
| *Hinton'/Hinton-way/Hynton'* | nos. **A16**, **A20** | *EPNS*, vol. 10, 54 |
| *Hollemor* | no. **A11** | *EPNS*, vol. 10, 278 |
| *Horsemor* | nos. **51**, **56**, **A6** | *EPNS*, vol. 10, 278 |
| *la Blakemore* | nos. **A16**, **A20** | |
| *la Hydeacre/la Hyde* | nos. **51**, **A6**, **A18** | |

26 MCA, EP/76/30.

27 It is both possible and plausible that *Smethnylle* in EP/76/30 is a variant of *Smethenhulle* (= Smanhill Covert in the parish of Aynho, King's Sutton Hundred).

Table 2.1 *continued*

| Place name | Recorded in | See also |
|---|---|---|
| *Langeford'* | no. **29**, Aynho 5 | |
| *le Blyndewell'/Blindewell* | no. **A12**, Aynho 5 | *EPNS*, vol. 10, 272, 278 |
| *le Breche* | no. **A11** | *EPNS*, vol. 10, 260, 278 |
| *le Estemede* | no. **A13** | |
| *le Heldernestock* | Aynho 56 | |
| *le Mores* | no. **A12** | |
| *le Smaleweye* | nos. **51**, **A6**, **A15** | |
| *Mortog/Moretoke/Morcok* | nos. **15**, **17**, **19** | |
| *Otindene* | no. **A17** | |
| *Radewellehoke* | nos. **A16**, **A20** | |
| *Refam/Rifam* | nos. **1**, **9** | MP/1/54(i) |
| *Rowelowe/Roulowe* | nos. **33**, **A16**, **A20** | *EPNS*, vol. 10, 51 |
| *Salterestrete* | no. **33** | *EPNS*, vol. 10, 5–6 |
| *Schortehanginde* | nos. **A16**, **A20** | |
| *Sefneacres* | nos. **51**, **A6** | |
| *Siche/le Syche* | nos. **55**, **A15** | |
| *Smalebrochulle/Smalebrokeill'* | nos. **56**, **A18** | |
| *Smethenhulle* | nos. **A16**, **A20** | *EPNS*, vol. 10, 48; EP/76/30 |
| *Stanihulle/Stanille* | nos. **56**, **A18** | *EPNS*, vol. 10, 277 |
| *Stenirul* | no. **9** | |
| *Swynestiforlong* | nos. **A16**, **A20** | |
| *Westbithebroc* | no. **A15** | *EPNS*, vol. 10, 274 |
| *Wetendene* | Aynho 5 | |
| *Withemorforlong* | Aynho 5 | *EPNS*, vol. 10, 278 |
| *þickeþorne* | no. **55** | |

What this table shows, even in the absence of specific geographic coordinates, is that the identifiable property locations recorded in the Aynho Cartulary and the extant original charters are concentrated pretty much exclusively – with the exception of *Bereford* (= Barford St John and St Michael, Bloxham Hundred, Oxfordshire) – in Northamptonshire's south-westernmost hundreds of King's Sutton and, to a lesser extent, Chipping Warden. At parish level, the four primary locations are Aynho, Brackley,

Croughton (all in King's Sutton), and Byfield (Chipping Warden). As the place names indicate, the hospital's diverse property portfolio in these locations was situated near meadows (-*mede*), hills (-*hulle*, -*ille*), roads (-*strete*, -*weye*), rivers and (small) bodies of water (-*broc*, -*ford*, -*mere*), and – perhaps most significantly – fields (-*aker*, -*furlong*, etc.).

As shown by Hall, almost all of Northamptonshire's thirteenth-century townships were 'two-field systems' (87%, compared to 100% in the twelfth century and 46% in the fourteenth century) whose arable lands had been laid out systematically in this manner since 1066, and possibly even pre-Conquest.[28] The hospital's charters and cartulary seem to conform and corroborate this system by recording multiple grants of land located in the northern field (*in campo aquilonari*) or the southern field (*in campo australi*), or both.[29] This division into a northern and a southern field, ideally of equal size and acreage to facilitate crop rotation, was a common practice not only in Northamptonshire but across later medieval England, one that ensured a consistent crop supply as long as there were no external factors (extreme weather, pests, etc.) reducing or destroying a given year's harvest.[30] However, Hall's more specific and in-depth study of Aynho's fields both before and after their partial enclosure in 1619 suggests that the northern/southern fields mentioned repeatedly in the hospital's earliest records probably 'do not fall into a simple type found in most parts of the county', meaning that their medieval designations were purely locational and as such 'did not relate to a two-field system'.[31] Aynho's furlongs (i.e., strips of ploughland measuring the length of the furrow, which commonly designated open-field divisions) also seem to have been unusual in that some (but not all) of them were 'bundled' into sets of ten or twelve. Instead of being given individual names, these adjacent furlongs became known collectively as, for instance, the cottagers' lands (*terrae cotariorum*), which is another rare example of a medieval place name connected to the hospital's estate and recorded in its cartulary (no. **8**) that, unlike most of the place names in the table above, can be located with unusual precision and, as demonstrated by Hall, can be traced continuously from the late twelfth/

28 Hall, *Northamptonshire*, pp. 51–3, 154.

29 See nos. **33**, **A11**, **A14**–**A17**, **A19**, and Aynho 5.

30 Hall, *Northamptonshire*, pp. 51–2; Hall, *England*, passim, esp. Chapters 1–2.

31 Hall, 'Aynho Fields', pp. 7, 9. On the enclosure(s) of Aynho's open fields in the seventeenth and eighteenth centuries, see also T. Partida, 'Drawing the Lines: A GIS Study of Enclosure and Landscape in Northamptonshire', unpublished PhD dissertation, University of Huddersfield, 2014, pp. 86–7, 307, with several maps (ibid., pp. 129, 166, 180, 191–2 = Figs. 3.8, 3.35, 4.4, 4.10–4.11).

early thirteenth through the fourteenth (1314; 1391) and into the first half of the seventeenth century (1617).[32]

Whether or not the open fields donated to Aynho Hospital during the period under consideration here adhered to a regular two-field or an irregular multi-field system (so-called 'variable fields'), their value to the hospital ultimately depended on their usage. In addition to cultivating the land themselves – a prospect that may well have proved challenging or altogether impossible, given what can reasonably be inferred about the hospital's permanent 'staff' (see Chapter 4) – Aynho's masters could and probably did rent it out to others to be cultivated in return for a payment/fee. Meanwhile, they would have made additional profit by selling the land's produce on the agricultural market, both at regional markets and fairs and, from 1207, at the hospital's very own fair, which was held for three days around the feast of its patron saint, St James (25 July).[33] Alternatively, land (mainly ploughland, but also woodland, vineyards, etc.) could be leased out long-term or sold off permanently to generate capital by liquidating the hospital's assets.[34] Like many medieval hospitals, much of Aynho's property, and especially the land acquired in the decades after its foundation from donations and bequests by benefactors other than its founders and, less frequently, via quittances, purchases, and exchanges, was bound up in fiefs, meaning its administrators would have been used to collecting rents and tithes from – and, in turn, owing them to – various external parties.[35]

Land was not the hospital's only source of rental income. Another lucrative revenue stream was the local property market, specifically rents from hospital-owned houses and tenements, ranging from single rooms to entire properties. We have seen good examples of this earlier in this section, specifically the various houses and tenements (nos. **31**, **A21** and Aynho 60–1, 67) in Aynho and Croughton given to Aynho Hospital as donations by members of landholding families. Between these buildings and the landed property in Aynho, Croughton, and a few other nearby locations, the hospital over the course of the thirteenth century built a fairly respectable estate in the locality, one which – while unable to rival the large estates of well-endowed monastic houses – would have allowed it to function and deliver care to the sick and needy on a daily basis, especially when combined with the various additional (yet unrecorded) resources and gifts it received through impromptu acts of charity. When the hospital was

32 See Hall, 'Aynho Fields', p. 9, with the relevant fourteenth- and seventeenth-century references.

33 For this market, see Chapter 1. For Northamptonshire's medieval fairs, see Goodfellow, 'Medieval Markets', pp. 305–23.

34 On these sources of income, cf. Davis, *Economy of Salvation*, pp. 166–74.

35 Davis, *Economy of Salvation*, pp. 185–6.

inspected by an archdeacon at the order of Bishop Oliver Sutton of Lincoln (1280–99) in the spring of 1282, soon after the resignation of its master, John of Gra(nt)ham (1269–82), the total property administered by John's direct successor, William of Occold (1282–94), was recorded as comprising four virgates minus one acre of land (= *c*.119 acres) plus the tithes from the aforementioned acre given by John de la Haye minus one lamb, one fleece, and one cheese pertaining to the church of Croughton.[36] All these resources, the inquest stipulated, were to be used wholly and exclusively for offering hospitality and shelter to the poor, disabled, and infirm who would come to the hospital (*ad hospitandum pauperes debiles ac infirmos illuc accedentes*), which from the beginning had been established for this very purpose (*fundatum fuit ab initio*).[37]

Unfortunately, the otherwise detailed report of the episcopal investigation does not specify the location(s) of the four virgates of land held by Aynho Hospital in 1282, nor does it tell us from whose pious gifts and charitable donations they were derived.[38] What we do know, however, is that the archdeacon's tally was rather less than what had been available in property and revenues to William's predecessors in the late twelfth and early thirteenth centuries from the collective donations by Roger Fitz Richard and his family during the first and second 'endowment waves' (see above), and certainly less – by some margin! – than what had been recorded in the Aynho Cartulary about two decades prior to Bishop Sutton's inquest (see Chapter 4 on the cartulary's likely date of production), even without taking into account the various original acts not copied in it. This serves as an important reminder that a medieval hospital's estate was no stable, safe, or self-perpetuating entity that, once established, would simply keep growing in size and value, but a fragile property portfolio that required management, networking, and continuous investment to counteract, as much as possible, loss, devaluation, or infringement by forces both internal (e.g.,

36 BL, MS Harley 6951, fol. 7r: '[I]n temporalibus et decimis quatuor virgatarum terre, una acra excepta[,] pariter cum minutis decimis de dominico Iohannis de Hay provenientibus, uno agno, uno vellere et uno caseo ad matricem ecclesiam de Crowelton' spectantibus exceptis'; edited in *Rolls of Sutton*, vol. 2, pp. 17–18, at p. 17, whose identification of 'magister Iohannes de Graham' (the same spelling as in the hospital's charters and cartulary) as 'John of Grantham' is adopted here. The inquest is dated 12 May 1282.

37 BL, MS Harley 6951, fol. 7r; *Rolls of Sutton*, vol. 1, p. 17.

38 Bishop Sutton's register also contains reports/letters issued following the deaths of William of Occold and his successor, Geoffrey of Croughton, on 16 February 1294 and 17 October 1298, respectively, but neither gives a tally of the hospital's property similar to that produced in 1282; *Rolls of Sutton*, vol. 2, pp. 107–8, 153–4.

mismanagement) and external (e.g., property disputes, conflicting claims, institutional rivalries, etc.).[39]

## INVESTMENT AND PRESTIGE IN THE SPIRITUAL ECONOMY

The previous section of this chapter used the combined evidence of the Aynho Cartulary and selected original charters to reconstruct the creation of the hospital's estate and explore the uses and benefits of charitable gifts and donations primarily from the perspective of the receiving institution (the hospital and its inhabitants), rather than that of the donating parties. As noted in a recent study, however, a peculiarity of many (in fact most) medieval hospitals is that 'we know much more about their donors than about their residents',[40] and Aynho is no exception. In this section, we thus invert the perspective by studying bequests to the hospital not as economic transactions, but as socio-political capital and – first and foremost – as spiritual investments in the medieval economy of salvation. The terms 'spiritual economy' and 'economy of salvation', though used widely in scholarship,[41] require some explanation. Attempts at offering concise working definitions include that by Frederick Paxton, who speaks of 'a system of exchanges among the living, the dead, and the court of the living God – a "medieval economy of salvation"', whose 'currency included tangible assets, like labour, land, and treasure',[42] as well as other worldly goods and services that were, in effect, traded for spiritual assistance in the afterlife through intercessory prayer, anniversary masses, almsgiving, and commemoration.

39 On the erosion and shrinking of hospital estates due to these and other factors, see the discussion, with several pertinent examples, in Watson, '*Fundatio*', pp. 222–239.

40 S. Inskip et al., 'Pathways to the Medieval Hospital: Collective Osteobiographies of Poverty and Charity', *Antiquity*, 97 (2023), 1581–97, at p. 1582.

41 Monographs carrying these terms prominently in their titles include Davis, *Economy of Salvation*; Sweetinburgh, *Role of the Hospital*. Also cf. the shorter (case) studies by G.E.M. Gasper, 'Economy Distorted, Economy Restored: Order, Economy and Salvation in Anglo-Norman Monastic Writing', *ANS*, 38 (2016), 51–66; G.E.M. Gasper, 'Bernard of Clairvaux, Material and Spiritual Order, and the Economy of Salvation', *JMH*, 45 (2019), 580–96; T.N. Bisson, 'A Micro-Economy of Salvation: Further Thoughts on the "Annuary" of Robert of Torigni', *ANS*, 40 (2018), 213–19; C. Lutter et al., 'Kinship, Gender and the Spiritual Economy in Medieval Central European Towns', *History and Anthropology*, 32 (2021), 249–70; F.S. Paxton, 'The Early Growth of the Medieval Economy of Salvation in Latin Christianity', in S.C. Reif et al. (eds), *Death in Jewish Life: Burial and Mourning Customs Among Jews* (Berlin, 2014), pp. 17–42; C. Florea, 'Beyond the Late Medieval Economy of Salvation: The Material Running of the Transylvanian Mendicant Convents', *Hereditas monasteriorum*, 3 (2013), 97–110.

42 Paxton, 'Early Growth', p. 17.

By localising medieval English hospitals within this system of mutual exchanges and expectations across the boundary between life and death, albeit without offering a similarly succinct definition, Sheila Sweetinburgh's influential book argues that – in one reviewer's helpful paraphrase – 'hospitals were not passive recipients of charity, but participants in a reciprocal *spiritual economy*, with the "gift", be it the initial endowment or later grants of money, land or goods, being part of an exchange', in which '[t]he "counter-gift", the other side of the exchange, usually took the form of prayers for the benefactor's soul'.[43] As the same reviewer points out, however, we should be mindful that '[t]he patron's calculation would often have encompassed the social, as well as spiritual, capital to be gained from the ostentatious distribution of charity', capital that, while of great significance, 'is more difficult to measure, since the terms of a grant of land, money or goods often specified the prayers and other services to be provided in return, but prestige has to be inferred'.[44] This important socio-political dimension of the medieval economy of salvation and spiritual gift-giving is also emphasised by Thomas Blanton, who observes that '[t]he gift [...] establishes a circle that, in the view of those that participate in it, unites the human and the divine, the terrestrial and the heavenly, in a system of social relations: worshippers give of themselves because their saviour first gave of himself', while 'those who have been saved' – and, perhaps more to the point, those *seeking* to be saved – 'willingly offer[ed] their tithes, their time, their thanksgiving, and their praise'.[45] Charity thus constituted a moral imperative for those in a position to give, and charitable giving to hospitals such as Aynho was part of a 'moral economy'.[46]

The above should not be taken to suggest that expectations towards salvation and the (trans)actions performed in its pursuit remained stable throughout the millennium conventionally designated as the European/Latin Middle Ages (*c*.500–1500). On the contrary, scholars have repeatedly drawn attention to the fact that the period under consideration here – the later twelfth and thirteenth centuries – marked an important milestone (if perhaps not quite a 'watershed') in the development of the medieval spiritual economy. Paxton, for instance, posits such a 'watershed' around the year 1100, separating what was, in his terminology, the early medieval 'gift economy' of rural landowners from the later medieval 'profit economy'

43 P. Fleming, 'Review of Sheila Sweetinburgh, *The Role of the Hospital in Medieval England: Gift-Giving and the Spiritual Economy*', *EHR*, 122 (2007), 471–3, at p. 471; our emphasis.

44 Fleming, 'Review of Sweetinburgh', p. 472.

45 T.R. Blanton IV, *A Spiritual Economy: Gift Exchange in the Letters of Paul of Tarsus* (New Haven, CT, 2017), p. 4; our interjection.

46 Inskip et al., 'Pathways', p. 1593.

concentrated in urban settings with mercantile activity.[47] While seemingly straightforward categories and distinctions such as these easily (and justifiably) attract scepticism,[48] the impact of commercial developments on later medieval cultures of charity and charitable gift-giving is widely acknowledged in scholarship. Davis thus identifies the twelfth and thirteenth centuries as 'a pivotal moment in European history when care for the sick and poor became popularized and institutionalized', a period when 'new commercial economy infused charitable giving and service with new social and religious meaning and a heightened expectation of reward', yet without – *contra* Paxton – 'eroding the power of the gift'.[49] Equally widely accepted is the role of urbanisation as a major contributing factor to and powerful catalyst for new hospital foundations in later medieval England and other parts of Europe, with Miri Rubin noting that '[t]he awareness of structural problems of urban life, the peculiarities of its complex social structure, and the importance of towns as venues for experimentation in social and political ideas [...] underlay an understanding of the ways in which new solutions to old problems were sought'.[50] The important and, in a sense, inseparable relationship between medieval community, commerce, and charity – each in their constantly evolving and developing formats – is epitomised by Rubin's conclusion that 'forms of charity and relief were thus re-evaluated and refashioned as the perception of the community's economic well-being and its religious and social aims changed'.[51] The communities and networks of which Aynho Hospital was a part and from which it benefited both spiritually and materially were no exception, and they can only be understood and studied fruitfully within these overarching parameters.

At the same time as belonging within this wider orbit of the medieval spiritual economy, Aynho Hospital is also different – and distinct – from many of the houses that underpin the field-shaping studies by Rubin, Davis,

47 Paxton, 'Early Growth', pp. 19–20.

48 See, for example, S.C. Reif, 'A Response to Professor Paxton's Paper', in S.C. Reif et al. (eds), *Death in Jewish Life: Burial and Mourning Customs Among Jews* (Berlin, 2014), pp. 43–50.

49 Davis, *Economy of Salvation*, pp. 5, 9.

50 M. Rubin, 'Development and Change in English Hospitals, 1000–1500', in L. Granshaw and R. Porter (eds), *The Hospital in History* (London, 1989), pp. 41–59, at p. 42. On the development of urban charity in medieval England, see also S. Watson, 'City as Charter: Charity and the Lordship of English Towns, 1170–1250', in C.J. Goodson et al. (eds), *Cities, Texts, and Social Networks, 400–1500: Experiences and Perceptions of Medieval Urban Space* (Farnham, 2010), pp. 235–62.

51 Rubin, 'Development and Change', p. 55.

Sweetinburgh, Watson, Clay, and others.[52] To begin with, its comparatively early date of foundation in the early 1170s (see Chapter 1) makes Aynho a rather precocious yet extraordinarily well-documented example of a phenomenon that, while traceable in post-Conquest England from about the 1080s, only took off in earnest during the second half of the twelfth and the first half of the thirteenth century.[53] As noted recently by Watson, '[n]o hospital is less known or less studied than the pre-1200 hospital', and while 'English hospitals appear in the records haphazardly before *c.*1180 [...] [t]he period 1085–1200 [nevertheless] witnessed the arrival of the hospital into every English county, and the foundation of hundreds of houses of a consistent and recognised form'.[54] Besides being founded at the very eve – and indeed slightly ahead – of this steep incline in English hospital foundations during the final decade and a half of the twelfth century, Aynho Hospital also sets itself apart from many (perhaps most) twelfth- and thirteenth-century houses that have left an equally rich documentary trail by being situated not in a town or burgeoning city, but within a decidedly rural setting. This rural setting of both the hospital itself and, as we saw above, its donated lands and properties, is significant in the context of the present discussion. Though derived from a study of hospitals located across the Channel in Champagne, Davis's pertinent observation that '[t]here was certainly a tendency for people to give to institutions that were nearby or to which they felt some connection, with people in the countryside [...] tending to give to country institutions and towns-people tending to give to urban institutions',[55] also applies, *mutatis mutandis*, to the localities of interest to us here. While the founding family had its origins and patrimony further north and east (mainly in Northumberland and Essex), the individuals and families who followed the lead of Roger and his sons by donating further property in Aynho, Croughton, and elsewhere during subsequent waves of endowment seem to have been of a much more local (or at least regional) background. Another – and possibly a significant – factor in the generosity shown to Aynho Hospital by successive generations

52 In addition to the studies already referenced in this chapter, see also Rubin, *Charity and Community*; Watson, *On Hospitals*; still useful is Clay, *Mediæval Hospitals*, though the figures and (some of the) interpretations presented therein must be taken with caution and are best read in conjunction with the important revisions by Orme and Webster, *English Hospital*.

53 The table 'Hospital statistics, *c.*1080–1530' in Orme and Webster, *English Hospital*, p. 11 lists no existing and 68 new houses for the period 1080–1150, followed by 61 existing/191 new houses in 1151–1200, 225/164 houses in 1201–50, 344/152 houses in 1251–1300, and 440/101 houses in 1301–50.

54 Watson, 'Origin of the Hospital', p. 77; also cf. Watson, 'Sources for Hospitals', p. 65.

55 Davis, *Economy of Salvation*, p. 127.

of twelfth- and thirteenth-century benefactors were the latter's connections across the Channel, particularly with the Low Countries. As discussed in Chapter 1, at least one family closely connected to the hospital (the de Wavres) probably hailed from the duchy of Brabant, and their important gift of the chapel of St Michael in Croughton (see above) might well have been intended to establish and help sustain Aynho Hospital as a place where fellow cross-Channel travellers would be assured of Christian burial, should they need it.[56] To help us understand the motivations of such 'investments' into Aynho Hospital – and the 'investment culture' of the medieval spiritual and moral economy more widely – we need to take a closer look at the language used in the hospital's acts of donation, both those copied in the Aynho Cartulary and those that survive in the original.

Unlike Roger's foundational bequest (no. **4**), the successive donations by others – beginning with the grants of Roger's sons, Robert (I) and William Fitz Roger – were issued not (or not primarily) *in elemosinam* but *pro anima*, a custom that, as noted elsewhere, is indicative of the significant spiritual power ascribed to hospital gifts at a time when *pro anima* clauses were falling out of fashion among monastic donors across Europe, who, from the thirteenth century, generally seem to have preferred to request intercessory prayers and, more desirable still, anniversary services from cloistered monks and nuns in return for their sponsorship.[57] William Fitz Roger donated solely 'for the salvation of the soul (*pro salute anime*) of Earl Geoffrey [(III) de Mandeville, †1166], lord of the fee (*domini fundi*), and the soul of my father, and [those] of my mother and all my relations alive and dead' (no. **5**), and, on the second occasion, 'for the salvation of my father's soul, and [the souls] of my mother, my lord Earl William [II de Mandeville], and all my friends alive and dead' (no. **6**). Robert (I), too, repeatedly employed the customary *pro anima* formula when granting property to the hospital 'for the salvation of my soul and the souls of all my ancestors' (nos. **7**, **9**), and, more specifically, 'for the salvation of the souls

[56] Recent study of the medieval burials at the hospital of St John the Evangelist in Cambridge has revealed 'strong genetic affinities with Dutch and Scandinavian populations', many of whom 'may never have lived in the hospital, but were simply buried there', with the hospital providing a crucial service to those who died far from their home and parish; Inskip, 'Pathways', pp. 1592–3; R. Hui et al., 'Medieval Social Landscape through the Genetic History of Cambridgeshire before and after the Black Death', *BioRxiv* (2023), <https://doi.org/10.1101/2023.03.03.531048>. As discussed in Chapter 1, Aynho's proximity to a major tournament site, its geographical location on a major throughfare, and the hospital's right to hold a three-day fair make it almost certain that it was a place visited regularly by those far from Aynho itself.

[57] Davis, *Economy of Salvation*, pp. 116, 131. Also cf. J. Burton (ed.), *The Cartulary of Byland Abbey* (Woodbridge, 2004), pp. lxi–lxii.

of my father Roger, my mother Alice, and my brother William, and for my own soul and [that] of my wife Margaret, and [those] of all my ancestors' (no. **8**). Unlike his brother, however, in each case he also adopted the more current and fashionable *in elemosinam* clause in line with his father's original grant (*in puram et liberam et perpetuam elemosinam*). Moving forward chronologically through the cartulary's contents, acts exclusively using *pro anima* clauses like the hospital's original endowment quickly begin to diminish in number and frequency, merely constituting *c.*12.5% of the total corpus (nos. **12–13, 17, 25, 30, 44**). Given that over the course of the thirteenth century *pro anima* gifts were gradually being replaced wholesale on both sides of the Channel by *in elemosinam* gifts,[58] one might expect to see a much higher proportion of the latter in the cartulary. This is not the case, however, with acts exclusively using *in elemosinam* clauses only accounting for *c.*12.5% of the cartulary (nos. **11, 22–4, 43, 58**). Rather, by far the largest portion (nearly 40%) of the donations received by the hospital and recorded in its cartulary are what can be considered a transitional or 'mixed' type, one which combines *both* formulae (*pro anima* and *in elemosinam*) similar to Robert (I) Fitz Roger's bequests.[59] An even clearer picture emerges from those Aynho Hospital charters not copied in the cartulary, five of which (nearly 25%) use the mixed type, three (*c.*15%) *in elemosinam* only, and none *pro anima* only.[60]

It is difficult to know why Aynho Hospital's benefactors seem to have 'bucked the trend' somewhat by persisting for longer than usual in their use of the *pro anima* formula without completely rejecting the increasingly widespread *in elemosinam* clauses either, opting instead for something of a 'halfway house' well into the final quarter of the thirteenth century (and quite possibly beyond). It is not implausible, however, that these third- and fourth- generation donors might have chosen – or perhaps were instructed by the beneficiary – to follow the precedent set in the late twelfth century by the founder's son and heir. Robert (I) Fitz Richard was a very influential

58 Davis, *Economy of Salvation*, pp. 131–9, with reference to the unpublished work of R.L. Keyser, 'Gift, Dispute, and Contract: Gift Exchange and Legalism in Monastic Property Dealings, Montier-la-Celle, France, 1100–1350', unpublished PhD dissertation, Johns Hopkins University, 2001. Also cf. A. Angenendt, '*Donationes pro anima*: Gift and Countergift in the Early Medieval Liturgy', in J.R. Davis and M. McCormick (eds), *The Long Morning of Medieval Europe: New Directions in Early Medieval Studies* (Aldershot, 2008), pp. 131–54; E. Magnani, 'Almsgiving, *Donatio Pro Anima* and Eucharistic Offering in the Early Middle Ages of Western Europe (4th–9th century)', in M. Frenkel and Y. Lev (eds), *Charity and Giving in Monotheistic Religions* (Berlin, 2009), pp. 111–24.

59 These are nos. **20–1, 26–7, 29, 31–7, 41–2, 45–6, 56–7**.

60 *In elemosinam*: nos. **A2, A15, A17**; mixed type: nos. **A3–4, A7, A10–A11**.

and well-connected patron – 'a man of some consequence',[61] to borrow one scholar's words – and association with him, if only through imitation, would have carried no small amount of prestige in the locality and even further afield. As we saw in Chapter 1, Robert, having inherited his father's original estates, expanded his powerbase through marriage into East Anglia before rising to the shrievalty of Norfolk and Suffolk, and subsequently Northumberland, with King John's reign marking the apex of his career. Robert was also a founder in his own right, having established and patronised Langley Abbey, where he would be buried in 1214. Given this monastic connection, it is perhaps no coincidence that Robert's grants to his father's hospital should introduce some terminology that, while only adopted gradually by hospital benefactors, were embraced much more readily and comprehensively, and from an earlier point, by patrons of monastic foundations. Thus, when the next wave of benefactors – represented by more modest aristocratic couples such as Robert de Beaumont and Melisende, Baldwin de Boulogne and Alice de Wavre, and Walter Chamberlain and Roeis – began to turn their attention and resources to Aynho Hospital, Robert (I) Fitz Roger was still very much alive and, as noted in the previous section of this chapter, had become if not the most generous, then certainly the hospital's most visible patron. These aspiring families could have done worse than to follow – and, importantly, be seen to follow – Robert's prominent example by fashioning themselves in his image and by mirroring, as much as possible, the terms of his donations in their own gifts, which they did by combining, as Robert had done, *pro anima* and *in elemosinam* formulae,[62] thereby ensuring maximum consistency with the local tradition and maximising the prestige and cultural capital of their investments.

It is not only the specific *modus* of gift-giving (*in elemosinam* vs. *pro anima*) that distinguishes the donations made to Aynho Hospital by its benefactors, but also the terminology used to describe their dedicatees. Given the hospital's lack of domestic scribal and documentary expertise (see Chapters 3 and 4), it seems likely that this choice of terminology lay with, first and foremost, the donors themselves. In his original bequest, Roger Fitz Richard had nominated God, St Mary, and the hospital's primary patron saint, St James (with St John acting as its 'co-patron' from the early-to-mid thirteenth century), as beneficiaries (*Deo et sancte Marie et sancto Iacobo*; no. **4**).[63] His son, Robert, then adopted this dedication in one of his bequests, merely adding the now established hospital as a dedicatee in its

61 Round, 'Early Sheriffs', p. 492.

62 See, for examples, nos. **20–1**, **36–7**, **45–6**.

63 The first act in the cartulary with a dedication to both SS James and John is no. **14** (*Deo et fratribus hospitalis beatorum apostolorum Iohannis et Iacobi de Hayno*), with similar dedications occurring regularly thereafter.

own right (*et hospitali*; no. **8**). Robert's second grant uses the same formula but (quietly) subsumes the patron saint under the hospital (*Deo et beate Marie et hospitali*; no. **9**), whereas his third grant names only the hospital (*hospitali*; no. **7**). Robert's brother, William, names either only the hospital (no. **5**) or the hospital and God (no. **6**) in his donations. The Almighty's prominence among the named beneficiaries of the hospital's early donations is worthy of note. As emphasised by Davis, 'Deo et hospitali' is 'a formulation that, while relatively rare in thirteenth-century charters, reflects the common association between pious gift and divine reward', with some benefactors 'conceiv[ing] of their gifts as gifts to God as much as to a hospital and its sick [inhabitants]'.[64] In a sense, couching gifts in these and similar terms provided an opportunity to 'cut out the middle man' by donating directly to God as a 'high-return investment' in one's own salvation. In addition, formulae such as 'Deo et hospitali' might have served as a kind of safeguarding mechanism. By being assigned and dedicated explicitly not just to the hospital and its appointed administrators (masters/proctors), but also and specifically to its saintly protectors and even to God Himself, the gifted land and resources effectively became 'shared property' that was protected, at least in theory, against future alienation, sale, or transferral, thereby guaranteeing, again in theory, their donors a relatively safe and long-term spiritual return on their temporal investments – the 'purchase of paradise', to adopt one scholar's colourful expression.[65] Rather than depending on intercession through prayers, anniversary masses, or other commemorative services performed by the hospital's inhabitants, these investments were registered directly with – and their returns distributed directly by – the highest spiritual authority ahead of the Last Judgement.

Such direct investment with the bank of God and requests for intercessory support from the hospital's staff and inhabitants were not mutually exclusive, of course. Indeed, one of the regular (and primary) functions of medieval hospitals – and an important motivator for their benefactors – was the provision of religious, liturgical, and commemorative services, from worship and prayer to pastoral care and burial.[66] The prospect of

64 Davis, *Economy of Salvation*, p. 132.

65 J.T. Rosenthal, *The Purchase of Paradise: Gift Giving and the Aristocracy, 1307–1485* (London, 1972).

66 Cf. Orme and Webster, *English Hospital*, pp. 49–56; Sweetinburgh, *Role of the Hospital*, pp. 37–8; N.R. Rice, *The Medieval Hospital: Literary Culture and Community in England, 1350–1550* (Notre Dame, IN, 2023), pp. 4–9; M. Carlin, 'Medieval English Hospitals', in L. Granshaw and R. Porter (eds), *The Hospital in History* (London, 1989), pp. 21–39, at p. 32; C. Rawcliffe, 'Communities of the Living and of the Dead: Hospital Confraternities in the Later Middle Ages', in C.N. Bonfield et al. (eds), *Hospitals and Communities, 1100–1960* (Bern, 2013), pp. 125–54. For a case

these services would have remained attractive to the benefactors of Aynho Hospital, including those who had made out their gifts to God with a view to being recompensed in the afterlife, some of whom also made specific provision for spiritual assistance in this world, often as a part of the same grant. William (II) de la Haye thus confirmed the two houses in Croughton given 'Deo et beate Marie et magistro et fratribus hospitalis beatorum apostolorum Iacobi et Iohannis de Eynno [...] in liberam, puram et perpetuam elemosinam' by his late father, Guy, 'for the sustenance of two wax candles to be burned during the daily mass of St Mary in their chapel at Aynho' (*ad sustentationem duorum cereorum ardentum ad missam beate Marie omnibus diebus scilicet in capella sua de Eynno*; no. **31**). Around the same time, the same William gave one acre of land in free, pure, and perpetual alms to God, Mary, and the master and brothers of the hospital at Aynho, which he expected – and earmarked explicitly in his charter – to provide not only for the salvation of his own soul and those of his ancestors and successors (*pro salute anime mee et animabus antecessorum et successorum meorum*), but also, and more specifically, 'for the anniversary [mass] of my father Guy, and [those of] my mother Amicia and my boys, to be celebrated annually in their church on the days marked with their names in the hospital's book of obits' (*per aniversarium Gwidonis patris mei et Amicie matris mee et puerorum meorum annuatim in ecclesia sua celebrandum in diebus quibus nomina eorum notantur in martilogio dicti hospitalis*; no. **33**). As with monastic houses, having one's name (and those of one's family) inscribed and marked for perpetual commemoration in a hospital's book of obits or 'book of life' (*liber vitae*) amidst its venerated saints, martyrs, patrons, and other high-ranking benefactors was a great privilege that carried considerable cultural capital and prestige.[67] When Thomas Newman (no. **56**) gave two acres and one rood of land 'Deo et beate Marie et magistro et fratribus hospitalis beatorum apostolorum Iacobi et Iohannis de Heyno' in free, pure, and perpetual alms (*in liberam et puram et perpetuam elemosinam*), he did so explicitly 'on the condition that the anniversary day of Margaret, countess of Kent, deceased, is celebrated for the salvation of her soul in the said hospital, each and every year, on the feast day of St Malo, bishop and

study, see C. Rawcliffe, "Gret criynge and joly chauntynge": Life, Death and Liturgy at St. Giles's Hospital, Norwich, in the Thirteenth and Fourteenth Centuries', in C. Rawcliffe et al. (eds), *Counties and Communities: Essays on East Anglian History Presented to Hassell Smith* (Norwich, 1996), pp. 37–55.

67 C. Rawcliffe, '"Written in the Book of Life": Building the Libraries of Medieval English Hospitals and Almshouses', *The Library*, 3 (2002), 127–62; M. Niederkorn-Bruck, 'Prosopographisches in Martyrologien', in R. Berndt (ed.), "*Eure Namen sind im Buch des Lebens geschrieben": Antike und mittelalterliche Quellen als Grundlage moderner prosopographischer Forschung* (Münster, 2014), pp. 205–28.

confessor' (*ita tamen quod omnibus et singulis annis celebretur anniversarius dies Margarete comitisse de* Kent, *defuncte, pro salute anime eius in dicto hospitali, die sancti Macuti episcopi et confessoris*). Countess Margaret was the daughter of William the Lion, king of Scots (1165–1214). Thomas's wish that she be commemorated on the feast of St Malo (15 November), whose cult was celebrated widely in medieval Brittany, Wales, and also Scotland,[68] might reflect an attempt to emphasise (and perhaps imitate) the Scottish dynastic connections of the hospital's founding family (see Chapter 1). Be that as it may, William (II) de la Haye, Thomas Newman, and others were keen to maximise the return on their investments in Aynho Hospital by making them work and pay dividends twice: first as a spiritual deposit with God to be 'cashed in' at the day of reckoning, and second as a temporal deposit with the hospital's present and future members that obliged them to render certain services for the donors and their kin. As with their strategic choice of using an idiosyncratic combination of *pro anima* and *in elemosinam* clauses, the hospital's later twelfth and thirteenth-century benefactors once again appear to have opted for a 'mixed economy' that combined various dedicatees (God, the saints, the hospital's inhabitants, etc.) and thus enabled them to get the best of *both* worlds: this one and the next.

As with these *pro anima/in elemosinam* formulae, the evidence from Aynho of gifts given 'to God and the hospital' seems to go against and/or anticipate some wider trends that scholars have identified across the map. Far from constituting an exception, the formula 'Deo et hospitali' continues to figure prominently in the acts that follow those of the founding family in the cartulary. No fewer than twenty (*c.*42.5%) of the acts copied after those by Robert (I) Fitz Roger employ this formula (or a variant thereof), including grants by the hospital's most prominent second-, third-, and fourth-generation donors from families like the Beaumonts, the de la Hayes, and the Newmans, with additional examples among the extant original charters.[69] As before, it is difficult to know what part (if any) the example of the hospital's founding family – specifically Robert (I) Fitz Roger – played in shaping a possible model for future generations of benefactors aspiring to follow in their footsteps and to fashion themselves as their peers. But we should not discard the possibility that the memory of these early grants, and the considerable prestige and socio-political currency attached to them, exercised a gravitational pull that continued to be felt strongly

68 See B.J. Lewis, 'St Mechyll of Anglesey, St Maughold of Man and St Malo of Brittany', *Studia Celtica Fennica*, 11 (2014), 24–38, at pp. 29–30; M. Hammond, 'Royal and Aristocratic Attitudes to Saints and the Virgin Mary in Twelfth- and Thirteenth-Century Scotland', in S. Boardman (ed.), *The Cult of Saints and the Virgin Mary in Medieval Scotland* (Woodbridge, 2010), pp. 61–85, at pp. 73–4.

69 See nos. **12–14**, **17–18**, **21–5**, **29**, **31–5**, **50**, **56–8**; Aynho 8, 39, 51, 66.

throughout the later twelfth and thirteenth centuries. As noted by Rubin, '[i]n the nature of institutional foundations which are meant to enhance prestige, the personal symbolic act of giving was always of vital importance in the charitable exchange'.[70] The endowments of Aynho Hospital studied and contextualised in this chapter are no exception. In the spiritual economy of the thirteenth century, being seen – and, ideally, being recorded for posterity – as giving alongside one's peers was of equal importance from a socio-political and socio-economic perspective as the gift itself, lending hospital donations a public and performative quality (not entirely dissimilar from modern-day charity fundraisers organised among society's most wealthy and well-connected).

The provision of a chapel formed an important element of this 'public' investment culture. Chapels fulfilled various key functions in the everyday life and activities of medieval hospitals, most fundamentally perhaps as sites of worship, community engagement, and for the performance of burial rites.[71] The right to be buried in a hospital's cemetery in proximity to its chapel was a privilege usually reserved for its primary patrons (the founders and their families) and the most generous benefactors as a powerful symbol of their elevated status and special attachment, one that could be considered on a par with other exclusive privileges such as the right to appoint the head of house.[72] The contemporary hospital at Brackley, which became a quasi-mausoleum for the de Quincy family, provides a pertinent comparison.[73] It was also a custom that brought hospitals into direct competition, and sometimes conflict, with diocesan bishops and local parish churches. It is no coincidence, therefore, that one of Innocent III's privileges for the hospital copied prominently at the opening of the Aynho Cartulary gives its masters 'the [right of] burial for the brothers and your family [or household], for the poor and guests, and for those who hand themselves over to your house, saving the rights of the mother church' (*sepulturam pro fratribus et familia vestra, pauperibus hospitibusque et hiis, qui se domui vestre reddiderint, salvo iure matricis ecclesie*; no. **1**). As we saw in the previous section, the earliest evidence for the presence of a hospital chapel at Aynho (or rather at nearby Croughton) comes from the first two decades

70 Rubin, 'Imagining Medieval Hospitals', p. 21.

71 See Fry, 'Hospitality', pp. 67–74. Recent scholarship dedicated to medieval hospital chapels includes I. Soden and D.J. Leigh, 'The Hospital Chapel of St John, Northampton', *Northamptonshire Archaeology*, 34 (2006), 125–38; L. Grant, 'The Chapel of the Hospital of Saint-Jean at Angers: *Acta*, Statutes, Architecture and Interpretation', in J.A. Franklin et al. (eds), *Architecture and Interpretation: Essays for Eric Fernie* (Woodbridge, 2012), pp. 306–14.

72 Davis, *Economy of Salvation*, pp. 123–4; Watson, '*Fundatio*', pp. 129–88.

73 See above, Chapter 1; also cf. Watson, 'A Mother's Past', pp. 244–8.

of the thirteenth century, when the hospital received, seemingly in quick succession, a series of grants whose donors included virtually all major benefactors who have accompanied us throughout this chapter – Robert de Beaumont and Melisende, Walter Chamberlain and Roeis, and Baldwin de Boulogne and Alice de Wavre, as well as the latter's sons, William (I) and Guy de la Haye, and grandson, William (II) de la Haye – each of whom was involved, in some capacity or another, in granting and/or confirming to the hospital the chapel of St Michael. The reason for this 'joint venture', which, as suggested above, seems to have been undertaken in the spirit of collaboration, rather than competition, might well have been the special combination of spiritual privilege and social prestige that the patronage of a hospital chapel offered to aristocratic investors seeking to make their mark on both the local economy and, perhaps more importantly, the medieval economy of salvation.

## CONCLUSION

This chapter has served a twofold purpose: first, it has used the primary evidence of the Aynho Cartulary alongside original charters for a quantitative and qualitative survey of Aynho Hospital's property, its major patrons and benefactors, and the development and expansion of its estate over the course of the later twelfth and thirteenth centuries. Doing so has enabled us to detect and distinguish successive phases or 'waves' of endowment, beginning with the foundational grants by the hospital's founding family – Roger Fitz Richard, his wife Alice, and their sons, Robert (I) and William Fitz Roger – and continuing with additional bequests on the part of the family's subsequent generations, including Roger's and Alice's grandson, John (I) Fitz Robert, and their great-great-grandson, Robert (II) Fitz Roger. Most property initially donated to the hospital by members of this family, especially its earliest generations, came from the family estate at and around Aynho, the manor of which they had inherited from Alice's lineage via her nephew, Earl William (II) de Mandeville. As the thirteenth century got underway and the benefactor's baton was gradually passed from the founding family to other aristocratic families, some of them more locally rooted than Roger and his heirs, the hospital's property portfolio broadened and diversified as a result, with the nearby vill of Croughton replacing Aynho as the primary location. Besides land, the hospital also acquired important assets and revenue streams in the form of houses (or parts thereof) that could be rented or leased out for profit on the local property market, again with a notable concentration in Croughton. Shifting its focus away from the temporal benefits enjoyed by the hospital as a consequence of charitable gift-giving to the spiritual advantages and rewards offered to its benefactors, the chapter's second purpose has been to explore the significance of these donations in the context of the medieval economy of salvation. At the same time as being located within a wider European landscape of charity, Aynho Hospital also provides us with important evidence of a more local culture of investment in the 'new' spiritual and moral economy of the twelfth and thirteenth centuries, with developments that sometimes confirm but at other times contradict the trends seen more broadly across the board.[74] As we saw, Aynho's successive generations of benefactors developed their own individual and sometimes idiosyncratic investment strategies and documentary customs, but they also were – and were keen to be seen as – part of an established tradition, allowing them both to maximise the spiritual returns on their investments and to garner the significant prestige and cultural capital attached to charitable donations to hospitals among their peers and in medieval society generally. Taken together, the analyses presented in this chapter have allowed us to establish a 'social taxonomy' of the individuals and families, who, through charitable gifts of property and/or resources, helped build Aynho Hospital's estate during a period that saw both transformative economic changes and, as argued in a recent study, 'the growing democratization of charity'.[75] Having situated the hospital within these networks of patronage, we can now turn our attention to other networks that, as the next chapter will show, were crucial to the documentary and scribal cultures that produced the Aynho Cartulary.

74 The recent interdisciplinary study of the medieval hospital of St John the Evangelist in Cambridge provides a particularly fruitful case for comparison; Inskip, 'Pathways', pp. 1593–5.

75 Davis, *Economy of Salvation*, p. 116; the term 'social taxonomy' is adopted from ibid., p. 11.

Table 2.2. Aynho Hospital's property according to the Aynho Cartulary.

| Property | Given by | Confirmed by | Act(s) |
|---|---|---|---|
| 2 × ½ hide of land in **Aynho** | Roger Fitz Richard | i. William Fitz Roger<br>ii. Robert Fitz Roger<br>iii. William de Mandeville<br>iv. Hugh [I], bp of Lincoln | **4–7, 10–11** |
| ½ hide of land in **Aynho** [same as above] | William Fitz Roger | William de Mandeville | **6, 10** |
| 1 messuage in **Aynho** | Robert Fitz Roger | Hugh [I], bp of Lincoln | **7, 11** |
| ½ virgate of land in **Aynho** | Robert Fitz Roger | | **8** |
| 1 meadow (*Refam*) and 1 demesne pasture (*Stenirul*) | Robert Fitz Roger | | **9** |
| 1 virgate of land and 1 messuage in **Aynho** | Ralph the clerk and Matilda | John Fitz Robert | **12–14** |
| 1 virgate of land in **Croughton** and 1 croft called *Mortog/Morcok* | Walter Chamberlain | i. Geoffrey de Loenhout<br>ii. Guy de la Haye | **15–19** |
| ½ virgate of land in **Croughton** | Robert de Beaumont and Melisende | i. Geoffrey de Beaumont<br>ii. Richard, son of Osbert | **20–1, 24–5** |
| 1 messuage in **Croughton** | Robert de Beaumont and Melisende | i. Geoffrey de Beaumont<br>ii. Richard, son of Osbert | **22–5** |
| 1 part of a courtyard in **Croughton** | Robert of Fritwell | Thomas [of Fritwell] | **26–7** |
| 2 acres of land in **Croughton** (at *Langeford'* and *Grundhole*) | Guy de la Haye | | **29** |
| 1 part of land in **Croughton** | William [II] de la Haye | | **30** |
| 2 houses in **Croughton** (1 cottage and 1 messuage) | Guy de la Haye | William [II] de la Haye | **31** |

Table 2.2. *continued*

| **Property** | **Given by** | **Confirmed by** | **Act(s)** |
|---|---|---|---|
| 2 half acres of meadowland in **Aynho** (in the meadow of Croughton) | William [II] de la Haye | | **32** |
| 2 × ½ acre of land in **Croughton** | William [II] de la Haye | | **33** |
| 1 house in **Croughton** | Reginald of Halse | | **34** |
| 1 virgate of land in **Byfield** | Baldwin de Boulogne and Alice | i. William [I] de la Haye<br>ii. Guy de la Haye | **36–9** |
| 1 chapel of St Michael in **Croughton** | Baldwin de Boulogne and Alice | i. William [I] de la Haye<br>ii. Guy de la Haye<br>iii. Hugh [II], bp of Lincoln<br>iv. Roger, dean of Lincoln | **41–4, 47–8** |
| 1 chapel of St Michael in **Croughton** [same as above] | Robert de Beaumont and Melisende | | **45** |
| 1 chapel of St Michael in **Croughton** [same as above] | Walter Chamberlain and Roeis | | **46** |
| 5 acres of land in **Croughton** | Robert of Sheering | | **49–50** |
| 3 acres of land in **Croughton** | Paulinus of Marlow | | **51** |
| 2 acres of land in **Croughton** | Robert of Sheering | | **55** |
| 2 acres and 1 rood of land in **Croughton** | Thomas [Newman] | | **56** |
| ½ virgate of land and 1 messuage in **Croughton** | William de Turville | | **57** |
| ½ virgate of land and 1 messuage in **Croughton** [same as above] | William de Turville | | **58** |

Table 2.3. Aynho Hospital's property according to acts not copied in the Aynho Cartulary.

| **Property** | **Given by** | **Confirmed by** | **Act(s)** |
|---|---|---|---|
| 1 messuage and courtyard in **Brackley** | … | | **A5** |
| ½ acre of meadowland in **Aynho** (in the meadow of Croughton) | William [II] de la Haye | | **A7** |
| 1 messuage in **Aynho** | … | | **A8** |
| [?] of land in **Croughton** | … | William Wakelin and Joan | **A9** |
| 2 × ½ acre of land in **Croughton** (at *Hollemor* and *le Breche*) | John de la Haye | | **A11** |
| 2 × 1 rood and ½ acre of land in **Croughton** (at *Astermere*, *Helkesden*, and *le Estemede*) | Richard de Beaumont | | **A13** |
| 1 acre of land in **Croughton** (above *Chereslawe*) | Robert of Sheering | | **A14** |
| 4 × ½ acre of land in **Croughton** (above *Coliers-forlong* and *le Syche*, beyond *le Smaleweye*, and at *Westbithebroc*) | Thomas Newman | | **A15** |
| 2 × ½ acre of land in **Croughton** (at *le Mores* and *le Blyndewelle*) | Thomas Newman | | **A12** |
| 4 acres of land in **Croughton** (at/near *Foxholeforlong*, *Roulowe*, *Swynestiforlong*, *le Blakemore*, *Hinton-way*, *Alnettesaker*, *Schortehanginde*, *Smethenhulle*, and *Radewellehoke*) | Richard de Beaumont | Alice le Beaumont | **A16**, **A20** |
| 2 × 1 acre of land in **Croughton** | Thomas Newman | | **A17** |

Table 2.3. *continued*

| Property | Given by | Confirmed by | Act(s) |
|---|---|---|---|
| 2 × ½ acre of land in **Croughton** (at *Smalebrokeill'* and *Stanille*) | Thomas Newman | | **A18** |
| 1 plot of land in **Brackley** with houses and 1 meadow | Roger [le Goer] | | **A19** |
| 1 tenement in **Croughton** | Thomas Newman | Margaret [Newman] | Aynho 47 |
| 1 messuage in **Brackley** | … | Richard [le Goer] | Aynho 11 |
| 1 walled fishpond in **Aynho** | John de Clavering | | Aynho 16 |
| 2 acres of land in **Croughton** (at *le Heldernestock*) | Agnes | | Aynho 56 |
| [?] of land and [?] tenements in **Croughton** | Paulinus, son of Roger Cook of Marlow | i. Lucy<br>ii. Imayna | Aynho 60–1, 67 |
| 2 × 1 acre and 3 × ½ acre of land in **Croughton** (at *Elkesdene*, *Wetendene*, *Withemorforlong*, *Blindewell*, *Hethermersforlong*, *Affegore*, *Langeford*, and *Blindewell*) | Geoffrey de Beaumont and Agnes | | Aynho 5 |
| 1 messuage and ½ virgate of land in **Croughton** | William de Turville | Nicholas de Turville | Aynho 54 |

# 3

# SCRIBAL PRODUCTION AND DOCUMENTARY CULTURE

Like the institution that produced it, the Aynho Cartulary can be placed in much wider contexts than the overwhelmingly local focus of its contents would at first suggest. Unlike many medieval cartularies, which have since been separated from the original charters on which they are based (either through loss or transfer to a separate repository), the Aynho Cartulary is highly unusual in that it can be studied both in tandem and in situ with most of the acts whose texts it contains, since these are also conserved in the archives of Magdalen College. This chapter therefore uses these documents, as well as contemporary charters produced for hospitals in Oxford and Brackley, which are also preserved at Magdalen, as a lens through which to examine and bring into focus the wider scribal and documentary culture(s) in Northamptonshire and neighbouring Oxfordshire during the second half of the thirteenth century. In doing so, we can contextualise the work of those scribes who specifically identify themselves as having written Aynho charters. We also show how a broader survey of Magdalen's medieval deeds allows for otherwise anonymous scribes responsible for producing Aynho acts to be named. Taken together, this chapter then situates the work of the main Aynho cartularist, who himself worked anonymously, within these wider scribal milieux, and examines the documentary resources that a rural hospital like Aynho could muster in-house or call upon from outside.

## MEDIEVAL HOSPITALS IN THE MAGDALEN ARCHIVE

Setting the Aynho Cartulary within its extended scribal and documentary contexts requires some preliminary commentary on the wider archive of which it now forms a part. As we saw in the Introduction, the records accumulated by Aynho Hospital over the course of its history were transferred to Magdalen College at the time of the hospital's acquisition in October 1483 by Magdalen's founder, William Waynflete. Aynho was not the only hospital to be annexed to Magdalen in this way. The current college site, located outside what would have been medieval Oxford's east gate, was previously occupied by another hospital, dedicated to St John the Baptist. When and by whom this hospital was founded is unknown (its earliest mention dates from 1170 × 1180), but by the 1230s it had secured royal patronage, receiving from Henry III new buildings and the land where Magdalen College now stands on which to erect them.[1] By the time of its acquisition by William Waynflete, to whom the patronage and advowson were granted by Henry VI (1422–61, 1470–1) on 27 October 1456,[2] the hospital of St John had amassed a substantial landed estate in the city of Oxford and wider Oxfordshire, with outlying manors in Northamptonshire, Buckinghamshire, and Warwickshire, as well as further holdings in Coventry, Bristol, and London.[3] As with Aynho, the hospital's administrative archive, which includes over 1,400 single-sheet charters for the city and county of Oxford alone, plus a late thirteenth-century cartulary,[4] was transferred to Magdalen's ownership. A similarly substantial archive came to the college from the hospital of SS James and John in Brackley, which had been founded by the earl of Leicester in 1166 × 1167/68.[5] Acquired around the same time as Aynho Hospital, its estates were located throughout Northamptonshire, with outlying possessions in Scotland, which came to the hospital through the earls of Winchester, to whose descendants the patronage had passed in the thirteenth century.[6] The Brackley archive, now held at Magdalen, includes almost 1,500 deeds, as well as a thirteenth-century cartulary.[7] It also contains records relating to Brackley's leper hospital of St Leonard.[8]

1 For the hospital's early years, see Salter (ed.), *Cartulary*, vol. 3, pp. v–xxii. The earliest mention of the hospital, which is alluded to by Salter but not given any precise citation, is found in A. Clark (ed.), *The English Register of Godstow Nunnery, Near Oxford, Written About 1450* (London, 1911), p. 382.

2 Davis, *William Waynflete*, p. 62.

3 For the hospital's landed estates, with a useful map of their location, see B. Durham et al., 'The Infirmary and Hall of the Medieval Hospital of St John the Baptist at Oxford', *Oxoniensia*, 56 (1991), 17–75, at pp. 24–6.

4 The cartulary is now MCA, MS 275. Despite the title of Herbert Salter's work cited above (p. 48 n. 5), this manuscript has never been edited. Salter's 'cartulary' is instead what francophone scholars would call a '*cartulaire factice*', being simply a transcription of the hospital's charters for the city of Oxford, arranged artificially together to form a 'cartulary'.

5 For the date of Brackley's foundation, traditionally said to have taken place around 1150, see Chapter 1.

6 For Brackley's possessions in Scotland, see Macray, *Notes*, p. 131.

7 MCA, MS 273.

8 The earliest mention of this hospital dates from the late thirteenth century: VCH, *Northampton*, vol. 2, p. 153.

Though they are not part of the analysis presented here, it is worth noting that the Magdalen archive also contains charters of the leper hospital of SS Stephen and Thomas in Romney, Kent, founded in the late twelfth century, the advowson of which William Waynflete acquired for his nascent college in September 1457.[9]

Together, these individual archives today form part of an internationally significant collection of some 13,000 medieval deeds relating to lands and properties across twenty English counties,[10] of which over 4,000 items date to the period before 1300. As noted in the Introduction, the first concerted effort to describe this collection took place in the early seventeenth century, when the President and Fellows of Magdalen endeavoured to produce comprehensive deed lists, which were then bound together in a volume that is today referred to as the 'Old Catalogue'.[11] The method they used was simple: properties were taken one by one and then deeds numbered as they were found, without close examination or any attempt at arrangement either by property or chronology. Large deed collections were divided at random, and each section numbered alphabetically, so that Brackley, for instance, has five such sections (i.e., Brackley and Brackley A–D). These sections have no archival significance, and it is evident that in creating the Old Catalogue items from separate collections were at times mistakenly listed together under the wrong heading, as was the case with eight Aynho acts, which were described and numbered in the sections for Brackley.[12] Such errors were largely corrected by William Macray when he compiled

9 Although acquired just before the issuance of Magdalen's foundation charter, the hospital at Romney was not formally annexed to the college until 1481: Davis, *William Waynflete*, p. 129.

10 The exact number of items in Magdalen's medieval muniment collection has never been precisely calculated (or, if it has, this figure has never been published). The unpublished *Guide to the Archives of Magdalen College, Oxford* mentions a collection of 'about 13,000 medieval deeds': <https://www.magd.ox.ac.uk/wp-content/uploads/2022/10/Magdalen_Archives_Guide_2022.pdf>. Macray himself speaks of working with 'nearly fourteen thousand' documents: Macray, *Notes*, p. vi. It is clear, however, that this number includes some of the early modern documents added to the original medieval series. Macray's unpublished calendar includes these post-medieval documents, while his system hides multiple documents under a single numbered entry, such that adding all his calendar numbers together would not produce an accurate total. This process would also not take into account any losses that have occurred since the nineteenth century. The ongoing retro-conversion of Macray's calendars (see above, p. 4 n. 4) should allow for a precise figure eventually to be calculated.

11 MCA, CP/3/31.

12 These are MCA, Aynho 81–88, which were once Brackley 127, Brackley 169, Brackley 171, Brackley 170, Brackley B130, Brackley B131, Brackley B237, and Brackley B243, respectively.

his calendar between 1864 and 1878. That said, the original of at least one Aynho act transcribed in the roll cartulary is still kept in the Brackley collection (no. **40**), while four originals relating to land in Wiltshire remain listed among the Aynho deeds by mistake.[13] The resulting archival landscape is therefore one in which any semblance of original medieval order has been lost. Moreover, while Macray's calendars give us a useful chronological overview of the collection, it is by the non-chronological numbering of the Old Catalogue that the collection is still physically arranged. Whatever these shortcomings, however, Magdalen's medieval muniments represent a veritable treasure trove of information with regard not only to each deed's contents, but also to the scribal activities of those who produced them. It is to these individuals and their identification in the specific context of the Aynho archive that we shall now turn.

## IDENTIFYING CHARTER SCRIBES AND THEIR WORKING MILIEUX

The process of identifying medieval charter scribes, and of contextualising their work more broadly, is one fraught with difficulties. In the first instance, unlike those individuals who produced and/or copied authorial and non-authorial works for institutional libraries, many of whom tell us their names and thereby 'published' their work for both medieval and modern audiences,[14] the parallel world of 'pragmatic writing' (*écriture pragmatique* in French; *pragmatische Schriftlichkeit* in German), which included the production of administrative documents such as account rolls and charters, is one in which the vast majority of scribes worked anonymously across the Middle Ages (both in terms of chronology and geography).[15] As this would suggest, however, and as we shall see later in this chapter, not every charter scribe kept their identity to themselves. That said, the techniques used to identify those who remain anonymous rely in large part on a series

13 These are MCA, Aynho 75–78, which make no explicit mention of Aynho Hospital. These acts instead relate to the medieval village of Widhill (*Northwydyhull'*/*Westwidihulle*), which lay about 2 km to the east of Cricklade (Wiltshire). These appear to be connected to the Aylmer family of Upper Widhill. There is no indication as to how they came into the Magdalen archive (Woolgar, 'Catalogue', vol. 3, p. 759).

14 For a useful summary of the current literature on the concept of medieval publishing, see B. Pohl, *Publishing in a Medieval Monastery: The View from Twelfth-Century Engelberg* (Cambridge, 2023), pp. 1–6.

15 On so-called 'pragmatic writing' (*écriture pragmatique*), see Bertrand, *Documenting the Everyday*, which is a translation of P. Bertrand, *Les écritures ordinaires: Sociologie d'un temps de révolution documentaire (1250–1350)* (Paris, 2015). Also cf. B. Pohl, 'Robert of Torigni's "Pragmatic Literacy": Some Theoretical Considerations', *Tabularia* (2022), <https://journals.openedition.org/tabularia/ 5576>.

of subjective assessments made primarily in relation to a scribe's handwriting (otherwise known as their 'script' or 'hand'). What is already quite a complicated landscape is made yet more so by the fact that experienced scribes are known to have been able to write using a range of scripts that differ either subtly or significantly from one another (what is called either 'digraphism', 'multigraphism', or 'polygraphism'), leading some to champion not the cataloguing of scribes, which will always necessitate the search for individuals, but only of 'hands' or 'profiles', whose coherent features allow for palaeographical commonality and change to be tracked over time.[16] Scholars working in the field of digital palaeography have looked to harness machine learning in an effort to improve scribal attribution in such circumstances,[17] but the corpus of texts used to inform these developments has been largely restricted to the world of medieval manuscript books, which, if not insignificant, survive in nowhere near the same numbers as medieval charters (nor, one might argue, with the same range of scripts). What is more, whenever individual charter scribes can be identified with any level of certainty, their work often tends to be subsumed by scholars within the institutional worlds of the 'chancery' and the 'scriptorium', two evocative terms that present as many difficulties in their all too frequent use as the means used to identify the scribes in the first place.[18]

As already noted above, however, not every medieval charter scribe chose to work anonymously. Those who do identify themselves (usually through witness list entries followed by such phrases as 'qui hanc cartam scripsit' or 'huius carte scriptore') are very much more the exception than the rule. The extent to which this is the case is vividly illustrated by the Magdalen deed collection. A survey of William Macray's calendars, which

16 This is the approach taken, for example, by Joanna Tucker (Tucker, *Reading and Shaping*, pp. 55–63) and by scholars working on the project 'Models of Authority: Scottish Charters and the Emergence of Government, 1100–1250' <https://www.modelsofauthority. ac.uk/blog/barrows-scribes/>. On scribal profiling, see also B. Pohl, 'Who Wrote MS Lat. 2342? The Identity of the *Anonymus Beccensis* Revisited', in F. Siri et al. (eds), *France et Angleterre: Manuscrits médiévaux entre 700 et 1200* (Turnhout, 2020), pp. 153–89; B. Pohl., 'A Reluctant Historian and His Craft: The Scribal Work of Andreas of Marchiennes Reconsidered', *ANS*, 45 (2023), 141–62.

17 For discussion, see P. Stokes, 'Scribal Attribution Across Multiple Scripts: A Digitally Aided Approach', *Speculum*, 92 (2017), 65–85.

18 On the use of the term 'scriptorium', see R.M. Thomson, 'Scribes and Scriptoria', in E. Kwakkel and R.M. Thomson (eds), *The European Book in the Twelfth Century* (Cambridge, 2018), pp. 68–84; for critical discussion, see Pohl, *Publishing*, pp. 7–16. On the 'chancery', see O. Guyotjeannin, 'Écrire en chancellerie', in M. Zimmermann (ed.), *Auctor et auctoritas: invention et conformisme dans l'écriture médiévale. Actes du colloque tenu à l'Université de Versailles-Saint-Quentin-en-Yvelines, 14–16 juin 1999* (Paris, 2001), pp. 17–35.

include full descriptions of the witnesses to each act, shows that of over 4,100 pre-1300 deeds only a little over seventy contain the name of the scribe responsible.[19] The rarity of such mentions is reflected in other large charter collections, including those compiled in relation to individuals or institutions known to have had a coterie of well-trained scribes at their disposal.[20] Despite such circumstances, those scribes who do give their names in the Magdalen collection furnish us with a key piece of information, one that not only allows us to say something about these individuals and their work but also to discover, in some instances, the identity of their anonymous counterparts. The technique used to do so, which involves comparing charters based on the last-named witness within them, is hardly novel,[21] but it is an approach that yields results of interest not just to Aynho itself but also to the wider documentary world(s) in which it was situated.

## AYNHO SCRIBES

Let us begin, however, by looking at those scribes who name themselves within the original deeds for Aynho Hospital. Alongside its roll cartulary, the Aynho archive at Magdalen College today contains a total of

19 By comparison with other deed calendars, produced either for other medieval muniment collections in Oxford or for those at national institutions, William Macray's descriptions are unusually detailed. They include a full account of each act's contents, sometimes stretching over multiple pages, retaining original place and personal name spelling throughout, and contain unabbreviated descriptions of the witness lists that note the precise status of each person (or their relationships to one another) as described therein.

20 For other examples in England, see J. Hodson, 'Medieval Charters: The Last Witness', *Journal of the Society of Archivists*, 5 (1974), 71–89, at p. 71. For examples in France, see R. Allen, 'Episcopal *Acta* in Normandy, 911–1204: The Charters of the Bishops of Avranches, Coutances and Sées', *ANS*, 37 (2015), 25–32; R. Allen, 'À la recherche d'un atelier d'écriture de la Normandie cistercienne: le scriptorium de l'abbaye de Savigny (XIIe–XIIIe siècles)', in A. Baudin and L. Morelle (eds), *Les pratiques de l'écrit dans les abbayes cisterciennes (XIIe–milieu du XVIe s.): Produire, échanger, contrôler, conserver* (Paris, 2016), pp. 31–54; R. Allen, 'Les chartes originales de Savigny des origines jusqu'au XIIIe siècle (1112–1202)', in V. Gazeau and B. Galbrun (eds), *L'abbaye de Savigny (1112–2012). Un chef d'ordre anglo-normand* (Actes du colloque de Cerisy-la-Salle, 3–6 octobre 2012) (Rennes, 2019), pp. 55–82; R. Allen, 'La production diplomatique des évêques de Bayeux et de Coutances (XIe–XIIIe siècles)', in G. Combalbert and C. Senséby (eds), *Écrire à l'ombre des cathédrales. Pratiques de l'écrit en milieu cathédral (espace anglo-normand et France de l'Ouest, XIe–XIIIe siècle)* (Actes du colloque de Cerisy-la-Salle, 8-12 juin 2016) (Rennes, 2024), pp. 25–41.

21 On the last-witness-as-scribe phenomenon, see S. Bond, 'The Attestation of Medieval Private Charters Relating to New Windsor', *Journal of the Society of Archivists*, 4 (1971), 278–84; Hodson, 'Last Witness', pp. 71–89.

eighty-seven documents, all of which date to the period before 1508.[22] Of these, a little over sixty are for the period before 1300, of which five make mention of the scribe responsible for their writing. Such a small number may at first appear to give us little to work with, especially since two of the scribes identify themselves by their first names only. The scribe called Thomas, however, who was responsible for writing an early thirteenth-century act later transcribed in the Aynho Cartulary (no. **16**), likely also wrote three contemporaneous charters for the hospital at Brackley, one of which identifies him as being the brother of a certain 'Master Robert'.[23] Unfortunately, this relationship does not allow us to identify Thomas with any further precision, but his activities across four charters for two different hospitals is illustrative of the sort of outside scribal resources on which a rural hospital like Aynho might rely. The same dynamic is likely at play with regard to the early thirteenth-century Aynho charter written by a certain Ernald the chaplain (no. **22**). He is perhaps the same as the chaplain of Brackley by that name, who appears among the witnesses of various Brackley Hospital acts in the late twelfth and early thirteenth centuries.[24] Chaplains have long been known to have played a key role in the production of charters,[25] and the medieval hospital was one type of institution in which such figures were to be found regularly, where they were often installed to celebrate obits, as was the case at Aynho itself (no. **A10**).[26] As we saw in Chapter 1, individuals with such rank might also be installed as a hospital's head of house. It is not impossible, therefore, that the scribe named Jordan, who identifies himself as the person responsible for one of the Aynho acts (no. **39**), is also the chaplain and future master of Aynho Hospital by that

22 This figure includes the act still in the Brackley collection but not Aynho 75–78 (see above, p. 86 n. 13). It also includes a bull of John XXII (1316–34), issued in December 1328, which has been artificially extracted from the Aynho collection to form part of the 'Chartae regiae' series at Magdalen, where it is unnumbered.

23 MCA, Astwick and Evenley 51 (the hand of this act also has a lot in common with that of a charter written by Alan, chaplain of Brackley Hospital: MCA, Brackley 161), Astwick and Evenley 68A (as brother of Master Robert), and Whitfield 155.

24 MCA, Brackley 54, Brackley B98, Brackley C52, Brackley D248.

25 C.R. Cheney, *English Bishops' Chanceries, 1100–1250* (Manchester, 1950), pp. 9–11; B.-M. Tock, *Une chancellerie épiscopale au XIIe siècle: le cas d'Arras* (Louvain-la-Neuve, 1991), pp. 188–9; J. Barrow, *The Clergy in the Medieval World: Secular Clerics, their Families and Careers in North-Western Europe, c.800–c.1200* (Cambridge, 2015), pp. 236–68.

26 At Brackley, on 30 January 1256, Roger de Quincy, earl of Winchester, established two chaplains to celebrate Mass for the souls of his late brother and wife (MCA, Brackley 4A), while an agreement reached between Ellen la Zouche and the hospital on 9 October 1279 made provision with regard to eleven chaplains who were supposed to celebrate for the souls of her ancestors (MCA, Brackley B67).

name.[27] Elsewhere, the dynamic that drove recruitment and benefactors to the hospital, wherein the expansion of Clavering influence brought with it individuals from outside Northamptonshire to Aynho (see Chapter 1), seems also to have played out in a scribal context, since one of the scribes to identify himself is a certain Robert of Colchester (*Colecestra*) (no. **29**), whose toponymic shows he hailed from Essex. That said, it is also clear that the hospital was able to call upon local expertise, since the clerk John, who identifies himself as the scribe of a charter not copied in the cartulary (no. **A9**), is almost certainly the clerk John of (King's) Sutton who appears at the end of a witness list of a cartulary act surviving in the original and written in the same hand (no. **51**) (**Fig. 3.1**).

A palaeographical analysis of the hospital's original charters also shows that some of them were written by the same scribe(s). In some instances, it is clear that a single individual was commissioned to write a series of acts relating to a single donation. This is the case, for example, with the charters issued by members of the de Wavre family. The act of Alice de Wavre, daughter of Geoffrey de Wavre (no. **37**), and those of her husband, Baldwin de Boulogne (no. **36**), and son, William (I) de la Haye (no. **38**), confirming to the hospital the grant of land in Byfield are all written in the same hand (**Fig. 3.1**), which is similar to that responsible for a near contemporaneous act issued by Turbert, son of Turbert, rector of Aynho (no. **A1**). The same is also true for two of the family's three charters concerning the chapel of Croughton (nos. **A2–A3**), the hand of which is paleographically close to the charter of Alice's and Baldwin's other son, Guy de la Haye, concerning the land at Byfield, which is written by the scribe above called Jordan (no. **39**). Seven Aynho original charters from the later thirteenth century are the work of two different scribes (Scribe 1: nos. **A15–A16**, **A19**; Scribe 2: nos. **52**, **A13–A14**, **A18**; **Fig. 3.1**), although each act concerns a different donation, suggesting that these individuals were simply called upon by the hospital as reliable practitioners of their trade. By the mid-thirteenth century, finding such people must not have posed too many difficulties, since even the small vill of Aynho did not lack for scribal expertise, being home to a clerk called John, who was the father of another clerk called Richard.[28]

Alternatively, the repeated use of the same few scribes might indicate that they were members of the hospital itself, especially since their distinctive hands have not yet been identified in charters for neighbouring institutions

27 He is certainly not the same, it would seem, as the clerk Jordan, who claims responsibility for writing an act of Brackley Hospital (MCA, Brackley D218), and whose script is paleographically different, although the two were working around the same time.

28 John the clerk appears in various other hospital charters (nos. **32**; **A7**), as does his son, Richard (nos. **A12**, **A15**).

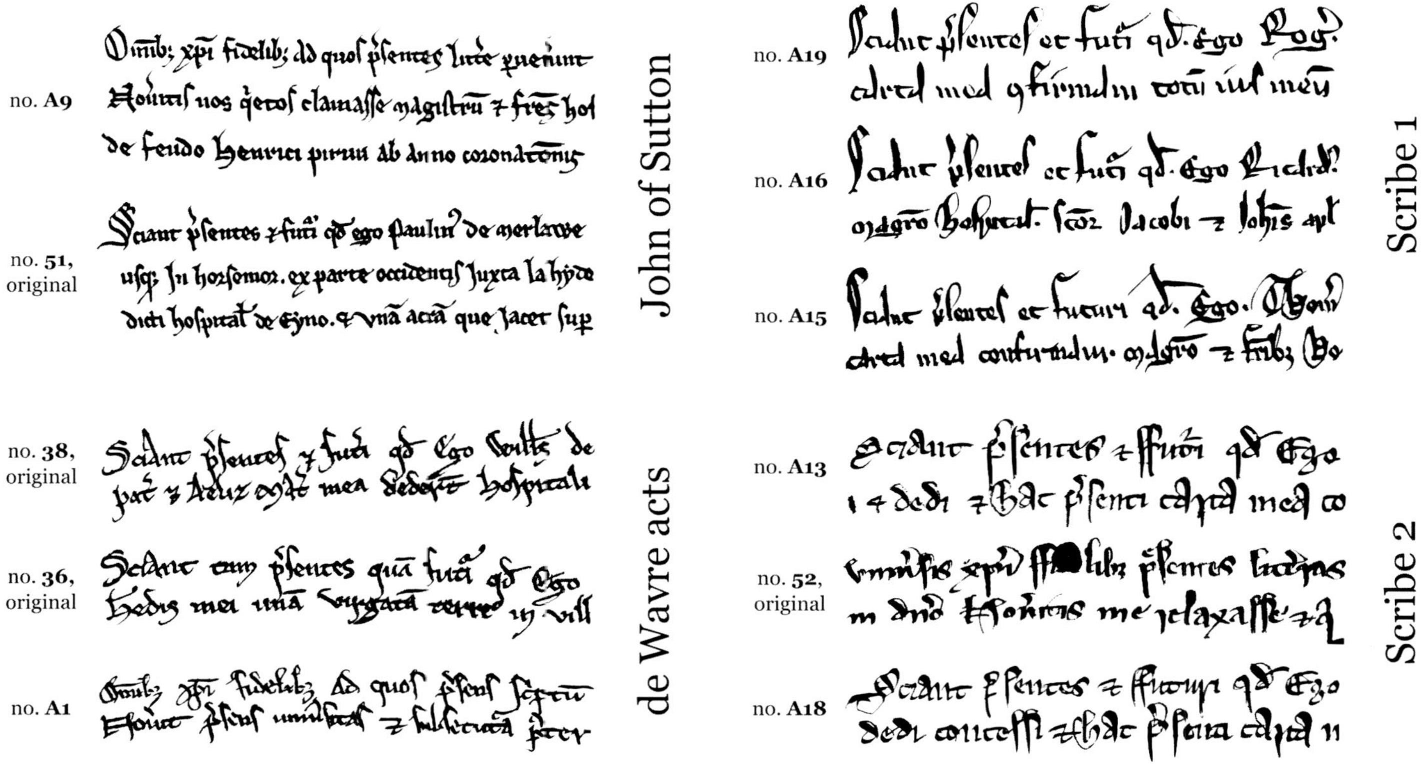


Fig. 3.1. Hands of John of Sutton, the de Wavre acts, and two Aynho Hospital charter scribes.

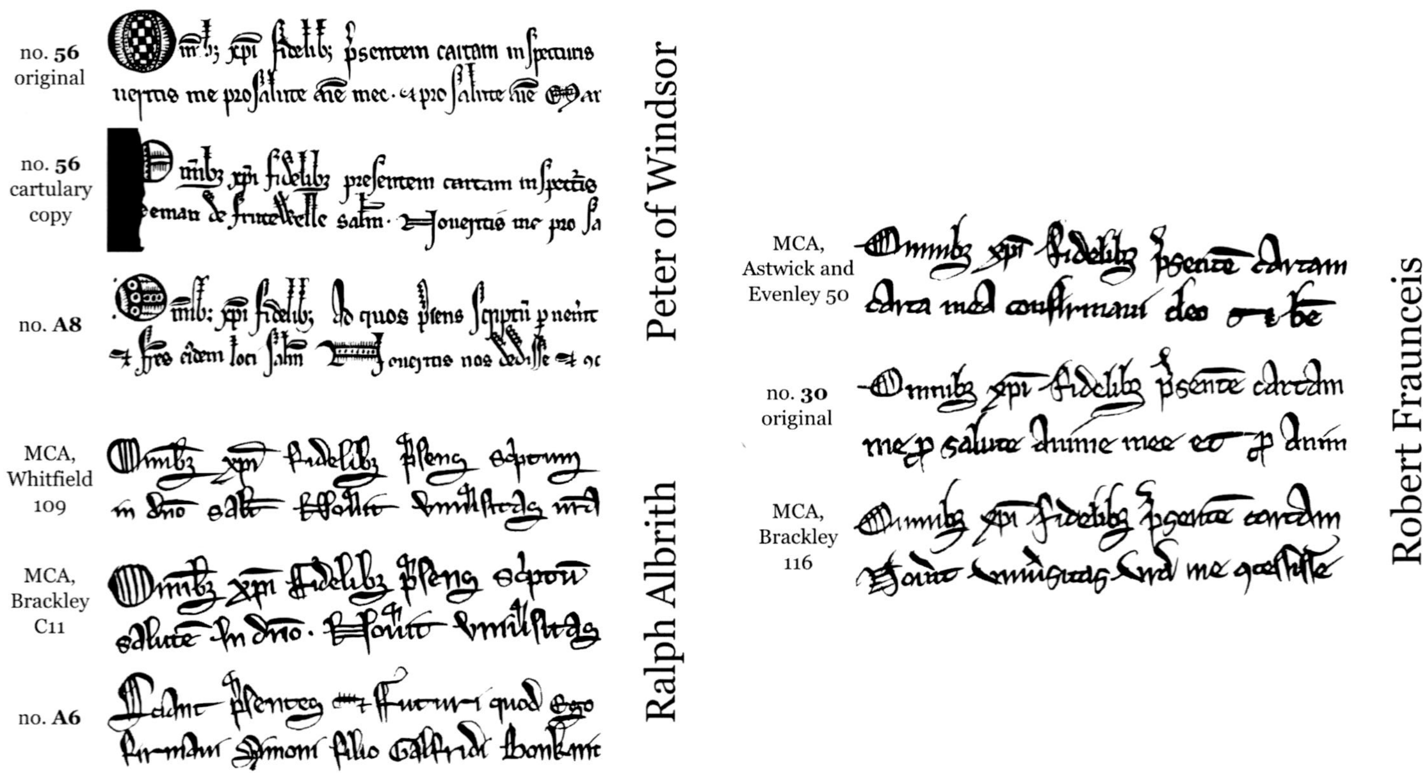

Fig. 3.2. Hands of 'Peter of Windsor', Ralph Albrith, and Robert Frauncei s.

within the Magdalen archive. The extent to which a rural hospital like Aynho was home to individuals with high literacy levels is difficult to determine,[29] but, as we shall see in Chapter 4, at least two of the Aynho Cartulary's continuators are also known to have written some of the hospital's extant original charters. The hand of one, Scribe B, can only be found in a single act issued *c.*1260 × 1270 (no. **32**), but the fact that he made just two additions to the cartulary (nos. **49–50**) makes it more likely that he was a hospital resident with ready and easy access to its domestic archive, rather than someone brought in from outside and specially commissioned to perform this task. The other continuator, Scribe E, transcribed four cartulary acts (nos. **55–8**) and also penned two surviving originals, one of which is among the very acts he copied into the cartulary (no. **56**). Interestingly, the other act (no. **A8**) is issued in the name of the hospital's then master, Peter of Windsor, making it the only such act to survive from this period. Like his predecessors, Peter probably held the rank of chaplain, meaning that he was almost certainly literate to a relatively high level.[30] The hand of Scribe E, meanwhile, is one notable for both its legibility and sophistication, especially with regard to its intricate decorative elements (ladder marks and loops on ascenders, chequerboard patterns in bowls, etc; **Fig. 3.2**), which suggests it belonged to someone who was not only accustomed to wielding a quill but who also wished to deploy such skills in relation to his own institution's written records (outside of which this distinctive hand has not yet been found). Whether the scribe in question was Peter of Windsor himself is a question that will likely remain unanswered, but the combination of facts presented by Scribe E's work is certainly enough to raise this as a possibility.

## AYNHO SCRIBES IN THEIR WIDER MILIEUX

Whether or not Aynho's masters ever put pen to parchment themselves to produce the hospital's charters, the resulting scribal profile for the hospital itself is one in which anonymity typically prevails. It is only by expanding any palaeographical survey to include those acts issued in relation to neighbouring institutions in Brackley and Oxford that we can both contextualise the work of those scribes responsible for producing Aynho charters and, in some instances, identify more of them by name. Such comparisons must

29 For literacy in late medieval urban hospitals, see Rice, *Medieval Hospital*.

30 Both of Peter's immediate predecessors, Adam of Stuchbury and Stephen, were chaplains: Hoskin (ed.), *Grosseteste*, nos. 608, 799, pp. 116, 148. Unfortunately, Peter was appointed at a moment in time for which we are lacking the episcopal institution rolls that contain the sort of details available for his predecessors (see above, p. 44, n. 166).

begin, naturally, with those scribes who identify themselves in Brackley and Oxford charters in the Magdalen archive. For the Oxford deeds, no scribe is known to have taken such a step, a point of interest to which we return below. As for Brackley, twenty-three individuals name themselves as the scribe of one of the hospital's acts (**Table 3.1**). Of these, only six claim responsibility for the writing of more than one act, of whom one (Thomas) also penned a charter for Aynho Hospital. Even if the remaining individuals only identify themselves on a single occasion, some of them can be shown to have been otherwise prolific charter scribes. As for their backgrounds, three of the twenty-three scribes give us their first names only, with a further three providing toponymics or family relationships without any indication of their social rank. Of the remaining seventeen, one was the hospital's own chaplain (*capellanus*), two were priests (*presbiteri*), and two deacons (*diaconi*), one of whom was particularly active. But the overwhelming majority – twelve, in total – were clerks (*clerici*). Why these individuals, like their counterparts in Aynho Hospital acts, sometimes broke their anonymity is a question discussed more fully elsewhere.[31] It is worth noting here, however, that it is often difficult to determine any logic to the practice, especially when a given scribe can be shown to have produced two exactly contemporaneous acts, naming himself in one but not the other.[32] It is also worth noting that while the total number of scribes named in Brackley charters is greater than those in Aynho ones, the percentage per act is greater at Aynho (around 8%, compared to approximately 5% at Brackley).

The scribes' backgrounds reveal nothing of any great surprise. That said, the act written by the chaplain Adam shows how individuals holding this rank within a medieval hospital might be entrusted with the writing of charters, as was argued above in relation to the Aynho acts produced by Ernald the chaplain and the scribe named Jordan. What the list of Brackley scribes shows above all else, however, is that even a large and relatively well-endowed hospital relied most often on outside expertise for the writing of its acts. In some instances, it is clear that the individuals who took credit for producing a Brackley charter were attached to large households that were themselves equipped with clerical staff able to perform administrative tasks. Such is the case, therefore, with the clerk Robert of Trafford, who identifies himself as the scribe of a single Brackley act, and who other hospital charters reveal was a clerk of Roger de Quincy, earl of Winchester

31 R. Allen, '"*Qui scripsit hanc cartam*": Charters and their Scribes through the Archives of Magdalen College, Oxford (*c.*1100–*c.*1300), *ANS*, forthcoming.

32 Take, for example, the case of Adam, son of Robert son of Randulf, who wrote two acts with identical witness lists, save for the fact that he identifies himself as the scribe in one but not in the other.

and constable of Scotland (†25 April 1264), a position he held alongside another clerk called Brian.[33] Similarly, in the one Brackley act for which he takes credit, Robert of Oxendon identifies himself as the clerk of a certain John of Oxendon, who appears elsewhere in hospital charters as a steward (*senescallus*) of Ellen la Zouche (†bef. 1296),[34] daughter of Roger de Quincy and wife of Alan la Zouche (†1270), a member of whose family married Robert (II) Fitz Roger, great-great-grandson of Aynho Hospital's founder, Roger Fitz Richard.[35]

What is more, even if the vast majority of Brackley scribes cannot be shown to have enjoyed such connections, their title of clerk nevertheless allows us to situate both them and their work within a wider and flourishing thirteenth-century scribal ecosystem. By the time of the Aynho Cartulary's creation, urban centres throughout England were not only increasingly home to clerical staff involved in the making and handling of documents, but they were also the place in which such administrative functions began to be professionalised, most notably in the office of town clerk, whose occupant ensured the creation and circulation of documents recording the social, economic, and legal life of the place in which he lived.[36] For Aynho, nearby Oxford was home by the thirteenth century to a small army of people dedicated to the production of the written word,[37] who worked both in relation to the needs of Oxford's burgeoning university and those of the town more generally, the municipal development of which required an

33 MCA, Brackley C109, Brackley C133.

34 MCA, Brackley B67, Brackley B239.

35 A genealogy of the founders of Horsham Priory, Norfolk, names Robert's wife as Margaret la Zouche ('*Margeriam de* la Souche'): Dugdale, *Monasticon*, vol. 3, p. 636. Her precise relationship to the la Zouche family has yet to be determined.

36 For the development of literacy outside religious institutions, see N. Orme, 'Lay Literacy in England, 1100–1300', in A. Haverkamp and H. Vollrath (eds), *England and Germany in the High Middle Ages* (Oxford, 1996), pp. 35–56. On provincial town clerks, see K. Bevan, 'Clerks and Scriveners: Legal Literacy and Access to Justice in Late Medieval England', unpublished PhD dissertation, University of Exeter, 2013.

37 Scholars have written at length on Oxford's scribal community, especially in relation to book production. See, for example, G. Pollard, 'The University and the Book Trade in Medieval Oxford', *Beiträge zum Berufsbewusstsein des mittelalterlichen Menschen. Miscellanea Medievalia*, 3 (1964), 336–44; M.B. Parkes, 'The Provision of Books', in J. Catto et al. (eds), *The History of the University of Oxford* (8 vols, Oxford, 1984–2000), vol. 2, pp. 407–83. The deeds in the Magdalen archive relating to the city of Oxford contain among their witness lists various scribes and other individuals involved in the production of the written word (parchment makers, bookbinders, copyists, illuminators, etc). In one striking example, a charter of *c*.1220 × 1230 is witnessed by no fewer than four scribes, two of whom are associated with particular areas within the town (St Giles and Holywell): MCA, St Peter's in the East 7A.

ever-increasing number of written records and the functionaries, including town clerks, needed to create them.[38]

We shall meet some of Oxford's professional scribes a little later. For now, let us note that, by the second half of the thirteenth century, Brackley seems to have had its own active network of professional clerks on whom institutions like the town's hospital routinely relied to write their acts. Of these individuals, two stand out: Ralph Albrith and Robert Fraunceis. Active at the same time as one another, they each take credit for the writing of just a single Brackley charter. Finding other acts in their hands within the Magdalen muniments might otherwise be a prohibitively laborious task, given that their system of arrangement, as noted above, is the one put in place in the early seventeenth century and thus entirely non-chronological. Armed with William Macray's detailed descriptions, however, it is possible to identify with relative ease the other acts in which Ralph and Robert appear as witnesses. What is more, extracting these acts and comparing them paleographically to one another reveals an important pattern: when either Ralph or Robert is the last-named witness, the act concerned is usually written in their hand (see **Table 3.2** and **Fig. 3.2**). The results show them to have been both prolific and active over a long period of time. Nothing is known about Ralph's background, although it is possible that he was the son (or some other relation) of the man named Albrit (*Albrittus*), whom a charter of 14 February 1256 shows was both dead and had owned a housed in Brackley.[39] With regard to Robert, he is identified in a hospital charter of 25 July 1262 as being the son of Hugh Fraunceis (*Frauncey*s),[40] who likewise had a house in Brackley.[41] It is likely that Robert was of some relation to Richard Fraunceis, who, by 6 February 1261, had been admitted as one of the hospital's brethren.[42] We know that the two were not siblings, however, since in an act written in Robert's hand, we find that Richard was the son of Geoffrey Tanewombe,[43] whose own brother was Master Reginald of Halse,[44] who was himself a benefactor of Aynho Hospital (no. **34**).

Whatever Ralph's and Robert's connection to other Brackley residents, or their formal positions (if any) within the town, the simple technique

38 On the development of Oxford's town clerks, see G. Pollard, 'The Medieval Town Clerks of Oxford', *Oxoniensia*, 43 (1966), 44–76.

39 MCA, Brackley 163.

40 'Hiis testibus: […], Roberto clerico filio Hugonis Fraunceys […]': MCA, Brackley C57.

41 MCA, Brackley D247.

42 MCA, Brackley 70A.

43 MCA, Astwick and Evenley 8.

44 MCA, Astwick and Evenley 108A. In a rare error, Macray's calendar mistakenly identifies Reginald as 'Richard of Hals' and omits his title.

by which their acts have been identified can be extended to include other Brackley Hospital charters in which no scribe otherwise identifies himself. Indeed, even a relatively quick survey of the Macray calendars reveals the same individual appearing as the final witness across multiple acts. When that individual also happens to be a clerk, the hand is almost always the same and can be ascribed with some degree of confidence to him. Such is the case, for example, with the charters in which we find the clerks Robert le Somenur and William Dodevile of Kemerton (*Kenemerton*), whose toponymic shows he hailed from Worcestershire (**Tables 3.3** and **3.4**; **Fig. 3.3**). Once identified, it is then possible to use this corpus of hands to attribute to a particular scribe the writing of an act in which he is not listed as a witness, as is the case with two Aynho charters produced by Ralph Albrith and Robert Fraunceis (and two acts written by Robert for Brackley Hospital). The results reveal a small but flourishing network of scribes based in and around Brackley, whose services might not only be called upon by the town's hospital (and no doubt its other institutions as well), but also those based in neighbouring vills such as Aynho. The extent and nature of their activities means that the clerks and scribes of Brackley, like their counterparts in provincial towns throughout thirteenth-century England, no doubt became the custodians of local memory and custom,[45] which is perhaps why the writing of particularly complicated hospital charters was entrusted to them, even though the act in question was being issued in the name of someone known to have had their own clerical staff, some of whom appear among the witnesses.[46]

## CONCLUSION

It is within the local documentary culture(s) and scribal milieux identified in this chapter that the work of the Aynho cartularist must be situated. Whether he was himself a local clerk or one of the hospital's inmates is a

45 Bevan, 'Clerks and Scriveners', pp. 150–74; E. Cuenca, 'Town Clerks and the Authorship of Custumals in Medieval England', *Urban History*, 46 (2019), 180–201.

46 Take, for example, the act by which Roger de Quincy established a chaplain at the hospital to pray for the soul of Richard de Yvetot, which is written in the hand of Robert Fraunceis: MCA, Brackley D247. The act lists eighty rents payable by various Brackley residents on their houses or other properties, and it is perhaps for this reason that Robert, the most active of Brackley's thirteenth-century clerks and thus one familiar with the town's intricate web of connections, was entrusted with its writing, rather than Roger's own clerk, Brian, who appears among the witnesses. It is also perhaps no coincidence that the penultimate witness of the act is Robert's contemporary, Ralph Albrith. Robert Fraunceis also wrote another act issued by Roger de Quincy in which the earl's own clerks appear as the last two witnesses: MCA, Brackley C133.

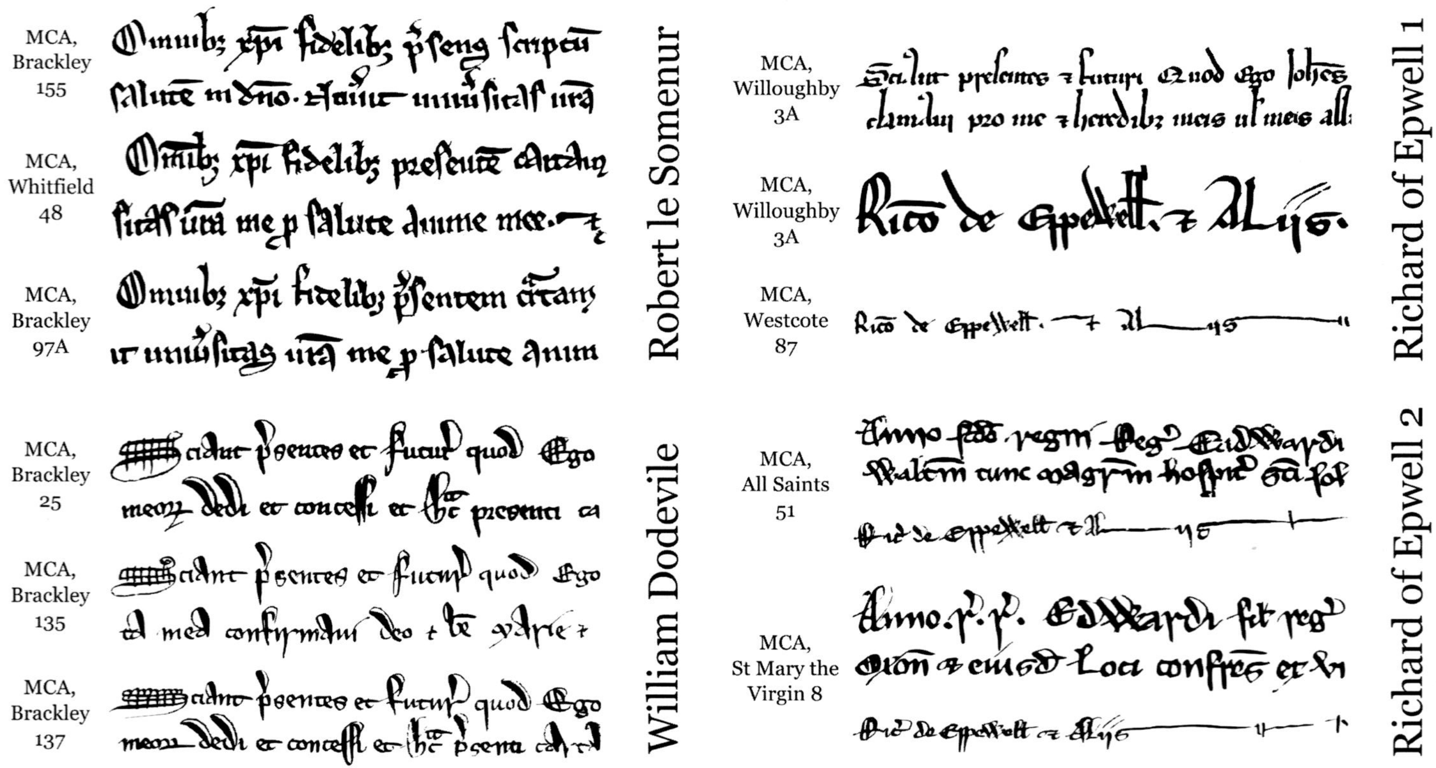


Fig. 3.3. Hands of Robert le Somenur, William Dodevile, and Richard of Epwell.

question that cannot be definitively answered, primarily because his hand has not yet been found anywhere else in the Magdalen archive (nor in any other charter collection, for that matter). The evidence from Brackley, however, vividly illustrates the extent to which the production of a hospital's written records depended on scribes active outside its walls. The same can also be said in relation to Oxford and its hospital of St John the Baptist. Many of Oxford's thirteenth-century scribes were first identified by Herbert Salter in the early twentieth century.[47] Unlike their Aynho and Brackley counterparts, these men never seem to have identified themselves as charter scribes, presumably because the comparative size and sophistication of Oxford's documentary culture did not require it. Of these individuals, at least one, Philip, is described specifically as 'the hospital's clerk' (*clericus hospitalis sancti Iohannis*).[48] Another, Geoffrey Belewe, whose hand can be found in various hospital acts,[49] lived in a house next to the river Cherwell on the present site of Oxford's Botanic Gardens and thus directly opposite what was the hospital of St John,[50] to whose inmates he would have almost certainly been a well-known figure. From our perspective, however, the most important scribe of thirteenth-century Oxford was Richard of Epwell (*Eppewelle*), whose toponymic shows he hailed from a small vill approximately 10 km due west of Banbury. Herbert Salter identified seven hospital charters as being in Richard's hand,[51] which is both paleographically and orthographically distinctive (Richard consistently spells 'parochea' with an 'e' rather than an 'i'). A wider survey of Oxford deeds, however, shows that he produced over thirty charters (**Table 3.5** and **Fig. 3.3**), making him the most prolific of the town's thirteenth-century scribes identified to date.[52] His reticence in identifying himself as a clerk is striking, even by Oxford standards, but his skills were clearly appreciated within the hospital, for

[47] Salter (ed.), *Cartulary*, vol. 1, pp. vi–ix, plus Plates III–IV, VII–XV, XVII.

[48] Salter (ed.), *Cartulary*, vol. 1, no. 22, p. 25. Philip also served as town clerk from 1261/5 to 1271/3: Pollard, 'Clerks of Oxford', pp. 61—2.

[49] Herbert Salter specifically attributes only a handful of charters to Geoffrey: Salter (ed.), *Cartulary*, vol. 1, no. 294, p. 293; vol. 2, no. 879, p. 357. For other examples, see MCA, Oddington 1A, Oddington 5A, Oddington 28A, Oddington 31A, Oddington 41, St Peter's in the East 46A. Geoffrey is the final witness in all these acts.

[50] Pollard, 'Clerks of Oxford', p. 61.

[51] Salter (ed.), *Cartulary*, vol. 1, nos. 34, 51, 141, 295, pp. 35–6, 52–3, 135, 294; vol. 2, nos. 567–8, 871, pp. 81–2, 350–1. Salter identifies an eighth act as being in Richard's hand (St Clement's 5 = Salter (ed.), *Cartulary*, vol. 1, no. 3, p. 4), but this is not the case.

[52] Of the town clerks identified by Graham Pollard, only Jordan, who was bailiff's clerk between 1235 and 1244/5, comes close to Richard in terms of the number of charters that can be attributed to him: Pollard, 'Clerks of Oxford', pp. 59–64.

which he not only produced so many single-sheet charters but also its cartulary.[53]

Had the Aynho Cartulary been similarly produced by a local clerk, especially a prolific one like Richard, then we might expect to see it written in the hand of someone like Ralph Albrith or Robert Fraunceis, both of whom had been called upon to produce the hospital's charters. As it stands, the fact that the main cartularist's hand cannot be found elsewhere, combined with his apparent difficulty in transcribing certain acts (see Chapter 4), suggests that the cartulary instead represents the work of a literate though not otherwise active member of Aynho Hospital's domestic community (although not, it would seem, its master, if the arguments above concerning Peter of Windsor are accepted). After all, employing a clerk was not cheap: Geoffrey Belewe was seemingly owed 12d for the writing of three charters for Reginald the mason (*cementarius*) at some point before 1261,[54] which, at a very rough cost estimate of 4d per act, means that the work of the main cartulary scribe might have cost as much as 16s, a considerable sum that would have likely stretched the hospital's meagre resources.[55] That said, an analysis of the charters in which we find Richard of Epwell as witness shows he wrote using two very different scripts, an example of polygraphism that has hitherto gone unnoticed with regard to Oxford's thirteenth-century scribes (**Fig. 3.3**).[56] It is therefore possible that the main hand of the Aynho Cartu-

53 For the cartulary, see above, p. 84, n. 4. For the identification of Richard as its scribe, see Salter (ed.), *Cartulary*, vol. 1, p. vii.

54 Pollard, 'Clerks of Oxford', p. 61.

55 The question of purchasing power in thirteenth-century England is a vexed one, with wages and prices fluctuating considerably across the decades: A.R. Bridbury, 'Thirteenth-Century Prices and the Money Supply', *The Agricultural History Review*, 33 (1985), 1–21.

56 The majority of Richard's acts, along with the cartulary of the hospital of St John the Baptist, are written in what might be considered his 'main hand', which is regular and upright. Of the five charters in which he appears as witness that are not in this hand, one (MCA, Westcote 33) is clearly by someone else. The other four, which are all chirograph charter notices (*chartes notices*), are in the same hand, of which some letter forms echo those of Richard's main hand. More importantly, three contain Richard's distinctive spelling of 'parochea': MCA, All Saints 51, St Giles 9, St Mary the Virgin 8; the fourth, All Saints 52, does not contain this word. It is possible, of course, that in all these instances a scribe was simply copying a text already established by Richard, but the chirograph form of each act makes this unlikely, unless we wish to envisage either two scribes producing one half each of the chirograph or the chirograph itself being produced in duplicate (i.e., resulting in four separate copies). Instead, it is possible that Richard used this hand, the ductus of which is much more angular than his main hand, when needing to write an act more than once and at speed. Interestingly, the same hand is found in MCA, Westcote 7, a non-chirograph act that is almost an exact copy of MCA, Westcote 6, which is in Richard of Epwell's

lary is simply one of a number used by this particular individual, meaning he may yet have been a local clerk. Whatever the case may be, the cartulary's creation represented a considerable investment of time and resources for a hospital like Aynho. The end result was a multi-dimensional material object that eventually involved the work of more than one individual, and which responded to various needs. It is this materiality, these needs, and the date at which the cartulary was written that we will now examine in Chapter 4.

Table 3.1. Brackley Hospital scribes.

| | |
|---|---|
| *Adam, son of Robert son of Randulf*[57] | |
| Astwick and Evenley 46* | [*c*.1215 × *c*.1220] |
| Astwick and Evenley 47 | [*c*.1215 × *c*.1220] |
| *Alan, chaplain of Brackley Hospital* | |
| Brackley 161 | [*c*.1190 × 1200] |
| *Alan* | |
| Syresham 28 | [*c*.1220 × 1230] |
| *Geoffrey, priest of Finmere* | |
| Brackley 174 | [*c*.1210 × 1220] |
| *Geoffrey, priest* | |
| Brackley D205 | [*c*.1220] |
| *Geoffrey, clerk* | |
| Whitfield 80* | [*c*.1220] |
| **Aynho 44** | [*c*.1220 × 1230] |

'main hand'. (The only difference between the two is the absence of Richard's name at the end of the witness list in Westcote 7.) It would be normal to assume that these acts were the work of two different scribes, but the evidence of the three acts above suggests that having produced Westcote 6 in his main hand, Richard was then asked to produce a copy, which he dashed off in his second. Whatever the case may be, it is certainly not unknown for scribes to have written in markedly different scripts which would otherwise be impossible to attribute to them if they did not claim responsibility: Hodson, 'Last Witness', pp. 71–2.

57 In the table, an asterisk next to a scribe's name denotes an identification based on palaeographical similarities between the script of each charter and the appearance of 'the scribe' as the final witness in the witness list (on which point, see the discussion above). An asterisk next to a reference number indicates that the individual specifically identifies himself as the charter's scribe. If an asterisk appears neither next to a scribe's name nor next to any reference number in the table, the individual specifically identifies himself as the scribe of every charter listed beneath his name.

Table 3.1. *continued*

| | |
|---|---|
| *Geoffrey of Farthinghoe** | |
| Brackley B110 | [*c*.1260] |
| Brackley 57 | [*c*.1260] |
| *Gilbert, clerk* | |
| Astwick and Evenley 102A[58] | [*c*.1220 × 1230] |
| Brackley 94A | [*c*.1220 × 1230] |
| Brackley B93 | [*c*.1240] |
| Brackley B201 | [*c*.1240] |
| Syresham 37 | [*c*.1240 × 1250] |
| *Gregory, clerk* | |
| Whitfield 26 | [*c*.1230] |
| *Henry son of Griffin* | |
| Brackley 203 | [*c*.1230 × 1240] |
| *John, deacon* | |
| Astwick and Evenley 13 | [*c*.1220] |
| Astwick and Evenley 77A | [*c*.1220] |
| Whitfield 107 | [*c*.1227/28] |
| Whitfield 104 and 166[59] | [*c*.1227 × 1230] |
| Whitfield 106 | [*c*.1228] |
| Whitfield 123 | [*c*.1240] |
| *John, clerk** | |
| Brackley D89 | [*c*.1270 × 1280] |
| Brackley D142 | [*c*.1270 × 1280] |
| Whitfield 41 | [*c*.1270 × 1280] |
| Whitfield 47 | [*c*.1270 × 1280] |
| Whitfield 91 | [*c*.1270 × 1280] |
| Brackley 59 | [*c*.1280] |
| Brackley D7 | [*c*.1280] |
| *Jordan, clerk* | |
| Brackley D218 | [*c*.1200 × 1220] |

58 In this and the subsequent act, Gilbert identifies himself by his first initial only.

59 This charter is heavily mutilated and was already in two parts when the Old Catalogue was compiled *c*.1610. William Macray did not notice that the two parts were related and also calendared each 'act' separately.

| | |
|---|---|
| *Lawrence, clerk* | |
| Whitfield 135 | [*c*.1210 × 1220] |
| *Lawrence, clerk of Brackley* | |
| Astwick and Evenley 95A* | [*c*.1220] |
| Syresham 52[60] | [*c*.1220] |
| Whitfield 3* | [*c*.1220 × 1227] |
| Whitfield 17* | [*c*.1220 × 1227] |
| *Michael, deacon* | |
| Brackley 131(a) | [*c*.1210 × 1220] |
| *Peter* | |
| Whitfield 16 | [*c*.1220] |
| Whitfield 161 | [*c*.1220] |
| *Ralph Albrith, clerk* (Hand 1) | |
| Brackley C43 | [*c*.1250] |
| Brackley C5 (as Ralph, clerk) | [*c*.1250] |
| **Aynho 59** | [*c*.1250] |
| Whitfield 109* | [*c*.1250 × 1260] |
| Brackley D40 | 30 Apr 1258 |
| Brackley C11 | [*c*.1260] |
| Brackley 47A | [*c*.1260] |
| Brackley D98 | [*c*.1260] |
| Brackley D243 | [*c*.1260] |
| Whitfield 73 | [*c*.1260] |
| Brackley C20 (as Ralph, clerk) | 25 Dec 1260 |
| *Ralph Albrith, clerk* (Hand 2) | |
| Brackley 142 | [*c*.1260] |
| Brackley 52 | [*c*.1260] |
| Brackley 51 | [*c*.1260] |
| Brackley D193 (as Ralph, clerk) | [*c*.1260] |
| Brackley D194 (as Ralph, clerk) | [*c*.1260] |
| Brackley 136 | [*c*.1260] |
| Brackley D201 | [*c*.1260] |

60 It is only in this act that Lawrence is referred to as 'Lawrence, the clerk of Brackley'. In all the others for which he takes credit, he refers to himself only as 'Lawrence, clerk'.

Table 3.1. *continued*

| | |
|---|---|
| Brackley D202 | [*c*.1260] |
| Brackley 23A | [*c*.1260 × 1265] |
| Brackley 141 | [*c*.1260 × 1265] |
| Brackley D133 | 24 Apr 1262 |
| Brackley 36A (as Ralph, clerk) | [*c*.1270] |
| *Ralph Albrith, clerk** (Hand 3) | |
| Brackley B50 | [*c*.1270] |
| *Richard de Cailly*[61] | |
| Whitfield 108 | [*c*.1230] |
| *Robert of Brackley, clerk**[62] | |
| Brackley B20 (as Robert, clerk) | [*c*.1270] |
| Brackley D17 (as Robert, clerk) | [*c*.1270] |
| Brackley 87A (as Robert, clerk) | [*c*.1270] |
| Whitfield 12 | [*c*.1270 × 1280] |
| Whitfield 18 | [*c*.1270 × 1280] |
| Whitfield 24 | [*c*.1270 × 1280] |
| Whitfield 40 | [*c*.1270 × 1280] |
| Brackley C36 (as Robert, clerk) | 22 Feb 1272 |
| Brackley C40 (as Robert, clerk) | 22 Feb 1272 |
| Brackley 82 (as Robert, clerk) | [*c*.1280] |
| Whitfield 32 | [*c*.1280 × 1290] |
| *Robert of Oxendon, clerk of John of Oxendon* | |
| Brackley B239* | 1 Aug 1279 |
| Whitfield 5[63] | [1279 × 1289] |
| Whitfield 100 | [*c*.1280 × 1290] |
| Brackley D182 | [*c*.1280 × 1290] |

61 Richard's toponymic derives from Cailly (Seine-Maritime, cant. Mesnil-Esnard) and is often rendered as Cayley in English.

62 The hand of these charters has much in common with that of the acts ascribed below to Robert le Somenur, such that these two Roberts may be one and the same person.

63 In both this and the subsequent act, Robert appears as the final witness as 'Robert of Oxendon, clerk'. John of Oxendon is the first witness in each act. John and Robert also appear as the first and last witness of another act (MCA, Brackley B60), which is not in the hand of the four acts attributed to Robert.

| *Robert Frraunceis, clerk* | |
|---|---|
| Brackley C133 (not named) | [*c*.1240] |
| Brackley 116 | [*c*.1240 × 1250] |
| Brackley D20 | [*c*.1240 × 1250] |
| Whitfield 144 | [*c*.1240 × 1250] |
| Whitfield 36 | [*c*.1245 × 1250] |
| **Aynho 26** | [*c*.1245 × 1250] |
| Brackley C134 | 2 Dec 1247 |
| Astwick and Evenley 50* | 10 Mar 1248 |
| Whitfield 110 | [before 1250] |
| Astwick and Evenley 56 | [*c*.1250] |
| Astwick and Evenley 106A | [*c*.1250] |
| Brackley C6 | [*c*.1250] |
| Brackley C74 | [*c*.1250] |
| Brackley C84 | [*c*.1250] |
| Brackley D4 | [*c*.1250] |
| Brackley B108 (not named) | [*c*.1250] |
| Brackley C46 | 2 Aug 1250 |
| Brackley 6A | [*c*.1250 × 1260] |
| Brackley B233 | [*c*.1250 × 1260] |
| Brackley D247 | [*c*.1250 × 1260] |
| Syresham 11 | [*c*.1250 × 1260] |
| Brackley 63A | [*c*.1250 × 1260] |
| Astwick and Evenley 52A | 29 Sep 1253 |
| Astwick and Evenley 107A | 1254 |
| Whitfield 61 | 8 Jun 1254 |
| Brackley 4A | 30 Jan 1256 |
| Brackley 152 | [? 1258] |
| Astwick and Evenley 8 | [*c*.1260] |
| Astwick and Evenley 11 | [*c*.1260] |
| Astwick and Evenley 61 | [*c*.1260] |
| Brackley 13 | [c 1260] |
| Brackley 63 | [*c*.1260] |
| Brackley B23 | [*c*.1260] |
| Brackley B154 | [*c*.1260] |

Table 3.1. *continued*

| | |
|---|---|
| Brackley B189 (as Robert, clerk) | [*c.*1260] |
| Brackley D163 (as Robert, clerk) | [*c.*1260] |
| Brackley D190 | [*c.*1260] |
| Brackley D239 | [*c.*1260] |
| Syresham 42 | [*c.*1260] |
| Brackley B63 | [*c.*1260 × 1265] |
| Brackley 89A | [*c.*1260 × 1265] |
| **Aynho 63** | [*c.*1260 × 1270] |
| Brackley B152 | [*c.*1260 × 1270] |
| Brackley D196 | [*c.*1260 × 1270][64] |
| Astwick and Evenley 63A | 1262 |
| *Robert le Somenur, clerk** | |
| Brackley 155 | [*c.*1250 × 1260] |
| Brackley D10 | [*c.*1250 × 1260] |
| Whitfield 48 | [*c.*1250 × 1260] |
| Brackley 97A | [*c.*1260 × 1265] |
| Brackley D22 | [*c.*1260 × 1270] |
| Brackley 87A | [*c.*1270] |
| Brackley D161 | [*c.*1270] |
| Brackley D17 | [*c.*1270] |
| Brackley C36 | 22 Feb 1272 |
| Brackley C40 | 22 Feb 1272 |
| *Robert of Trafford, clerk* (Hand 1)[65] | |
| Brackley C135 | [*c.*1220 × 1230] |
| Whitfield 122 | [*c.*1230 × 1240] |
| Astwick and Evenley 64A* | [*c.*1240 × 1245] |
| Astwick and Evenley 2 | [*c.*1250] |
| *Robert of Trafford, clerk** (Hand 2) | |
| Brackley C114 | [*c.*1240] |

64 Macray dates this act [*c.*1280 × 1290], but since it is written in Robert's hand, who does not otherwise appear in acts beyond the 1260s, it seems more likely to have been issued in the period *c.*1260 × 1270.

65 The hand of MCA, Whitfield 126 is very similar to that of these four charters, although Robert does not appear among the witnesses.

| | |
|---|---|
| Brackley 10 | [*c*.1240 × 1250] |
| Brackley C109 | [*c*.1255 × 1260] |
| *Robert of Trafford, clerk** (Hand 3) | |
| Brackley B106 | [*c*.1250] |
| Brackley C108 | [*c*.1250 × 1260] |
| *Thomas* | |
| Astwick and Evenley 51[66] | [*c*.1200] |
| **Aynho 52*** | [*c*.1200 × 1205] |
| Astwick and Evenley 68A* | [*c*.1200 × 1210] |
| Whitfield 155* | [*c*.1210] |
| *William, clerk** | |
| Whitfield 4 | [*c*.1270] |
| Whitfield 21 | [*c*.1270 × 1280] |
| Whitfield 23 | [*c*.1270 × 1280] |
| Whitfield 79 | [*c*.1270 × 1280] |
| *William Dodevile of Kemerton, clerk** (Hand 1) | |
| Brackley D37 | [*c*.1240 × 1250] |
| Brackley 150 | [*c*.1250 × 1260] |
| Brackley C2 | [*c*.1260] |
| *William Dodevile of Kemerton, clerk** (Hand 2) | |
| Brackley 135 | [*c*.1260] |
| Brackley 137 | [*c*.1260] |
| Brackley 138 | [*c*.1260] |
| Brackley D24 | [*c*.1260] |
| Brackley D91 | 14 Jun 1260 |
| Brackley 25 | [*c*.1260 × 1270] |
| Brackley 70A | 6 Feb 1261 |
| Brackley 165 | 30 Apr 1262 |
| Brackley 179 | 31 May 1263 |
| *William Dodevile of Kemerton, clerk** (Hand 3) | |
| Brackley D203 | 16 Mar 1264 |

66 The hand of this act also has a lot in common with that of a charter written by Alan, chaplain of Brackley Hospital, tabled above.

Table 3.1. *continued*

| | |
|---|---|
| *William of Pilton, of Brackley, clerk* | |
| Brackley 9A | [*c.*1250 × 1260] |
| Whitfield 2* | 7 Oct 1263 |
| *William le Tannur of Brackley, clerk* | |
| Brackley 85A[67] | [*c.*1270] |
| Brackley 88A | [*c.*1270] |
| Brackley B92* | [*c.*1280] |
| Brackley 49A* | [*c.*1290] |

Table 3.2. Ralph Albrith in Brackley Hospital charters.

| **Act** | **Date** | **Name** | **Last in witness list (Y/N)** | **Act in hand (Y/N)** |
|---|---|---|---|---|
| Brackley C9 | [*c.*1240 × 1250] | Ralph, the clerk | Y | N |
| Brackley C43 | [*c.*1250] | Ralph Aylbrit | Y | Y |
| Brackley 58 | [*c.*1250] | Ralph, the clerk | Y | N |
| Brackley C5 | [*c.*1250] | Ralph, the clerk | Y | Y |
| Brackley D247 | [*c.*1250 × 1260] | Ralph Aylbryht | N | N |
| Brackley 163 | 14 Feb 1256 | Ralph Ailbrit | N | N |
| Brackley D102 | 25 Nov 1256 | Ralph Aylbrith | Y | N |
| Brackley D40 | 30 Apr 1258 | Ralph Aylbruth | Y | Y |
| Brackley D141 | 17 Jan 1260 | Ralph Aylbryth | N | N |
| Brackley D91 | 14 Jun 1260 | Ralph Aylbrith | N | N |
| Brackley C20 | 25 Dec 1260 | Ralph, the clerk | Y | Y |
| Brackley B110 | [*c.*1260] | Ralph Aylbryth | N | N |
| Brackley C11 | [*c.*1260] | Ralph Aylbrit, clerk | Y | Y |
| Brackley 47A | [*c.*1260] | Ralph Aylbrith, clerk | Y | Y |
| Brackley 57 | [*c.*1260] | Ralph Aylbrith | N | N |
| Brackley D98 | [*c.*1260] | Ralph Albrith | Y | Y |
| Brackley 142 | [*c.*1260] | Ralph Aybrit, clerk | Y | Y |
| Brackley D243 | [*c.*1260] | [...] [...]it, clerk | Y | Y |
| Brackley 52 | [*c.*1260] | Ralph Aylbrith, clerk | Y | Y |

67 It is only in this act that William is referred to as a clerk.

| Act | Date | Name | Last in witness list (Y/N) | Act in hand (Y/N) |
|---|---|---|---|---|
| Brackley 51 | [*c*.1260] | Ralph Aylbrith, clerk | Y | Y |
| Brackley D194 | [*c*.1260] | Ralph, the clerk | Y | Y |
| Brackley D193 | [*c*.1260] | Ralph, the clerk | Y | Y |
| Brackley 136 | [*c*.1260] | Ralph Aylbrit, clerk | Y | Y |
| Brackley D201 | [*c*.1260] | Ralph Aylbrith, clerk | Y | Y |
| Brackley D202 | [*c*.1260] | Ralph Aylbrith, clerk | Y | Y |
| Brackley 23A | [*c*.1260 × 1265] | Ralph Aylbruth, clerk | Y | Y |
| Brackley 141 | [*c*.1260 × 1265] | Ralph Aylbrit, clerk | Y | Y |
| Brackley D133 | 24 Apr 1262 | Ralph Aylbrit, clerk | Y | Y |
| Astwick and Evenley 80A | [*c*.1260] | Ralph Aylbrith | N | N |
| Whitfield 109 | [*c*.1250 × 1260] | Ralph Aylbrit, the writer of this deed | Y | Y |
| Whitfield 73 | [*c*.1260] | Ralph, the clerk | Y | Y |
| Brackley 36A | [c 1270] | Ralph, the clerk | Y | Y |
| Brackley B50 | [c 1270] | Ralph Aylbrite, clerk | Y | Y |

Table 3.3. William Dodevile in Brackley Hospital charters.

| Act | Date | Name | Last in witness list (Y/N) | Act in hand (Y/N) |
|---|---|---|---|---|
| Brackley D37 | [*c*.1240 × 1250] | William Dodevile, clerk | Y | Y |
| Brackley 150 | [*c*.1250 × 1260] | William Dodevile of Kemerton, clerk | Y | Y |
| Brackley C2 | [*c*.1260] | William Dodevile of Kemerton, clerk | Y | Y |
| Brackley 137 | [*c*.1260] | William Dodevile of Kemerton, clerk | Y | Y |
| Brackley 138 | [*c*.1260] | William Dodevile | Y | Y |
| Brackley 135 | [*c*.1260] | William Dodevile of Kemerton, clerk | Y | Y |
| Brackley D24 | [*c*.1260] | William Dodevile | Y | Y |
| Brackley D91 | 14 Jun 1260 | William of Kemerton, clerk | Y | Y |

Table 3.3. *continued*

| Act | Date | Name | Last in witness list (Y/N) | Act in hand (Y/N) |
|---|---|---|---|---|
| Brackley 25 | [*c.*1260 × 1270] | William Dodevile, clerk | Y | Y |
| Brackley 70A | 6 Feb 1261 | William Dodevile, clerk | Y | Y |
| Brackley 165 | 30 Apr 1262 | William Dodevile of Kemerton, clerk | Y | Y |
| Brackley 179 | 31 May 1263 | William, the clerk | Y | Y |
| Brackley D203 | 16 Mar 1264 | William Dodevile of Kemerton, clerk | Y | Y |

Table 3.4. Robert le Somenur in Brackley Hospital charters.

| Act | Date | Name | Last in witness list (Y/N) | Act in hand (Y/N) |
|---|---|---|---|---|
| Brackley 155 | [*c.*1250 × 1260] | Robert le Somenur, clerk | Y | Y |
| Brackley D10 | [*c.*1250 × 1260] | Robert Sumonitore | Y | Y |
| Whitfield 48 | [*c.*1250 × 1260] | Robert le Somenur, clerk | Y | Y |
| Brackley 97A | [*c.*1260 × 1265] | Robert le Somenur, clerk | Y | Y |
| Brackley D22 | [*c.*1260 × 1270] | Robert le Somenur, clerk | Y | N |
| Brackley 87A | [*c.*1270] | Robert, the clerk | Y | Y |
| Brackley D161 | [*c.*1270] | Robert le Somenur, clerk | Y | Y |
| Brackley D17 | [*c.*1270] | Robert, the clerk | Y | Y |
| Brackley C36 | 22 Feb 1272 | Robert, the clerk | Y | Y |
| Brackley C40 | 22 Feb 1272 | Robert, the clerk | Y | Y |

Table 3.5. Richard of Epwell in Oxford deeds.

| **Act** | **Date** | **Name** | **Last in witness list (Y/N)** | **Act in hand (Y/N)** |
|---|---|---|---|---|
| St Mary Magdalene 3 | [*c*.1260] | Richard of Epwell | Y | Y |
| Willoughby 3A | [*c*.1264 × 1270] | Richard of Epwell | Y | Y |
| Westcote 87 | [*c*.1265 × 1270] | Richard of Epwell | Y | Y |
| Willoughby 56 | [c.1265 × 1275] | Richard of Epwell | Y | Y |
| Westcote 33 | [c.1265 × 1278] | Richard of Epwell | Y | N |
| Chipping Norton 2 | [1267 × 1277] | Richard of Epwell | Y | Y |
| Chipping Norton 4 | [1267 × 1277] | Richard of Epwell | Y | Y |
| South Newington 11A | [*c*.1270] | Richard of Epwell, clerk | Y | Y |
| South Newington 12A | [*c*.1270] | Richard of Epwell, clerk | Y | Y |
| Thornborough 19 | [*c*.1270] | Richard of Epwell | Y | Y |
| Thornborough 40 | [*c*.1270] | Richard of Epwell, clerk | Y | Y |
| Thornborough 85 | [*c*.1270] | Richard of Epwell, clerk | Y | Y |
| Cowley 7 | [1270 × 1278] | Richard of Epwell | Y | Y |
| St Martin's 8 | [? 1272/3] | Richard of Epwell, clerk | Y | Y |
| St Peter's in the East 76 | [1273/4] | Richard of Epwell | Y | Y |
| Holywell 9 | [1273/4] | Richard of Epwell | Y | Y |
| All Saints 52 | 9 Oct 1273 | Richard of Epwell | Y | Y (Hand 2) |
| All Saints 51 | 30 Nov 1273 | Richard of Epwell | Y | Y (Hand 2) |
| St Peter's in the East 47 | [*c*.1274/5] | Richard of Epwell | Y | Y |
| Westcote 6 | [*c*.1274] | Richard of Epwell, clerk | Y | Y |
| Garsington 22 | 20 Aug 1274 | Richard of Epwell, clerk | Y | Y |

Table 3.5. *continued*

| | | | | |
|---|---|---|---|---|
| Oxford, Lincoln College, EL/OXF/D/5 | [*c*.1275] | Richard of Epwell, clerk | Y | Y |
| St Peter's in the East 74 | [1275/6] | Richard of Epwell | Y | Y |
| St Peter's in the East 20B | [1275/6] | Richard of Epwell | Y | Y |
| Cowley 2 | 19 Mar 1275 | Richard of Epwell | Y | Y |
| St Peter's in the East 50 | 1 May 1276 | Richard of Epwell | Y | Y |
| South Newington 2A | 24 Jun 1276 | Richard of Epwell | Y | Y |
| St Giles 9 | 18 Aug 1276 | Richard of Epwell | Y | Y (Hand 2) |
| St Martin's 7 | 8 Aug 1277 | Richard of Epwell | Y | Y |
| St Mary the Virgin 8 | 29 Sep 1277 | Richard of Epwell | Y | Y (Hand 2) |
| St Peter's in the East 62C | [1278/9] | Richard of Epwell | Y | Y |
| St Peter's in the East 51D | [1278/9] | Richard of Epwell | Y | Y |

# 4

# DATE, DESIGN, AND MATERIALITY OF THE AYNHO CARTULARY

Through studying the foundation and early history of Aynho Hospital, its patronage networks and benefactors, and its participation in local documentary cultures and scribal milieux, the previous chapters have established the wider contextual picture and historical framework of our analysis. It is now time to turn to the artefact at the very heart of this book: the Aynho Cartulary (MCA, EP/137/1). While Part II of this book provides an edition and translation of the cartulary's text alongside a photographic facsimile, the present chapter introduces the reader to the physical object in which this text is preserved by exploring in detail the cartulary's format, design, material composition, and scribal preparation. It also proposes a new date for the cartulary's initial creation, showing that it is among the earliest roll cartularies to survive from both England and France, and the only one known to have been produced by a medieval hospital anywhere in Britain and Ireland prior to the fourteenth century.

## FORMAT

The first thing to notice (and note) about the Aynho Cartulary is its unusual format.[1] Unlike most cartularies produced across medieval Europe, especially those made in Britain and Ireland,[2] the example from Aynho does not

1 We use the term 'format' interchangeably with 'form' to denote the cartulary's physical size and shape in keeping with Robinson, 'Format of Books', p. 41, n.*.

2 For a principal overview, see still *Cartularies*; prior to its revised version, Davis's catalogue (originally published in 1958) had received several addenda: P. Hoskin, 'Medieval Cartularies of Great Britain: Amendments and Additions to the Davis Catalogue', *MRB*, 2 (1996), 1–12; I.C. Cunningham, 'Medieval Cartularies of Great Britain: Amendments and Additions to the Scottish Section of Davis', *MRB*, 3 (1997), 1–6; N. Vincent, 'Medieval Cartularies: Additions and Corrections', *MRB*, 3 (1997), 7–38; N. Vincent, 'Medieval Cartularies: Further Additions', *MRB*, 4 (1998), 6–12;

take the conventional form of a bound book (codex), but that of a roll. As noted by one of the editors of a volume on rolls in late medieval England and France, '[i]f a poll were carried out to establish which form of manuscript, the codex or the roll, the public associated more with the Middle Ages, the result would probably see the codex taking most votes', despite the fact that '[r]olls were also widespread in the Middle Ages and there was hardly anything that could not be written on them',[3] including cartularies. The use of rolls alongside – and often in lieu of – codices is well-known, and well-studied, in contexts of later medieval bureaucracy and administration, especially (but not exclusively) in royal government.[4] Roll cartularies, by contrast, have only very recently become a dedicated subject of coordinated and collaborative scholarship. In recent years, scholars across the Channel have led the charge with the major research project ROTULUS (2019–22), co-funded by the Agence Nationale de la Recherche and the Centre de Recherche Universitaire Lorrain d'Histoire, which has resulted in a suite of events (conferences, workshops, exhibitions), publications (print

N. Vincent, 'Medieval Cartularies: Further Additions II', *MRB*, 5 (1999), 26–28. Also cf. the recent discussion by Tucker, *Reading and Shaping*, pp. 12–13, arguing that 'understanding the cartulary [as a phenomenon] requires us to remain open to the variety of forms it can take and avoid unnecessary presumptions about structure, content, or purpose'.

3 Peltzer, 'The Roll in England and France', p. 1. For similar observations with a plea for looking beyond the codex – and towards the roll – as a primary medium of medieval literacy, see N. Kössinger, 'Gerollte Schrift: Mittelalterliche Texte auf Rotuli', in A. Kehnel and D. Panagiotopoulos (eds), *Schriftträger–Textträger: Zur materialen Präsenz des Geschriebenen in frühen Gesellschaften* (Berlin, 2015), pp. 151–68.

4 On the use of rolls as instruments of royal, aristocratic, and institutional administration in medieval England, see principally M.T. Clanchy, *From Memory to Written Record: England 1066–1307*, 3rd edn (Malden, 2013), pp. 137–46; N. Vincent, 'Why 1199? Bureaucracy and Enrolment under John and His Contemporaries', in A. Jobson (ed.), *English Government in the Thirteenth Century* (Woodbridge, 2004), pp. 17–48; also N. Vincent, 'Enrolment in Medieval English Government: Sickness or Cure?', in J. Peltzer et al. (eds), *The Roll in England and France in the Late Middle Ages: Form and Content* (Berlin, 2020), pp. 103–45; most recently A. Armstrong, *The Materiality of Medieval Administration in Northern England* (Turnhout, 2024), pp. 69–105. On what is perhaps the most prominent form of rolls in medieval English government, the Pipe roll, see now R. Cassidy, *Approaching Pipe Rolls: The Thirteenth Century* (Abingdon, 2023). Scholars have also studied the roll as a format for historical writing and illustration, again with a focus on England; S. Drimmer, 'The Shapes of History: Houghton Library, MS Richardson 35 and Chronicles of England in Codex and Roll', in J.F. Hamburger et al. (eds), *Beyond Words: Illuminated Manuscripts in Boston Collections* (Toronto, ON, 2021), pp. 253–68; L. Cleaver, 'From Codex to Roll: Illustrating History in the Anglo-Norman World in the Twelfth and Thirteenth Centuries', *ANS*, 36 (2014), 69–90.

and online), and freely available Open-Access tools for future research.[5] Their ongoing activities are released on a blog,[6] and their online database 'Rotuli/Inventaire des cartulaires-rouleaux médiévaux français' comprises (as of 2023/4) nearly two hundred roll cartularies (or cartulary rolls) made in France prior to 1501,[7] by far the largest and most diverse concentration anywhere in the medieval Latin West.

The numbers from England are rather modest by comparison, with fewer than two dozen examples from the twelfth to sixteenth centuries. Most come from religious houses, including Dieulacres Abbey (Stafford, William Salt Library, MS 539), Flaxley Abbey (BL, MS Add. 49996), Holme Cultram Abbey (Oxford, Bodleian Libraries, MS Norfolk Rolls), Hulme Abbey (BL, Cotton Roll XVI.51–52), Kirkstall Abbey (BL, Add. Roll 17121), Kirkstead Abbey (BL, Harley Roll G.21, L.20, and O.5),[8] Westminster Abbey (BL, Add. Roll 15895), Barnwell Priory (Cambridge, Christ's College, Muniments, Bourn E), Bullington Priory (BL, Harley Roll A.28–A.29), Holme Priory (BL, Add. Roll 24879), Lenton Priory (York, University of York–Borthwick Institute for Archives, CP.F.112),[9] Nuneaton Priory (BL, Add. Roll 47398), Stone Priory (BL, Cotton Roll XIII.6), West Dereham Priory (Norwich, Norfolk Record Office, Hare 624 188 x 1), Ely Cathedral Priory (BL, MS Cotton Vespasian A XIX, fols. 52r–54r), Exeter Cathedral Priory (BL, MS Add. 52729), and York Minster (York, York Minster Library and Archives, P 1/1/9), plus the two rare non-monastic – in fact, secular – examples of the 'Gaunt Roll' (Brighton, East Sussex and Brighton and Hove Record Office, GLY/1139) and the cartulary roll of Peter of Savoy, Lord of Richmond

5 See <https://crulh.univ-lorraine.fr/recherche/projets-anr-en-cours/anr-rotulus>.

6 <https://rotulus.hypotheses.org>.

7 <https://rotuli.univ-lorraine.fr>. Missing from this commendably comprehensive database is the thirteenth-century roll cartulary of Asprières (Chicago, Newberry Library, MS Greenlee 39), on which see R. Clemens and T. Graham, *Introduction to Manuscript Studies* (Ithaca, NY, 2007), pp. 238–9.

8 These rolls from Kirkstead constitute something of a case apart, as Kathryn Dutton has recently shown two of them (G.21 and L.20) to be precursors to the abbey's book-shaped cartulary also made in the thirteenth and expanded well into the fourteenth century (BL, MS Cotton Vespasian E XVIII), thus representing what Dutton calls 'a preliminary stage of archival consolidation', whereas the third (O.5) – dubbed the '*chirographa perpetua* roll' by Dutton – was probably produced 'by the [cartulary's] compiler himself to organize these chirographs prior to entering them into the cartulary': Dutton, 'Cartulary', pp. 91–2. See also Dutton's forthcoming book-length study and edition of the Kirkstead Cartulary and related archival materials.

9 On the Lenton roll, see J.E. Burton, 'A Roll of Charters for Lenton Priory', *Borthwick Institute Bulletin*, 2 (1979), 13–26; Hoskin, 'Medieval Cartularies', p. 6.

(1240–68).[10] There is also the roll cartulary from Reading Abbey's priory on the Isle of May, in the Firth of Forth, Scotland (BL, Add. Roll 19631), and several roll cartularies from Margam Abbey in South Wales, which have received much attention.[11] But there are, to our knowledge, only half a dozen examples of roll cartularies from medieval English hospitals besides Aynho. These take the shape of two fourteenth-century rolls from the leper hospitals in Ickburgh, Norfolk (Norwich, Norfolk Record Office, BRA 833/14/1, 669X1) and Lowcross, Yorkshire (Durham, University Library–Archives and Special Collections, Loc. III: 6),[12] plus a very badly damaged fragment of a fifteenth-century roll of St Edmund's Hospital, Sprotbrough (Sheffield, City Archives and Local Studies Library, CD433) and three rolls from the two hospitals of SS John the Baptist and Mary Magdalene, Exeter (Exeter, Devon Record Office, ECA/MR 64 and ECA/MAG 69 and 99), which were produced around the very end of the Middle Ages.[13] Moreover, all but six of the abovementioned cases (Flaxley, Hulme,

10 On the latter, see now H. Ridgeway, 'An English Cartulary Roll of Peter of Savoy, Lord of Richmond (1240–1268): Archives, Interests and Servants of an Alien Favourite of King Henry III', in N. Saul and N. Vincent (eds), *English Medieval Government and Administration: Essays in Honour of J.R. Maddicott* (Woodbridge, 2023), pp. 203–28.

11 R.B. Patterson, *The Scriptorium of Margam Abbey and the Scribes of Early Angevin Glamorgan: Secretarial Administration in a Welsh Marcher Barony,* c.*1150*–c.*1225* (Woodbridge, 2001); *Cartularies*, pp. 129–30 (= nos. 649.1–15); Papin, 'Cartulaires'; Papin, 'Cartulaires-rouleaux'.

12 The latter is edited in W. Brown Davis (ed.), *Cartularium prioratus de Gyseburne* (2 vols, Durham, 1889–94), vol. 1, pp. 171–96; *Cartularies*, pp. 100, 126 (= nos. 499.1, 633.2).

13 E. Peacock, 'A Mutilated Roll of Instruments Relating to the Hospital of St. Edmund, at Sprotborough, near Doncaster', *Archaeologia*, 42 (1870), 398–404; *Cartularies*, pp. 80, 186–7 (= nos. 393.1, 395–96, 924.3). Though originally founded as hospitals in the twelfth century, Cockersand (Premonstratensian), Creake (Augustinian), Anglesey (Augustinian), and Elsham (Augustinian) had all ceased operating in this capacity and been re-founded as priories by the time their respective roll cartularies were produced in the later Middle Ages; ibid., pp. 3, 54, 59, 73 (= nos. 12.2, 265, 286, 356.1). The so-called 'cartularies' of St Nicholas' Hospital, Clitheroe/Edisford (Preston, Lancashire Record Office, DDTO/box AA), St Bartholomew's Hospital, Oxford (TNA, C 47/9/7), and St Mary's Hospital, Castleton (TNA, DL 41/125) are single membranes that contain copies of two, three, and eight acts, respectively; ibid., pp. 53, 73, 149, 186 (= nos. 263.1, 742, 924.3). Likewise, the roll from St Leonard's (*olim* St Peter's) Hospital, York made in 1287 (Lichfield, Cathedral Library, QQ.1) and referred to as a 'roll of extents' can hardly be classified as a cartulary *stricto sensu*; ibid., p. 227 (= no. 1108). The 'tenor cartarum' of St Wulfstan's Hospital, Worcester from *c.*1500 (Birmingham, Archives and Heritage Service, 403957 [IIR.33]) merely provides abstracts on two membranes; ibid., p. 219 (= no. 1079). The roll of charters relating to St Leonard's Hospital, Kirkby and its 'mother house' of Conishead

Kirkstead, May, Margam, and Stone) date from between the mid-fourteenth and early sixteenth centuries, meaning the Aynho Cartulary – produced in the second half of the thirteenth century, likely the third quarter (see below) – claims a place of special distinction as being not only among the earliest roll cartularies from England and Britain,[14] but also the only one produced by/for an English hospital before the fourteenth century. There are, moreover, only two known parallels across the Channel (Cambrai and Limoges; see below), which further underscores the Aynho Cartulary's considerable historical significance and the need for a full contextual, codicological, and palaeographical study like the one offered here.

The twelfth and thirteenth centuries are widely recognised as a period of increased documentary productivity and innovation on both sides of the Channel, one that generated large numbers and varieties of archival sources (genuine and forged) in ecclesiastical and secular milieux.[15] The rising number of cartularies, most of them codices, and their increasingly widespread use during this period, can plausibly be linked to important socio-political and socio-economic developments in medieval European cultures of literacy, accountability, and administration – developments in which Aynho and its hospital no doubt took part, and in which the making of its cartulary finds its locus.[16] At the same time as firmly belonging within this wider European context, the Aynho Cartulary's unusual format offers us the unique opportunity, certainly within an English/British setting, to

(Augustinian) was only produced during/after its dissolution in the early sixteenth century; ibid., p. 56 (= no. 274.4).

14 The three late-eleventh-century cartularies of Worcester Cathedral Priory are widely held as the earliest English/British examples, though none of them takes the form of a roll; *Cartularies*, p. xv; N.R. Ker, 'Hemming's Cartulary: A Description of the Two Worcester Cartularies in Cotton Tiberius A. XIII', in R.W. Hunt (ed.), *Studies in Medieval History, Presented to Frederick Maurice Powicke* (Oxford, 1948), pp. 49–75. The abovementioned roll cartulary of Stone Priory dates from the twelfth century.

15 Case studies of rolls from Anglo-Norman and Angevin religious houses include H. Dewez, 'Le Rouleau comme support des comptes manoriaux au prieuré cathédral de Norwich (mi-XIIIe–mi-XIVe siècles)', *Comptabilités*, (2011), <https://journals.openedition.org/comptabilites/400>; T. Jarry, 'Évaluer, inventorier, exploiter: Le *Rotulus de denariis* de l'abbaye Saint-Étienne de Caen (XIIIe siècle)', *Tabularia* (2006), <https://doi.org/10.4000/tabularia.876>; for a cross-Channel view on forgeries, see R.F. Berkhofer III, *Forgeries and Historical Writing in England, France, and Flanders, 900–1200* (Woodbridge, 2022).

16 Bertrand, *Écritures ordinaires*; R.F. Berkhofer III, *Day of Reckoning: Power and Accountability in Medieval France* (Philadelphia, PA, 2004); Chastang, 'Cartulaires'; see also the contributions to H. Dewez and L. Tryoen (eds), *Administrer par l'écrit au Moyen Âge (XIIe–XVe siècle)* (Paris, 2019); H. Dewez (ed.), *Du nouveau en archives: Pratiques documentaires et innovations administratives (XIIIe–XVe siècle)* (Saint-Denis, 2019).

investigate in detail the means of production and documentary culture of a small and relatively obscure hospital operating in a rural (if not altogether remote) locality in proximity to two other hospitals – SS James and John, Brackley, and St John the Baptist, Oxford – of which neither has left us with a roll cartulary.

Before turning to analyse the cartulary's materiality and the work of its scribes, we should first give some consideration as to why this particular format was chosen. In other words, why decide to produce a roll cartulary rather than a codex? Could it have been a pragmatic choice, an economical concern even, one that had to do more with necessity or availability than with preference, or did the roll format perhaps offer something more specific and desirable that the codex did not? More generally still, is there a connection between form and content, between format and purpose? Much attention has been paid to these and similar kinds of questions, and there is no need to rehearse these debates here.[17] Suffice it to say, in the absence of a straightforward association, much less a universal correlation, between a cartulary's format and its intended use(s), there are certain characteristics which are widely acknowledged as distinguishing rolls – and, by extension, roll cartularies – from their bound and book-shaped counterparts. On the one hand, those of particular interest to the present discussion, and which are worthy of renewed consideration, concern the costs and complexities involved in a cartulary's initial production and its subsequent continuation or redaction, and, on the other hand, the ease of handling, storage, and transportation.

Beginning with the matter of costs and resources, there can be little doubt that rolls were, on average, quicker/cheaper to produce and easier to continue than codices.[18] For a relatively small and moderately endowed institution like Aynho Hospital, this probably would have been an important consideration. The main resource for the cartulary's creation was, of course, parchment. Even if the quality of the parchment required for this task did not have to match that needed to make a codex, this still meant resourcing at least two or three skins from which to cut the cartulary's seven membranes. As Bruce Holsinger points out in his recent book on the history of parchment, thinking of parchment simply as a by-product of husbandry that was available to more or less any institution with livestock, large or small, is inaccurate, 'and in any case the very notion of a byproduct is largely foreign to the economies of scarcity that characterized much of

17 Good summaries of the *état présent* are provided by Peltzer, 'The Roll in England and France'; Kössinger, 'Gerollte Schrift'; Robinson, 'The Format of Books'.

18 Kössinger, 'Gerollte Schrift', pp. 163–4; also cf. the concise discussion of the practical advantages of rolls by Clemens and Graham, *Introduction*, p. 250.

the medieval world'.[19] We know from acts copied in the cartulary (nos. **3**, **4**, **8–9**, **14**, **18**, **20–1**, **24**, **36–7**, **57**) and the charters surviving alongside it (Appendix) that the hospital's lands included a fair amount of pasture, and we may infer that this was used not only for oxen and horses (no. **9**), but also for sheep whose skins could, in theory, have been used to make the cartulary. That said, holding sheep as livestock and skinning them at the point of slaughter is not the same as turning these skins into parchment, and we should not assume that one always or necessarily involved the other. Even if the cartulary's membranes did come from the hospital's own flock, it still seems unlikely that the parchment making took place in-house, and more likely that it was done by external specialists, presumably for a fee. The alternative is, of course, that the parchment was purchased from an external source to begin with and paid for with domestic funds.

Either way, the costs and efforts involved in sourcing and preparing the cartulary's parchment would have marked a considerable investment for an institution such as Aynho, but they were still lower than those of producing or commissioning a codex. Rather than having to acquire a fixed number of sheets (*bifolia*) to produce regular quires/gatherings with a certain minimum of pages that could be bound into a book or booklet, thus possibly ending up with some unused and superfluous pages, the advantage of a roll cartulary was that it could be composed from any number of membranes, however small or odd, without the same risk of surplus. What is more, sewing together the roll's membranes would have required neither great skill nor special equipment, even when done in 'chancery fashion',[20] whereas binding a codex – even one with a limited number of quires – was a much more involved undertaking that demanded expertise, bespoke materials, and specialised tools like a sewing station.[21] Finally, a roll, unlike a codex, required no wooden boards or additional leather/skin wrappings to serve as protective covers and prevent its pages from expanding and warping due to changes in temperature or humidity, though it might well have had a physical storage container (see below). From a purely material

19 B. Holsinger, *On Parchment: Animals, Archives, and the Making of Culture from Herodotus to the Digital Age* (New Haven, CT, 2022), p. 21. This 'economy of scarcity' is also reflected in the conscientious re-use, repair, and recycling of parchment as a way of saving resources; cf. H. Ryley, *Re-using Manuscripts in Late Medieval England: Repairing, Recycling, Sharing* (York, 2022).

20 The term used by Woolgar, 'Two Cartularies', p. 498; also cf. our discussion below.

21 On the basic process and the materials/equipment involved, see J.A. Szirmai, *The Archaeology of Medieval Bookbinding* (Farnham, 1999); R.M. Thomson et al., 'Technology of Production of the Manuscript Book', in N.J. Morgan and R.M. Thomson (eds), *The Cambridge History of the Book in Britain. Vol. 2: 1100–1400* (Cambridge, 2008), pp. 75–109, especially pp. 95–109 ('Bookbindings').

perspective, therefore, a roll cartulary offered a 'budget option' that was more economical and less involved than the bound equivalent.

Human resources were just as important as material ones, if indeed not more so. Unfortunately, we know next to nothing about the hospital's permanent residents – its 'staff', so to speak. Given the numbers of staff recorded at other medieval English hospitals of roughly equivalent size, wealth, and status, especially non-leper houses, it seems unlikely that Aynho would have had many literate inhabitants besides the domestic priest responsible for the care of souls, the chaplain (we will recall the institution of a chaplain at Aynho to pray for Euphemia of Dunbar and the presence of a chapel in Croughton from *c.*1210; Chapter 2), and the proctor/master (*procurator/magister*) himself, let alone a steady domestic supply of trained and experienced scribes.[22] A far cry from the largest and wealthiest hospitals acting as centres of literacy, learning, and sometimes book production in their own right,[23] Aynho's domestic capacity and expertise probably would have been extremely limited in this regard. Unlike many of England's monasteries – the largest and most prolific of which had access to in-house scribes who, with the licence of their heads of house, could be exempted from routine tasks to produce books, charters, and other documents at considerable speed and without remuneration – a small-scale rural hospital such as Aynho needed to invest in staff as much as it had to invest in materials.[24] To do so, Aynho's heads of house had two options. First, like many other institutions, including those with access to domestic scribes, they could hire professionals active within the locality or from further afield to visit Aynho

22 In their national survey of medieval English hospitals in the period *c.*1070–1570, Nicholas Orme and Margaret Webster observe that '[m]ost hospitals were far more modest in size [than the likes of St Bartholomew, Gloucester with a dozen or so clergy and numerous lay brothers/sisters caring for nearly a hundred inmates]: a single master, a few brothers and sisters, and a dozen or so long-term inmates or sick patients', to the extent that '[a]t small hospitals [...] the master might virtually be the only officer': Orme and Webster, *English Hospital*, pp. 36, 80; on the social and educational backgrounds of these hospitals' heads of house, see ibid., pp. 77–8. Relatively low levels of literacy among some heads of house may be explained by the fact that they had been appointed by the hospital's aristocratic patrons from among their own family and secular associates with little (or no) concern for education or literary activity: Sweetinburgh, *Role of the Hospital*, pp. 37–8. On the different forms and degrees of medieval (il)literacy, cf. F.H. Bäuml, 'Varieties and Consequences of Medieval Literacy and Illiteracy', *Speculum*, 55 (1980), 237–65; B. Stock, *The Implications of Literacy: Written Language and Models of Interpretation in the Eleventh and Twelfth Centuries* (Princeton, NJ, 1983).

23 See the examples in Orme and Webster, *English Hospital*, pp. 64–6.

24 On the appointment of monastic scribes with the licence and permission of their head of house, see Pohl, *Abbatial Authority*, pp. 99–103, 169–91.

and do the work in situ, meaning these professionals had to be paid for their services, supplied with writing materials, and, for the duration of the assignment, provided with board and lodging inside the hospital, thereby placing additional strains on what were likely limited domestic funds.[25] Alternatively, they could commission these professionals to undertake the work *extra muros* to save the costs of their accommodation and subsistence. This, however, would have meant reimbursing them for all materials and transporting the domestic archives to them, rather than *vice versa*, a prospect that, especially in the case of the hospital's most valuable charters and papal privileges (nos. **1–2**), might have seemed too risky or logistically complicated. If nothing else, and depending on the scribes' working speed, it would have meant parting with the hospital's archives for several months or more.[26]

Roll cartularies continued to offer certain advantages beyond the circumstances of their production. For example, adding content to them at a later point was more straightforward than enlarging a codex, as it simply entailed stitching further membranes onto the end (or beginning) of the roll, with no need to interfere with, undo, or compromise the integrity of the existing material structure. By contrast, dismantling and re-assembling a bound volume was a materially difficult task to achieve, especially in the absence of proper bookbinding facilities and domestic expertise. It has been suggested that rolls – and, by extension, roll cartularies – also offered some concrete benefits in terms of their usability, such as by facilitating the more economical reading mode of 'scrolling'.[27] Whether such speedy reading and enhanced navigability were of concern to the Aynho Cartulary's makers and users is difficult to know, but it is not implausible, given that the cartulary would likely have served, among other functions, as an

25 Pohl, *Abbatial Authority*, pp. 218–33. On professional scribes in medieval England, see R. Sharpe, *Libraries and Books in Medieval England: The Role of Libraries in a Changing Book Economy (The Lyell Lectures for 2018–19)*, ed. J. Willoughby (Oxford, 2023), pp. 71–2; M. Gullick, 'Professional Scribes in Eleventh- and Twelfth-Century England', *English Manuscript Studies 1100–1700*, 7 (1998), 1–24; L.R. Mooney, 'Professional Scribes? Identifying English Scribes who had a Hand in More than One Manuscript', in D. Pearsall (ed.), *New Directions in Later Medieval Manuscript Studies: Essays from the 1998 Harvard Conference* (Cambridge, 2000), pp. 131–42.

26 On the speed of medieval domestic and professional scribes, cf. E.A. Overgaauw, 'Fast or Slow, Professional or Monastic: The Writing Speed of Some Late-Medieval Scribes', *Scriptorium*, 49 (1995), 211–27; J.P. Gumbert, 'The Speed of Scribes', in E. Condello and G. de Gregorio (eds), *Scribi e colofoni: Le sottoscrizioni di copisti dalle origini all'avvento della stampa* (Spoleto, 1995), pp. 57–69; M. Gullick, 'How Fast Did Scribes Write? Evidence from Romanesque Manuscripts', in L.L. Brownrigg (ed.), *Making the Medieval Book: Techniques of Production* (London, 1995), pp. 39–58.

27 Kössinger, 'Gerollte Schrift', p. 164.

important 'reference tool' in both internal and external contexts, from the hospital's domestic administration, the management of its estate and revenues, and the commemoration of its patrons and benefactors, to episcopal visitations, property disputes, court cases, etc. As such, the cartulary might have had to be taken outside the hospital on occasion, which is when its format would have once again revealed itself as advantageous, with rolls being easier to transport than codices due to their compact nature and the natural stability provided by their physical shape.[28] Indeed, the way in which the Aynho Cartulary is stored today for conservation conceals its noteworthy compactness. Rolled loosely around a toilet-roll-sized cardboard tube to stop the innermost membrane(s) from curling too tightly and to facilitate easy access to their contents, the document's current heft and circumference are deceptive. Without the tube (or anything) at its core, the cartulary could have been rolled up much more tightly into the shape and size of a large cigar. In this compact state, it would have fitted comfortably into a small container such as an oblong wooden box, a cloth bag, or – like a cigar – a slim metal cylinder (usually made from lead or tin), the use of which for storing archival documents and protecting them from accidental damage and the elements is well documented in religious houses.[29] There is precedent for this in the rolling of individual charters, sometimes including their seals, a practice known particularly (but not

28 Kössinger, 'Gerollte Schrift', p. 164; Vincent, 'Why 1199?', p. 42; Kössinger, 'Enrolment', pp. 125–6. Though calling into question the material advantages (weight, size, etc.) of rolls versus codices identified by these and other scholars, Stefan Holz upholds the validity of their logistical benefits in the light of medieval transportation practices; S.G. Holz, 'The *Onus Scaccarii* Rolls Under Edward I (1272–1307)', in J. Peltzer et al. (eds), *The Roll in England and France in the Late Middle Ages: Form and Content* (Berlin, 2020), pp. 167–96, at p. 185.

29 At La Trinité de Caen, for example, the abbey's archives were stored in wooden trunks, while the most precious documents – foundation charters and rolls (the latter perhaps now-lost roll cartularies?) – were placed inside tin cylinders first to provide an additional layer of protection (*les tubes de fer-blanc qui renfermoient les chartes de fondation et de rôles historiques*). This proved a wise (if ultimately futile) choice when Caen's last abbess, Marie VI de Pontécoulant (1787–92), buried the archives inside the abbey church lest they be found by French revolutionaries, only for the trunks to rot away over time and the cylinders – now exposed to rainwater – to corrode to such an extent that their contents were reduced to shreds (*lambeaux*); for references and discussion, see Pohl, *Abbatial Authority*, pp. 305–7; on the extant cartulary (codex) and documentary production of La Trinité, see C. Letouzey-Réty, 'Le cartulaire de l'abbaye de la Trinité de Caen (fin XIIe–début XIIIe siècle)', *Tabularia* (2009), <https://doi.org/10.4000/tabularia.482>; C. Letouzey-Réty, 'Administrer par l'écrit dans une grande abbaye de femmes anglo-normand: La Sainte-Trinité de Caen (XIIe–XIIIe siècles)', in H. Dewez and L. Tryoen (eds), *Administrer par l'écrit au Moyen Âge (XIIe–XVe siècle)* (Paris, 2019), pp. 23–40. On archival storage

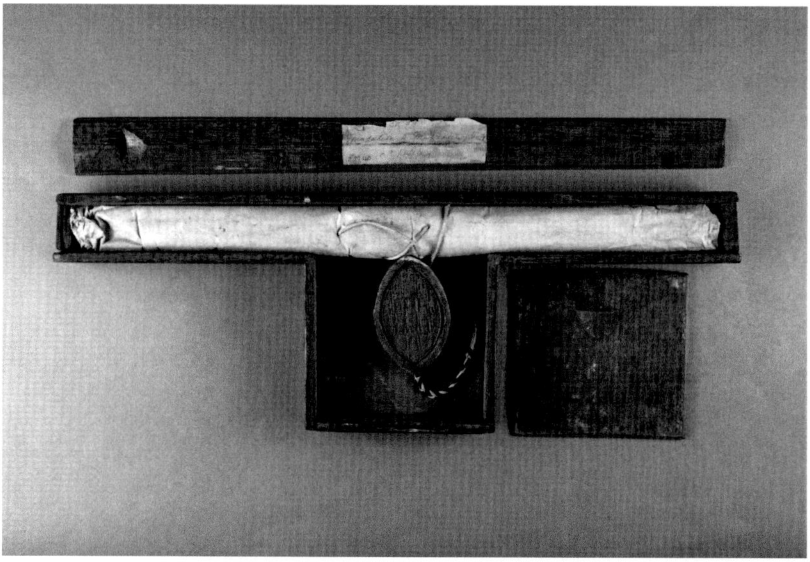

Fig. 4.1. MCA, Chartae Regiae 50.5.

exclusively) from later medieval England.[30] An instructive example in the collections of Magdalen College itself is the 'foundation deed' of Magdalen Hall (Magdalen College's predecessor),[31] dated 28 August 1448, which is still rolled up and stored in a custom-built wooden box with a separate compartment for its seal (**Fig. 4.1**).

Ultimately, we cannot know for certain whether the unusual format of the Aynho Cartulary is the result of choice or necessity, or both. As the discussion above has demonstrated, the roll format offered some concrete material and practical advantages that suggest a certain amount of deliberation on the part of its makers, quite possibly with a view towards the cartulary's future use(r)s. Economic considerations probably played at least as big a part in this as did design, and the constraints faced by a small institution such as Aynho Hospital in terms of both material and human resources would certainly have demanded a fair degree of pragmatism. It seems highly plausible, therefore, that the cartulary's format marks a compromise between managerial aspirations on the one hand, and logistical and financial realities on the other. With these reflections in mind, let us now turn to the cartulary's material composition and scribal preparation.

---

and record keeping, cf. Olney, *English Archives*, passim; Burton (ed.), *Cartulary*, pp. xxxiv–xlvii, with regard to the monastic archives of Byland Abbey.

30 W. Wattenbach, *Das Schriftwesen im Mittelalter*, 3rd edn (Leipzig, 1896), p. 171.

31 MCA, Chartae Regiae 50.5.

## MATERIAL COMPOSITION

The Aynho Cartulary is comprised of seven sheets (membranes) of parchment that gradually increase in length while maintaining a width of *c.*17.5 cm. The first and shortest membrane – added not long after the document's initial composition to provide a list of contents (see below) – measures 16 cm in length. Membrane 2, the beginning of the cartulary proper, measures 51.5 cm, with a writing space of 49 cm; membrane 3: 52.6 cm (50.7 cm); membrane 4: 57.4 cm (55.4 cm); membrane 5: 58.8 cm (56.7 cm); membrane 6: 61.7 cm (59.0 cm); membrane 7: 63.3 cm. Taken together, this gives the cartulary (including the contents list) a total length of *c.*361.3 cm when fully extended. The obverse (text side) of all the membranes (except membr. 1) has been ruled uniformly with a lead point (membr. 2: 68 lines; membr. 3: 67 lines; membr. 4: 76 lines; membr. 5: 79 lines; membr. 6: 80 lines; membr. 7: 87 lines), as have membranes 3v and 4v. This was done before they received their respective contents (nos. **53–4** and **55–8**). The membranes have been sewn together continuously (head to tail) using a medium-gauge, light-coloured (once white, now yellowed with age) thread with broad zig-zag stitches – a format typically referred to as 'chancery style' or 'chancery fashion'.[32] The overlap between membranes averages *c.*1.5–2 cm, with the beginning of a membrane (head) sewn on top of the previous membrane's end (tail) – except for membrane 1, the tail of which was sewn on top of membrane 2's head when it was prefixed to the original cartulary.

Intriguingly, there are traces of former zig-zag stitching at the head of membrane 1. While the thread (and whatever was once attached with it) has gone, the tell-tale needle holes are still perfectly visible, and the segments of thread running between these holes have left their physical and visual imprint on the face of the parchment. The likely explanation for this reveals itself on the reverse of membrane 2: here, we can detect traces of secondary stitching – again in the shape of needle holes – underneath (and therefore predating) the stitches that today attach the head of membrane 2 to the tail of membrane 1. The zig-zag pattern connecting these earlier needle holes runs contrary to that of the current stitching, and it is a close-enough match to the imprint on the head of membrane 1 to suggest that the two membranes were originally sewn together not head to tail like the remainder of the cartulary, but tail to tail – a decision that, for reasons unknown, was then reversed. From a practical perspective, it might have made sense to attach the contents list upside down so it could be consulted quickly by holding the cartulary by its thick (rolled-up) end and rolling out

[32] Woolgar, 'Two Cartularies', p. 498; Peltzer, 'The Roll in England and France', p. 3; Dewez, 'Le Rouleau', n. p. [pp. 3–5]; also cf. Vincent, 'Enrolment', passim.

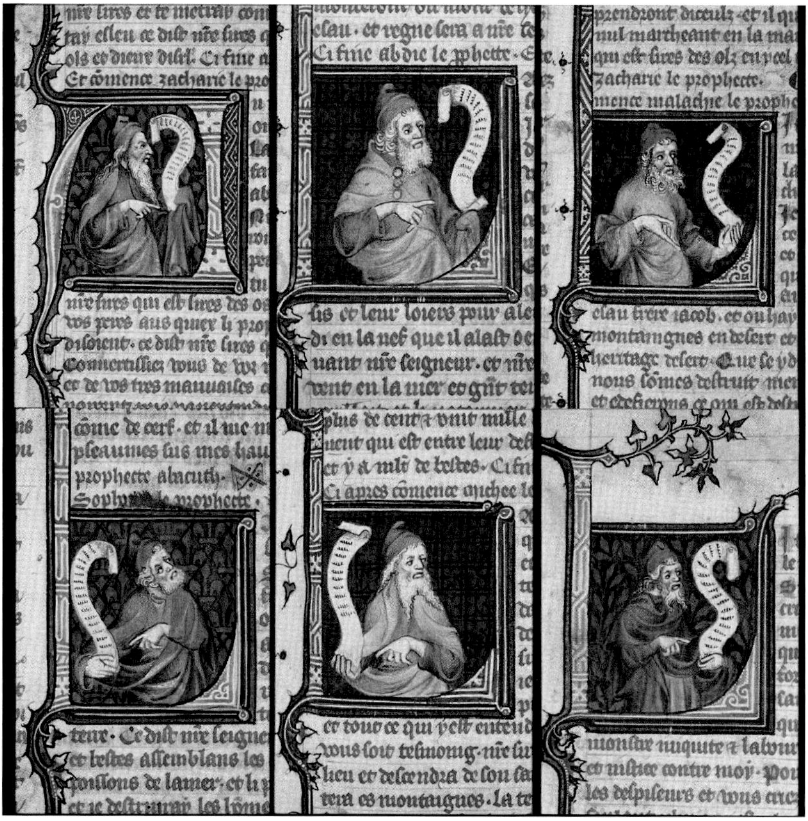

Fig. 4.2. The Hague, Museum Meermanno, MS 10 B 23, fols. 433r, 434r, 436v, 437r, 438v, 441v (detail).

the list from the bottom. This practice is known from the papyrus rolls of antiquity and is found with some regularity in medieval iconography, especially in depictions of the Prophets – for instance, in an inhabited miniature of Isaiah in the second volume of the famous twelfth-century Bury Bible,[33] on the frontispiece of a fourteenth-century manuscript of the works of John of Legnano showing the Old Testament's Minor Prophets,[34] and throughout a Bible Historiale illuminated by Flemish artist, Jan Boudolf, in 1372 (**Fig. 4.2**) – and in portraits of secular medieval rulers like the image of Countess Gunnor, mistress/wife of Richard I of Normandy, in the much celebrated twelfth-century cartulary of Mont Saint-Michel (**Fig. 4.3**).

33 Cambridge, Corpus Christi College, MS 2II, fol. 220v.

34 Vatican, Biblioteca Apostolica Vaticana, MS Vat. lat. 2639, fol. 2v.

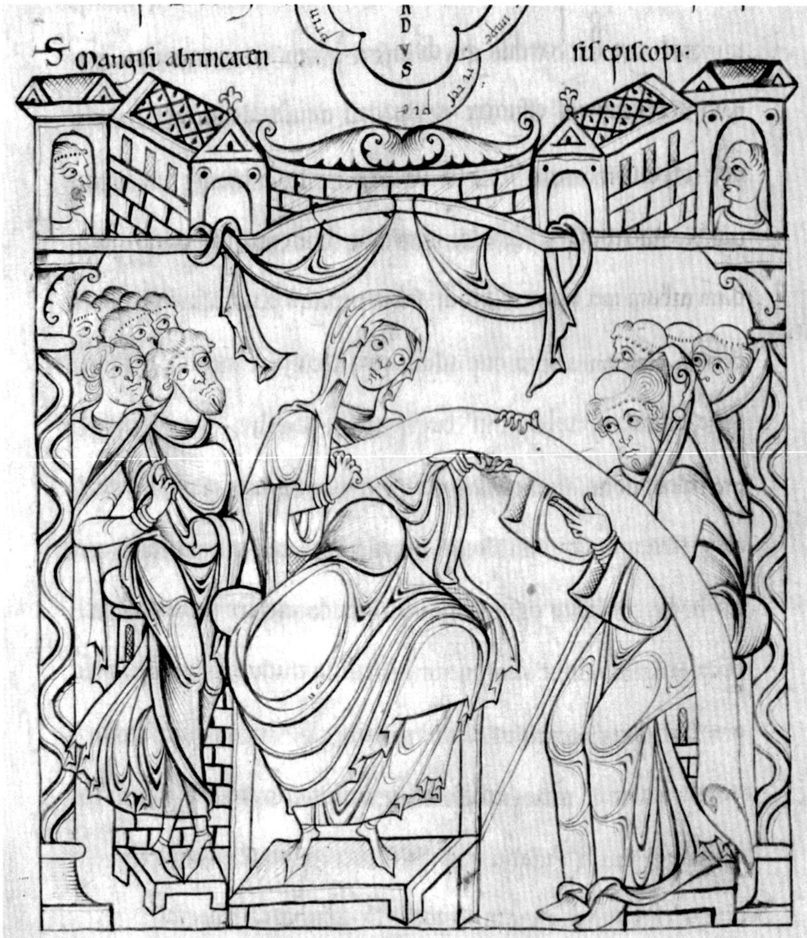

Fig. 4.3. Avranches, Bibliothèque patrimoniale, MS 210, fol. 23v (detail).

The cartulary's parchment – almost certainly sheepskin – is of low quality, perhaps constituting surplus stock that was cut to size, rather than skins that were made to measure and sourced especially for the task at hand. There are some material imperfections predating the writing process, including two holes on membrane 5 (measuring *c.*3.0 cm and *c.*4.0 cm in diameter, respectively) that result from minor physical injuries sustained while the animal was still alive, probably caused by an insect bite or a minor surface-level wound. Unsuitable for the manufacture of book pages or other high-quality/status writings, the skins from which the cartulary's membranes were made had most likely been intended for administrative records or other products of 'pragmatic literacy' generated within the context of the hospital's internal governance and everyday life.[35] The parchment has since sustained further and more serious damage in places, with membranes 2–4 affected so heavily around the right-hand edges (likely as a result of rodents gnawing away at it) as to cause lacunae in the text of some of the acts they contain. Ascertaining when this fraying occurred is impossible, but it appears to have been caused by improper storage conditions, rather than by simple wear and tear.

Signs of the cartulary's regular non-invasive use in the later thirteenth century and thereafter are few. There are some later medieval annotations in the document's margins (none on membr. 1r–2r; one on membr. 3r; eight on membr. 4r; three on membr. 5r; one on membr. 6r, five on membr. 7r) and no more than a handful of corrections to the text itself, all of which are the work of the cartulary's original scribe(s) (for example, no. **1**, l. 4; no. **26**, l. 2; no. **31**, l. 3; no. **34**, l. 2, no. **36**, l. 7.). There were clearly some occasions on which the document was consulted by the inhabitants (and leaders) of Aynho Hospital and/or the members of its subsequent institutional owner, Magdalen College – and, possibly, by some of its rivals and associates – in the period between its creation and the end of the Middle Ages, but determining precisely when and where this happened, and in what context(s), is impossible given the annotations' limited number, brevity, and formulaic nature (*maniculae*, nota marks, etc.). What can be established with much greater precision, however, is the cartulary's scribal preparation.

## SCRIBAL PREPARATION

The Aynho Cartulary is the work of six scribes, all of whom remain anonymous. For ease of reference, we will refer to them – in order of their appearance, if not their relative chronology (see below) – as Scribes A–F. Scribe A is the primary/main scribe, and it is to his hand that the cartulary owes fifty of its fifty-eight acts (86%; nos. **1–48**, **53–4**) as well as their rubrics. Judging from the palaeographical evidence, Scribe A penned acts nos. **1–48** during a single writing campaign with about half a dozen writing stints, stopping sporadically at the end of (and sometimes halfway through) an act to sharpen or replace his writing tool and refresh his ink (for example, membr. 2r, lines 8, 29; membr. 3r, line 15; membr. 5r, line 19; membr. 6r, lines 10, 49). Two acts written by Scribe A (membr. 3v; nos. **53–4**) are not part of this campaign, and the fact that they are inferior duplicates of nos.

35 On these kinds of documents and their proliferation in the thirteenth century and beyond, cf. Bertrand, *Écritures ordinaires*, passim; M.C. Howell, 'Documenting the Ordinary: The "Actes de la Pratique" of Late Medieval Douai', in A.J. Kosto and A. Winroth (eds), *Charters, Cartularies, and Archives: The Preservation and Transmission of Documents in the Medieval West* (Toronto, ON, 2002), pp. 151–73.

**1–2** marked (and marred) by numerous mistakes suggests a 'false start', with the scribe opting to abandon his 'botched' work, start over on a fresh sheet of parchment (membr. 2r), and re-cycle the still-usable reverse (membr. 3r; nos. **7–15**) later in the process.[36] Scribe A's work terminates about halfway through membrane 7 (line 40). The next two acts (nos. **49–50**) are the work of Scribe B, followed by a single act penned by Scribe C (no. **51**) and another by Scribe D (no. **52**), the latter of which completes the membrane and marks the end of the cartulary's obverse. Turning the document over, the first two acts on its reverse are the obsolete duplicates produced by Scribe A (nos. **53–4**), which are succeeded, on the next membrane, by four acts (membr. 4v; nos. **55–58**) copied by Scribe E. The lower part (*c.*¼–⅓) of this membrane and the next three membranes (membr. 5v–7v) remain blank. The list of contents that now marks the beginning of the cartulary (membr. 1r) is the work of Scribe F, whose hand does not appear anywhere else in the document.

As noted above, the order in which Scribes A–F appear in the cartulary does not correspond – or at least not entirely – to the sequence of their respective activity. Establishing the relative chronology of their work requires consideration of the palaeographical, textual, and contextual evidence of both the cartulary itself and the original acts that survive alongside it, some (but not all) of which are copied in the cartulary. Based on what has been established so far, there can be no doubt that the earliest scribal contribution – that which produced the cartulary's original version – belongs to Scribe A. If our interpretation of nos. **53–4** as discarded first attempts superseded by superior (if not quite perfect) versions of the same acts (nos. **1–2**) is correct, then the date of issue of the more recent of these papal privileges (no. **54**) provides a *terminus a quo* for Scribe A's activity: 27 November 1215.[37] This *terminus a quo* can be moved forward significantly once we turn to the dates of the more recent acts copied by Scribe A on the cartulary's obverse (nos. **3–48**). Two of these acts (nos. **21**, **25**) were issued *c.*1220 × 1230, one (no. **26**) *c.*1250 × 1260, and three (nos. **27**, **31–2**) as late as *c.*1260 × 1270.[38] Even if these last three acts were issued at the earlier end of their approximate date range, this means that Scribe A cannot have finished his writing campaign before *c.*1260 at the earliest. The fact that his

[36] In fact, there is evidence to suggest that nos. **1–2** resemble the scribe's third attempt at copying these two acts following a second failed attempt on the top of what is now membrane 2v, which – for reasons no longer obvious – was aborted after just two words ('Innocentius episcopus').

[37] The earlier privilege (no. **53**) was issued on 25 October 1202.

[38] There is a possibility that no. **27** might have been issued slightly earlier in *c.*1250 × 1260; there is also no. **28**, which was issued *c.*1212 × *c.*1235, and no. **29**, which was issued *c.*1220; cf. Appendix.

handwriting shows minimal variation/change between nos. **53–4** (reverse) and nos. **1–48** (obverse) further suggests that these were copied around the same time, giving us a similar *terminus a quo* for both. (If, conversely, these handwriting specimens were separated by several decades – let alone half a century, assuming Scribe A even lived that long – we surely could expect to see some signs of ageing such as the deterioration of fine motor skills.[39])

Moving on to Scribe B, we arrive at a similar date of activity. Unlike with Scribe A, however, this time the *terminus a quo* is given not by the two acts he copied where Scribe A had left off (nos. **49–50**), both of which are undated and have no known corresponding originals, but by the survival (in Magdalen College Archives) of an original charter also written in Scribe B's hand. Documenting the grant of two half acres of meadowland in Croughton to the hospital by William (II) de la Haye, this charter (Aynho 27) was issued *c.*1260 × 1270. What is more, it is among the acts previously copied into the cartulary by Scribe A (no. **32**), suggesting that the two scribes were in fact contemporaries working within a few years of each other, if not around the same time, and perhaps as part of a team. Whether the same is true for Scribe C is difficult to establish, given that he contributed only a single act to the cartulary and has left no corresponding specimens of his handwriting among the corpus of extant original charters. The cartulary act in question (no. **51**) dates from *c.*1250 × 1260, meaning it is not impossible, and perhaps probable, that Scribe C was working around the same time and within the same scribal milieu as – and perhaps even alongside – Scribes A

39 As observed recently by James Willoughby in relation to the handwriting of Ralph of Coggeshall, '[t]here is no reason to expect to see a tremor in an elderly [scribe's] hand, but one might plausibly expect a larger module and some inconsistency in duct'; J. Willoughby, 'The Chronicle of Ralph of Coggeshall: Publication and Censorship in Angevin England', in S. Niskanen and V. Rovere, *The Art of Publication from the Ninth to the Sixteenth Century* (Turnhout, 2023), pp. 131–66, at p. 151. We are grateful to the author and editors for giving us access to this study prior to its publication. Scholarship on the effects of ageing and age-related impairment on the handwriting of medieval scribes (and artists) is limited, though some important preliminary work has been produced in recent years, for example, D.E. Thorpe and J.E. Alty, 'What Type of Tremor Did the Medieval "Tremulous Hand of Worcester" Have?', *Brain: A Journal of Neurology*, 138 (2015), 23–31; D.E. Thorpe, 'Tracing Neurological Disorders in the Handwriting of Medieval Scribes: Using the Past to Inform the Future', *Journal of the Early Book Society for the Study of Manuscripts and Printing History*, 18 (2015), 241–48; K.E. Kennedy, 'Aging Artists and Impairment in Fifteenth-Century England', *Different Visions: New Perspectives on Medieval Art*, 10 (2023), 1–30; previously D. Rosand, 'Style and the Ageing Artist', *Art Journal*, 46 (1987), 91–3. Benjamin Pohl is currently preparing a new research project to investigate systematically the phenomenon of ageing scribes in medieval Latin Europe.

and B.[40] Palaeographically, and judging from the stylistic features of Scribe C's hand, this is certainly a plausible scenario, and one that hints at the remarkably short timeframe in which the Aynho Cartulary was produced with the hospital's relatively limited resources (see below).

The next stage in the chronology of the cartulary's scribal preparation was not the addition of further acts, but the appendage of a list of contents by Scribe F. This involved prefixing the existing document with a sheet of parchment (now membr. 1) and populating it with a brief summary description of every act. For acts nos. **1–48**, this was – or at least ought to have been – a rather straightforward task that required little more than simply copying the rubrics supplied by Scribe A (see above). Indeed, this is precisely what Scribe F set out to do, albeit with limited success. Not only did he skip over (possibly due to eye slip) four rubrics (nos. **7**, **31–2**, **35**) that are consequently missing from the list of contents, but he also misidentified the benefactor of no. **30**, William (II) de la Haye, as the latter's late father, Guy (*Carta Wydonis de Haya*, instead of *Carta Willelmi de la Haye*), who is in fact the donor of the cartulary's preceding act (no. **29**). While these all seem to have been genuine mistakes, perhaps indicating a lack of attention or experience (or indeed literacy) on the copyist's part, there is one instance (no. **1**) in which Scribe F appears to have second-guessed Scribe A's work. Rather than copying the papal privilege's existing rubric (*Privilegium Innocentii tertii*), he replaced it with a more specific one that reflects the content of the pope's confirmation (*Confirmatio capelle de Crowltone*).

For the remaining acts contained in the list of contents (nos. **49–51**), the task was somewhat more involved, given that, unlike Scribe A, the cartulary's two earliest continuators, Scribes B and C, had not provided rubrics for them. One possibility is that the entries in the list of contents corresponding to these three acts were copied from the endorsements of the originals kept in the hospital's archives or deed chest.[41] Though impossible to establish for two of these acts (nos. **49–50**) due to the loss of their respective originals, the fact that there was no endorsement on the reverse of the extant original of no. **51** in the thirteenth century (the only endorsement there today was added in the fifteenth century) shows that Scribe F composed this entry (and possibly those for nos. **49–50**, too) from scratch. The fact that the last act listed by Scribe F is no. **51** securely places him

40 Though cartulary act no. **51** does have a corresponding original (Aynho 58), the hand in which the latter is written certainly does not belong to Scribe C.

41 On the significance of endorsements to our understanding of medieval archival organisation and practice, see now R. Allen and B. Pohl, 'Mills, Manuscripts, and Monastic Archives: The Phillipps Charters of Mont Saint-Michel', *Bulletin of the John Rylands Library*, 100 (2024), 1–37.

after Scribe C in the cartulary's scribal chronology with a *terminus a quo* of *c.*1260 × 1270 (see above), while the absence of entries for nos. **52**, **55–8** suggests that he worked before these acts were added by Scribes D and E, respectively. If we want to determine the *terminus ad quem* for Scribe F's work, we thus need to turn to these continuators.

While so far it has been possible to establish the respective dates of activity and working sequence of the cartulary's Scribes A, B, C, and F with relative certainty, attempting the same for Scribes D and E proves rather more difficult. Scribe D only copied a single act (no. **52**), dated *c.*1270 × 1280, the surviving original of which (Aynho 55), though written in a different hand (see below), was endorsed by him in the process. The palaeographical similarities – in style as well as in ductus – between Scribe D's hand and the hand of Aynho 55 are strong enough to suggest contemporaneity and, quite plausibly, training within the same scribal milieu. The only other trace of Scribe D's hand is the endorsement of another original Aynho charter (no. **A14**), also dated *c.*1270 × 1280, which has not been copied into the cartulary. Meanwhile, the hand of **A14** is the same as that of both Aynho 55 and two more acts (**A13** and **A18**), which likewise date from *c.*1270 × 1280 (see Chapter 3). Moreover, a third hand that penned two extant acts (**A11** and **A17**, the former dated *c.*1270, and the latter *c.*1270 × 1280) is similar enough to both these hands to suggest that all three scribes were working within a few years of – if not indeed around the same time as – each other, possibly in a common location. Even if these notable parallels do not permit us to narrow down the window for Scribe D's activity further than the abovementioned date of no. **52** itself, they do seem to indicate strongly that Scribe D likely copied this act into the cartulary not long after it was issued, quite possibly closer to 1270 than to 1280.

Given this hiatus of at least a few years (and potentially as much as two decades) between the respective work of Scribes F and D, the final question must be whether the four acts copied by Scribe E on the reverse of the cartulary (nos. **55–8**) were appended within this interim period or after Scribe D had filled the last few lines of the cartulary's obverse (membr. 7r, lines 78–85) with a copy of no. **52**. None of the acts copied by Scribe E has a date of issue, but we know that one (no. **56**) – the only one of the four with a corresponding original (Aynho 36), which was produced by Scribe E himself – must have been issued after 25 November 1259. Scribe E also penned an original Aynho charter not copied in the cartulary, which is dated *c.*1260 (no. **A8**). As we saw in Chapter 3, he was likely someone attached to (or resident at) the hospital, possibly even its then master (and chaplain), Peter of Windsor. In the absence of more concrete dates, it is just possible that act no. **56** (along with nos. **55**, **57–8**) was copied into the cartulary before Scribe D added act no. **52** at some point after 1270, particularly if Scribe C (no. **51**) and Scribe F (list of contents) had indeed completed their work in or around 1260 (see above). The space left by Scribe C on the bottom of the cartulary's final obverse membrane would have been too small comfortably to accommodate any one – let alone all four – of the acts Scribe E set out to copy, and, rather than attempting to cram one of them (or parts thereof) into this space, he may have preferred to copy them *en bloc* on the cartulary's reverse at the beginning of the first clean membrane after the aborted first attempt of Scribe A. (Scribe E would have had no reason to suspect that nos. **53–4** are obsolete duplicates.) This lack of space was of no concern to Scribe D. Quite the opposite: the space available to him at the bottom of membrane 7r was more than sufficient to accommodate act no. **52**; if anything, the text was slightly too short, thus causing the copyist to lengthen the final word ('aliis') artificially to fill the remainder of the line. Scribe D therefore had no reason to make any use of the extra space offered by the cartulary's mostly empty reverse, even if Scribe E had done so before him – after all, acts nos. **52**, **55–8** all pertain to different subject matter, and they were not, as far as we know, copied in strict chronological order. Ultimately, this must remain conjecture, and while we can be certain that Scribes D and E are indeed the last two scribes to contribute to the cartulary, the order of their activity remains unknown.

In sum, the chronology of the cartulary's composition and scribal preparation can be reconstructed as follows: at some point during the 1260s, possibly as early as *c.*1260, Scribe A set out to create a new cartulary that comprised a total of forty-eight acts, starting – as was customary – with two of the hospital's most authoritative and valued privileges, that is, those issued by the papacy (in this case Innocent III). His first attempt (nos. **53–4**) was unsuccessful, with the mistakes introduced by Scribe A perhaps indicating that he was unaccustomed to reading papal chancery hand. He therefore started over from scratch on a new membrane (nos. **1–2**) before adding the other non-papal acts (nos. **3–48**), the most recent of which had been issued *c.*1260 × 1270, perhaps towards the earlier end of this range. Not long afterwards, if not indeed around the same time, three more acts were appended by Scribe B (nos. **49–50**) and, in turn, Scribe C (no. **51**), soon followed (likely before 1270) by a list of contents written on a separate membrane and prefixed to the existing document by Scribe F. Finally, the cartulary's five remaining acts were added to the end by Scribes D (no. **52**) and E (nos. **55–8**) at some point after *c.*1270, possibly even in that year, with a possibility – albeit one impossible to corroborate at present – that Scribe E's contribution preceded that of Scribe D. This reconstructed chronology suggests the scribal sequence ABCFED; or, alternatively, ABCFDE.

The reason why this matters, and why it is useful to discuss the working relationship of the cartulary scribes and their relative chronology at some length, is that it enables us to revisit and revise the document's date of production established in previous scholarship and push it back by perhaps as much as two decades. Philippa Hoskins' addendum (1996) to Godfrey Davis's short catalogue of medieval British cartularies (1958) simply dates the Aynho Cartulary to the thirteenth century, as does Rosemary Hayes's introductory report on a project on the records of medieval religious houses (1999).[42] The revised version of Davis's catalogue, produced by Claire Breay and others in 2010, lists it as 'late 13th cent.'.[43] The only scholar so far to have proposed a more concrete date is Christopher Woolgar, who, in 1981, concluded that 'the date of its [the cartulary's] compilation must be *c.*1280'.[44] Woolgar further hypothesised that the cartulary was produced in the context of an investigation into the hospital's affairs carried out in 1282 at the direction of Oliver Sutton, bishop of Lincoln (1280–99), which, according to Woolgar, involved an 'examination' of the hospital's deeds, for which the cartulary might have been produced with the dual purpose both 'to guide the inquiry and for the benefit of the new master of Aynho'.[45] While compelling in its contextualisation, Woolgar's confident dating of the cartulary *c.*1280 is at odds with the more granular chronology established in the present chapter. With Scribe A possibly working as early as *c.*1260 (certainly during the period *c.*1260 × 1270), the cartulary in its original form – that which comprised at least acts nos. **1**–**48**, and possibly also nos. **49**–**51** appended by Scribe A's close contemporaries, Scribes B and C – was produced more than a decade (if not two) before the episcopal investigation of 1282, meaning that the latter must be discarded as a possible catalyst for the document's creation.

Indeed, there is no compelling reason to believe, as Woolgar did, that the Aynho Cartulary must have been produced in response to (or even in anticipation of) a specific event, nor that its creation was necessarily 'triggered' by external scrutiny of the hospital's possessions, legal or jurisdictional challenges, or other forms of crisis. As observed elsewhere, the tendency to focus on (and foreground unduly) the role of such crises in medieval historiographical and documentary production 'can lead to historians creating or exaggerating crises solely to provide an explanation for why groups of religious wrote'.[46] Cartularies constitute no exception. In fact,

[42] Hoskins, 'Medieval Cartularies: Amendments', p. 2; R. Hayes, 'The Historical Manuscripts Commission's Project on the Records of Medieval Religious Houses', *MRB*, 5 (1999), 1–26, at p. 4.

[43] *Cartularies*, p. 5 (= no. 16.1).

[44] Woolgar, 'Two Cartularies', p. 498.

[45] Woolgar, 'Two Cartularies', p. 498.

[46] D. Talbot, 'Review of Charles C. Rozier, *Writing History in the Community of St Cuthbert, c.700–1130: From Bede to Symeon of Durham*', *History*, 106 (2021), 477–8, at p. 478.

recent research into medieval cartularies and their production has moved away from this default position of a presumed 'crisis mode' by exploring other (and more varied) possible 'triggers' for their composition.[47] More often than not, it appears that the creation of cartularies like that of Aynho may well have been motivated, first and foremost, by internal administrative processes and developments with the genuine objective to 'take stock' of what kinds of possessions, rights, and privileges a given institution held at a given point in time (and by whose donation and confirmation). This could (but did not have to) coincide with administrative transformations and changes in institutional leadership such as the appointment of a new head of house, who, especially in the case of external candidates, might have commissioned a cartulary as a convenient managerial tool for governing, safeguarding, and, ideally, enlarging the domestic estate. At Aynho, the arrival of Peter of Windsor as the hospital's new master (*magister*) *c.*1260 (see **Table 1.1**) might have presented just such an occasion.[48] What is more, the mounting political tensions that just a few years later culminated in the Second Barons' War (1264–7) might have generated anxieties around the hospital's rights and possessions that lent a certain sense of timeliness – and perhaps even urgency – to the cartulary project, especially as the earl of Leicester, Simon de Montfort (1239–65), whose potentially harmful actions at least one hospital benefactor took pains to allay (no. **58**), was a notable landholder in the vicinity, including at Croughton.[49] Last but not least, the creation of the cartulary almost exactly ninety years (three generations) after the hospital's foundation in 1170/1 closely coincided with a chronological threshold that in Cultural Memory Studies – and, more recently, in medieval studies – is recognised as the point of transition from the oral realm of communicative (or social) memory to the written media of cultural memory.[50] Adopting the terminology of Jan and Aleida Assmann,

47 For examples of such 'triggers', see the recent discussion by Tucker, *Reading and Shaping*, pp. 14–16 and the references provided therein.

48 The earliest surviving charter issued by Peter in his capacity as Aynho's master (no. **A8**) is dated *c.*1260.

49 J. Sadler, *The Second Barons' War: Simon de Montfort and the Battles of Lewes and Evesham* (Barnsley, 2008); I.F. Treharne and I.J. Sanders (eds), *Documents of the Baronial Movement of Reform and Rebellion* (Oxford, 1973), pp. 1–60. On the Second Barons' War as a catalyst not just of documentary, but also of literary production, see J.A. Jahner, 'The Poetry of the Second Barons' War: Some Manuscript Contexts', in A.S.G. Edwards and O. Da Rold (eds), *English Manuscripts before 1400* (London, 2012), pp. 200–22.

50 J. Assmann, 'Communicative and Cultural Memory', in A. Erll at al. (eds), *Cultural Memory Studies: An International and Interdisciplinary Handbook* (Berlin, 2008), pp. 109–18; A. Assmann, 'Four Formats of Memory: From Individual to Collective Constructions of the Past', in C. Emden and D. Midgley (eds), *Cultural Memory and*

the making of the cartulary would therefore have marked an act of 'cultural formation',[51] one that codified the memory of the grants and donations made to the hospital in the first ninety or so years of its existence (*c.*1170/1–1260) and preserved them, on a single roll of parchment, for the knowledge of future generations. Whether it was composed at Master Peter's initiative, or in anticipation of the volatile environment of the Second Barons' War, or because of the ninety-year/three-generation memory juncture, the Aynho Cartulary seems to have been executed at some speed, quite feasibly in the space of a single year or less. Its completion was marked by appending a list of its contents as is common for medieval cartularies.[52] Within a decade or two, the document acquired its present shape thanks to the supplementation of a handful of further acts, possibly under Peter's successor, John of Gra(nt)ham, meaning that it was long complete by the time this same John resigned from office in 1282 (to be succeeded by William of Occold) ahead of Bishop Sutton's inspection.[53]

This chronology corresponds very well with the palaeographical evidence. While notably different and distinguishable from one another due to their respective idiosyncrasies, idiom, and personal ductus, the individual hands of Scribes A–F all conform with what one might expect to see – in terms of letter forms, ligatures, abbreviations, etc. – in English cursive documentary (and, to a degree, book) script (sometimes referred to as *cursiva Anglicana*) in the period *c.*1250–1300.[54] While Scribe A's hand is the most conservative stylistically and harks back to developments closer to the middle of the thirteenth century, perhaps indicating his age or lack of confidence (or both), the hands of his contemporaries, Scribes B and C, are rather more

*Historical Consciousness in the German-Speaking World since 1500* (Oxford, 2004), pp. 19–38; fruitful applications of this 'three-generation model' in medieval studies include E.M.C. van Houts, *Memory and Gender in Medieval Europe, 900–1200* (Basingstoke, 1999), pp. 6–7; B. Pohl, *Dudo of Saint-Quentin's* Historia Normannorum*: Tradition, Innovation and Memory* (York, 2015), pp. 6–17.

51 J. Assmann and J. Czaplicka, 'Collective Memory and Cultural Identity', *New German Critique*, 65 (1995), 125–33, at p. 127; J. Assmann: 'Introduction: What Is Cultural Memory?', in J. Assmann and R. Livingstone (eds), *Religion and Cultural Memory: Ten Studies* (Stanford, CA, 2006), pp. 1–30, at p. 8.

52 See *Cartularies*, p. xiv.

53 See Table 1.1. The outcome of Aynho's episcopal inspection of 1282 was recorded in Bishop Sutton's register, edited in *Rolls of Sutton*, vol. 2, pp. 17–18.

54 For pertinent examples and discussion of the most common features, cf. Clemens and Graham, *Introduction*, pp. 159–61; M.P. Brown, *A Guide to Western Historical Scripts from Antiquity to 1600* (London, 1990), pp. 92–7 (= nos. 33–5); M.B. Parkes, *Their Hands before Our Eyes: A Closer Look at Scribes* (Aldershot, 2008), pp. 33–53 and 101–25; M.B. Parkes, *English Cursive Book Hands, 1250–1500*, rev. edn (Ilkley, 1979).

progressive in their embracing of stylistic features (or 'trends') that sit more firmly and comfortably within the second half, specifically the third quarter, of the century. Even the two most recent hands, those of Scribes D and E, belong in this period, thus further cementing the likelihood that the Aynho Cartulary as it survives today was completed within the short timeframe of a decade or two by half a dozen scribes, quite possibly professionals, all of whom were active, and had perhaps been trained, within a common milieu – and some of whom, just like the scribes we met above in Chapter 3, might well have been working also at the commission of local institutions other than Aynho Hospital.

## CONCLUSION

The significance of the Aynho Cartulary for the history of cartulary production and documentary culture in later medieval England – and Latin Europe more widely – cannot be overstated. It is one of only six complete roll cartularies from a medieval English hospital, and the only one produced earlier than the fourteenth century.[55] Even *outre-Manche* there are only two cases for comparison: one from Cambrai (Cambrai, Le Labo/Archives hospitalières, IX B 55–56), which is held to have been made *c.*1255 × 1300 and thus strictly contemporary,[56] and the other from Saint-Martial's Hospital in Limoges (Limoges, Archives départementales de la Haute-Vienne/Archives hospitalières, A 2–3), which was composed two centuries earlier (*c.*1056 × 1100),[57] making it the earliest recorded example from continental Europe. In terms of its physical length, Aynho's cartulary (*c.*361.3 cm) sits between those of Cambrai (*c.*143 cm) and Limoges (*c.*382 cm). Even when taking into account roll cartularies produced by British and Irish religious houses other than hospitals, the Aynho Cartulary

55 The fifteenth-century fragment from Sprotbrough Hospital and the three late medieval/early modern rolls from Exeter have already been mentioned above.

56 'Cartulaire-rouleau de l'office des Grands Chartriers de Cambrai (1)', ROTULI–CRULH, Université de Lorraine, <https://rotuli.univ-lorraine.fr/s/rotuli/item/4509>; 'Cartulaire-rouleau de l'office des Grands Chartriers de Cambrai (2)', ROTULI–CRULH, Université de Lorraine, https://rotuli.univ-<lorraine.fr/s/rotuli/item/4510>; also cf. 'Cartulaire de l'hôpital des Grands Chartriers de Cambrai [indéterminés 1 et 2]' in cartulR–Répertoire des répertoires médiévaux et modernes, <https://telma-repertoires.irht.cnrs.fr/cartulr/notice-entite/6980>, where an earlier date of production (*c.*1101 × 1200) is proposed.

57 H. Stein, *Bibliographie générale des cartulaires français, ou relatifs à l'histoire de France* (Paris, 1907) p. 299 (= nos. 2183–84); also cf. <https://rotuli.univ-lorraine.fr/s/rotuli/item/4555>; a reproduction (microfilm) is available online via the *Bibliothèque virtuelle des manuscrits médiévaux* (BVMM), <http://medium-avance.irht.cnrs.fr/ark:/63955/md52j6733507>.

is still among the earliest of its kind, being preceded only by the examples from Stone Priory (twelfth century), Kirkstead Abbey (late twelfth/early thirteenth century) and Margam Abbey (*c.*1205–10), with the two cartularies from Flaxley Abbey and May Priory dating roughly around the same time, if not slightly later. Given that these monastic houses were considerably larger in size and more generously endowed than Aynho Hospital, it is no real surprise to find that some of their cartularies are much longer than the Aynho Cartulary, with Flaxley's roll measuring almost twice as much in length (*c.*630 cm). That said, the Kirkstead rolls (*c.*99 cm and *c.*115 cm) are both notably shorter than Aynho's, possibly due at least in part to their precursory nature and supplementary function in the production of the abbey's more extensive codex cartulary,[58] which suggests that there is not always or necessarily a correlation between a cartulary's length and the size or wealth of its hosting institution. In terms of its materiality and scribal preparation, the Aynho Cartulary certainly offers one of the most intriguing and insightful examples of a hospital's documentary and archival culture both in England and the wider medieval Latin West.

[58] See above, p. 115, n. 8.

# CONCLUSION

Having studied the thirteenth-century roll cartulary of Aynho Hospital in its wider historical and documentary contexts, Part I of this book has made an original contribution to knowledge in three fields of scholarship that, despite their cognate nature, are rarely brought into dialogue: medieval cartularies, medieval rolls, and medieval hospitals. Here we have used the Aynho Cartulary and the corpus of original charters surviving alongside it in the muniments of Magdalen College both as a lens and as a gateway through which to view and gain access to the important social, political, economic, spiritual, and scribal networks within which this modest and relatively obscure medieval hospital was situated, and from which it benefited in various ways. The discussions and analyses presented across this book's chapters together have revealed a rich and diverse 'microcosm', one which encompasses not just the upper echelons of medieval English society, but which also simultaneously records and amplifies the voices of groups who are typically marginalised or altogether silenced in cartularies produced by larger and wealthier institutions (e.g., professional scribes, local clerks and witnesses, women, and, to a lesser extent, the nameless travellers, sick, poor, and impaired who constituted the hospital's residents). The respective agency of – and the relationships between – the various people connected to Aynho Hospital, who have left their traces in the documentary records studied and edited here for the first time, reveal processes of everyday life and community building in a rural locality that was at once relatively remote and remarkably well-connected.

Focusing on the foundation and early history of Aynho Hospital (*c.*1170–*c.*1280), Chapter 1 has shown how establishing, endowing, and sustaining even such a comparatively small and seemingly unassuming institution, which was situated close to two urban centres that were themselves home to hospitals (Oxford and Brackley), relied on a network of relationships and obligations that stretched far beyond the vill of Aynho and its immediate vicinity. The hospital's founder, Roger Fitz Richard, and his wife,

Alice of Essex, whose backgrounds and genealogies have been established more comprehensively and with greater precision here than in previous scholarship, enjoyed connections with some of the foremost aristocrats of twelfth-century England but were themselves of more modest aristocratic rank. For them and their peers, founding even a rural institution such as Aynho Hospital was an ambitious and aspirational enterprise that allowed them to fashion themselves after first-tier aristocrats such as the earls of Leicester, who just a few years earlier had founded a hospital in nearby Brackley. If Alice herself played a formative role in the venture, as is entirely possible since Aynho Hospital was established on her dower lands, then she may have seen it as a means by which to ensure her dynastic future, as Watson has shown was the case with the female patrons of hospitals located elsewhere, including at Brackley.[1]

This is not to imply, however, that either the founding family's influence or the landscape within which the hospital was established were otherwise insignificant during the later twelfth and thirteenth centuries. Far from it. Aynho's proximity to the river Cherwell made it a suitable place for habitation and a regular thoroughfare for travellers, who could cross that river using an alms bridge not far from Aynho. The nearby tournament site to Aynho's east, located between Brackley and Mixbury, which was in use from the late twelfth century onwards, would have also generated a fair amount of lucrative (if seasonal) traffic. A popular destination with knights, nobles, and sometimes even royalty, these public tournaments would have attracted substantial numbers of potential hospital benefactors from among England's wealthiest and most influential individuals (and their retinues). Moreover, just as Roger Fitz Richard perhaps sought to emulate his aristocratic superiors by founding Aynho Hospital, so those with whom he shared feudo-vassalic links looked to imitate his performative largesse towards it. This was true not just in terms of the material donations themselves, but also, as we have shown in Chapter 2, in the language used to record them. In this regard, Aynho Hospital's thirteenth-century donors bucked some of the trends seen elsewhere in England and on the Continent. Not only did most of them issue their grants using a 'mixed-type' formula that combined traditional with more current and fashionable terminology of charitable gift-giving, but they also made out their gifts to both God and the hospital: a stylistic choice which harked back to – and perhaps deliberately imitated – the foundational grants by Roger and his sons. As the founding family's influence grew, reaching its zenith during King John's reign, the individuals they managed to attract to Aynho – and, more specifically, to their patronised hospital – began to come from outside Northamptonshire.

1 Watson, 'Mother's Past', pp. 213–49.

In the case of the descendants of Geoffrey de Wavre, it has been possible to show that they had even more far-flung connections beyond England's shores, in Brabant.

These cross-demographic and multi-generational support structures resulted in the creation of an extensive (if patchwork) local property portfolio maintained by a sophisticated patronage network, both of which were the subject of Chapter 2. Over the course of the later twelfth and thirteenth centuries, the hospital's estate was extended gradually through several successive 'waves' of endowment, the first of which was driven by the founder and his sons, Robert (I) and William Fitz Roger. Though subsequent generations of the founding family also contributed to the hospital's upkeep, by the mid-thirteenth century, at the latest, the main initiative had passed to other families with more local roots and resources, specifically in and/or around the vill of Croughton. As a result, Croughton soon replaced Aynho itself as the hospital's main source of property and income. Besides land, the hospital also acquired buildings (or parts thereof) that could be rented or leased out for profit. By studying this diversification of the hospital's patronage network, and the resulting shifts and re-calibrations of its property portfolio, we have been able to identify different yet compatible – and often complementary – investment strategies and documentary traditions, which together account for the Aynho Cartulary's richness and significance as a witness of both changing local customs and wider trends and developments in medieval English and European cultures of hospitality, spirituality, and charity.

It was not just Aynho Hospital's growing estate that relied on such local support networks, but also its documentary production, which, in an environment of limited domestic scribal expertise, depended fundamentally on the work of professional scribes from outside its walls, some of whom also worked for other institutions in the vicinity and, perhaps, further afield. The scribal milieux of which Aynho was a part have been mapped out in Chapter 3, using a substantial corpus of original charters relating to both Aynho Hospital itself and the nearby contemporary hospitals at Brackley and Oxford. Very few of these charters have ever been subject to detailed scholarly examination, and those relating to Aynho are edited in the Appendix of this book. By bringing these documents into conversation with each other, and through a forensic comparative analysis of their witness lists and scribal hands, we have been able to identify for the first time, sometimes even by name, several of the otherwise anonymous scribes active in the wider milieux around Aynho in which the work of the hospital's anonymous cartularist also finds its locus. In doing so, we have not only better contextualised the Aynho Cartulary as a documentary object itself but have shown how the study of professional medieval scribes, especially those active outside major towns and in rural milieux, is an area of research that, despite some recent headway, stands to benefit from more comprehensive treatment. It is our hope, therefore, that the present book will help infuse this area of research with renewed energy and momentum. Indeed, what we have offered here amounts to more than a simple case study of a specific archival corpus, but instead provides a methodology for identifying scribal milieux and local documentary cultures, the principles of which can – and, we hope, will – be applied to other medieval cartularies and charter corpora produced within similarly circumscribed localities by multiple contemporary scribes.[2]

Moreover, if it has proven impossible to determine with certainty whether the main Aynho cartularist was himself a member of the hospital proper or a local clerk, there can be little doubt that the cartulary's creation required a considerable investment of both time and resources. The latter were typically in short supply for small-scale hospitals such as Aynho, which underscores the sense of importance and priority – and perhaps even urgency – that must have marked the cartulary's production in the second half of the thirteenth century. What motivated and expedited the cartulary's creation has been investigated more fully in Chapter 4. Its revised date of production (*c.*1260), which we have established here on the basis of a full palaeographical and codicological study of both the Aynho Cartulary itself and the corresponding original acts in the collections of Magdalen College, coincides closely with Peter of Windsor's appointment as the hospital's new master. It also coincides, more broadly, with the political and economic tensions that culminated in the Second Barons' War (1264–7). The resulting upheaval may have resonated particularly strongly at Aynho, located, as it was, near holdings in the Leicester fee (including one at Croughton), making the cartulary project seem especially apposite and timely. As previously noted (Chapter 4), however, one should be careful not to over-rely on models of explanation using experiences of crisis or change as catalysts of documentary and literary production. The way in which the cartulary was assembled, its material preparation, and, not least, its scribal execution all suggest that it was produced at some speed and completed in its original form (subsequent additions by a further five scribes notwithstanding) within a single year at most. What is more, the main cartularist himself can be shown to have been an individual who, while sufficiently literate to undertake the project, seems to have had relatively little calligraphic training and limited experience in dealing with charters of more unusual

2 Indeed, we are ourselves currently preparing a new collaborative research project that will apply this methodology to an even larger archival corpus.

form (papal bulls in particular), a lack of expertise that caused him to make some notable mistakes.

The Aynho Cartulary's material evidence has also been used to answer various important questions. Its unusual roll format appears to have been chosen due to a combination of economic (material and human resources) and practical concerns (usability, portability, storability, etc.), meaning the cartulary's peculiar design, while relatively rare across medieval Europe (certainly in later medieval England), is very unlikely to be accidental. The Aynho Cartulary is one of only seven roll cartularies to survive from medieval English hospitals, and the only one dating from before the fourteenth century. Roll cartularies are rare even among England's medieval monastic houses, very much despite the fact that these communities were typically significantly larger and better endowed than Aynho Hospital, and that several of them had access to in-house scribal workforces. For a small and rural hospital like Aynho to have produced such an artefact is a rarity. Its survival alongside many of the acts from which it was compiled (as well as others that also relate to matters treated in it) has given us an even rarer opportunity to study up-close the intriguing dynamics of charter and cartulary production in a type of institution, and in a kind of locality, that is hardly ever made the subject of scholarship on medieval documentary cultures.

As we hope to have shown in our detailed discussion of the Aynho Cartulary and charters, Michael Johnston's recent important observations concerning the often neglected rural milieux of later medieval English book production – namely that 'England's remoter parts supplied scribal labour', and that 'scribal collaborations tended to bring together those from the same vicinity'[3] – also hold true, *mutatis mutandis*, for the prolific scribal milieux and documentary culture(s) that in the twelfth and thirteenth centuries existed outside major urban centres and produced major pieces of 'pragmatic writing' like the Aynho Cartulary. Calling the cartulary 'pragmatic' is by no means intended to downplay its significance, nor indeed its conceptual design, as a medium of institutional and communal memory. Compiled ninety or so years after Aynho Hospital's foundation and thus at the critical three-generation juncture between oral and written memory, the Aynho Cartulary brought together and preserved for posterity vital information not only about the hospital's local lands and properties, but also, and importantly, about its most generous – and thus most faithfully remembered and commemorated – patrons and benefactors, many (but not quite all) of whom were firmly based in its environs. As

[3] M. Johnston, *The Middle English Book: Scribes and Readers, 1350–1500* (Oxford, 2023), pp. 158, 160.

we have shown in the historical and contextual discussions of the first two chapters, these included multiple generations of the hospital's founding family, as well as local aristocratic families, landlords, and townsfolk, all of whom 'invested' in the medieval economy of salvation through charitable donations to Aynho Hospital, and who, in return for their investment, expected spiritual rewards.

Taken together, this book's findings show how medieval hospitals such as Aynho's were part not just of one but of several interrelated communities. These included the living and the dead; the rich and the poor; the healthy and the sick; benefactors and beneficiaries; and scribes, clerks, and other professionals active in the vicinity. In a scholarly landscape dominated by studies of urban hospitals, this book has also demonstrated the importance of focusing more closely on their counterparts in small medieval towns and villages. Even at the most basic level, our close analysis of Aynho Hospital, its thirteenth-century roll cartulary, and its wider documentary culture has shown how many common assumptions about rural hospitals are in serious need of revisitation and revision, from their actual dates of foundation and the backgrounds of their founders, to the coverage and composition of their estates, their immersion and embeddedness in various and often wide-ranging networks, and – of particular interest here – their dependence on and contribution to local documentary cultures. The photographic facsimile, critical edition, and translation of the Aynho Cartulary provided in Part II of this book, and the editions of further Aynho charters in the Appendix, encourage readers to engage directly with the primary evidence for both research and teaching. If other rural hospitals and their archival heritage were afforded the same detailed treatment that Aynho and its cartulary have been given here, this would almost certainly generate similar findings and resources, which would, in turn, transform our state of knowledge about when, how, by whom, and why these institutions, which dotted the medieval English landscape and were well-known to princes and paupers alike, were established.

# PART II

# FACSIMILE, TEXT, AND TRANSLATION

# PHOTOGRAPHIC FACSIMILE

*RECTO*

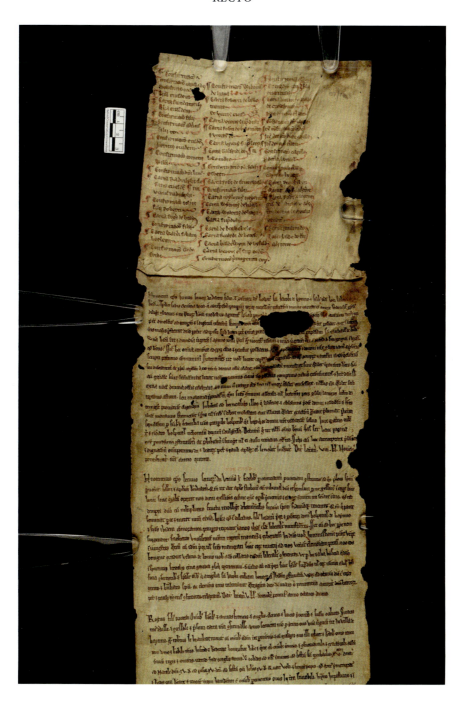

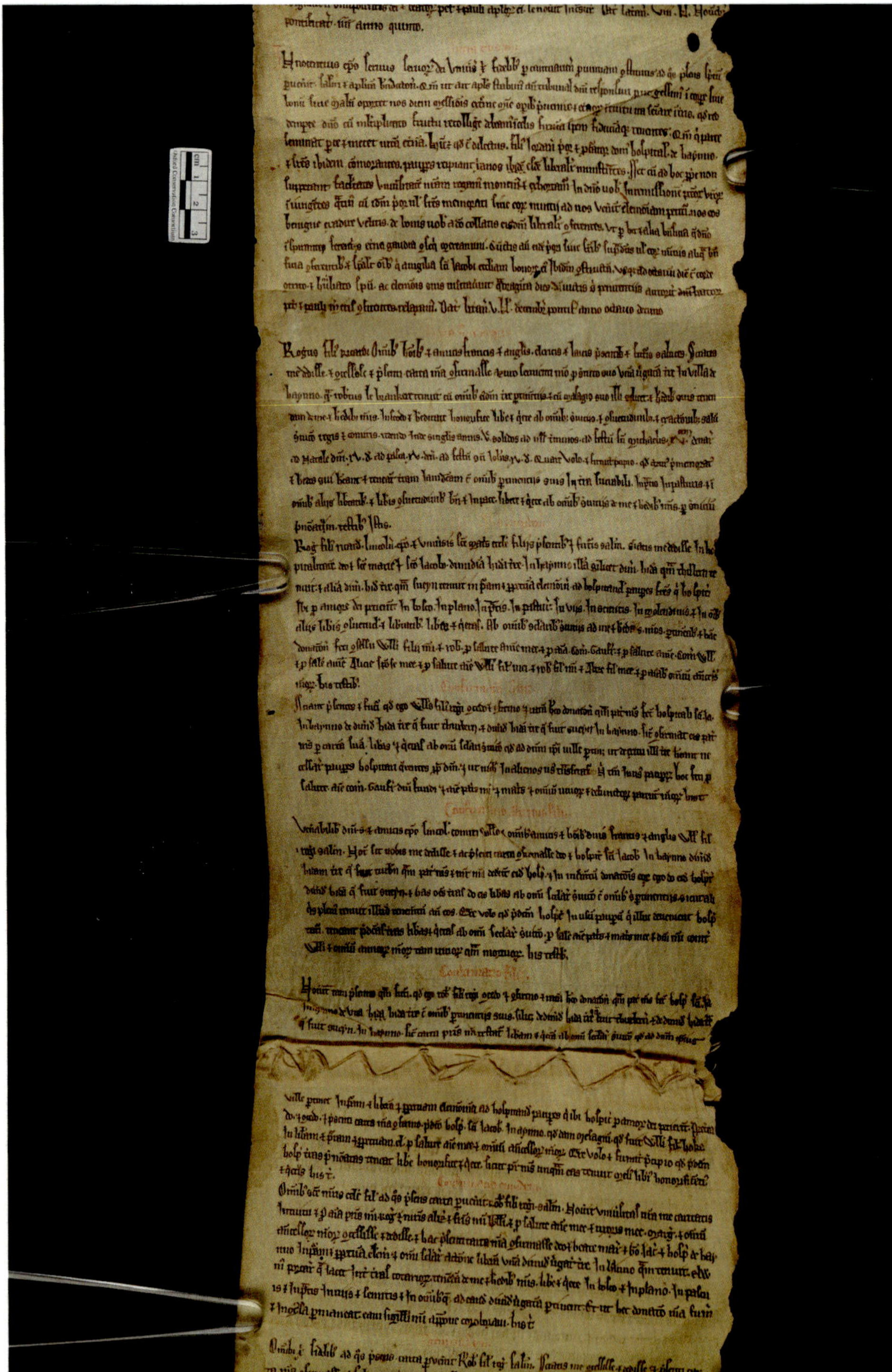

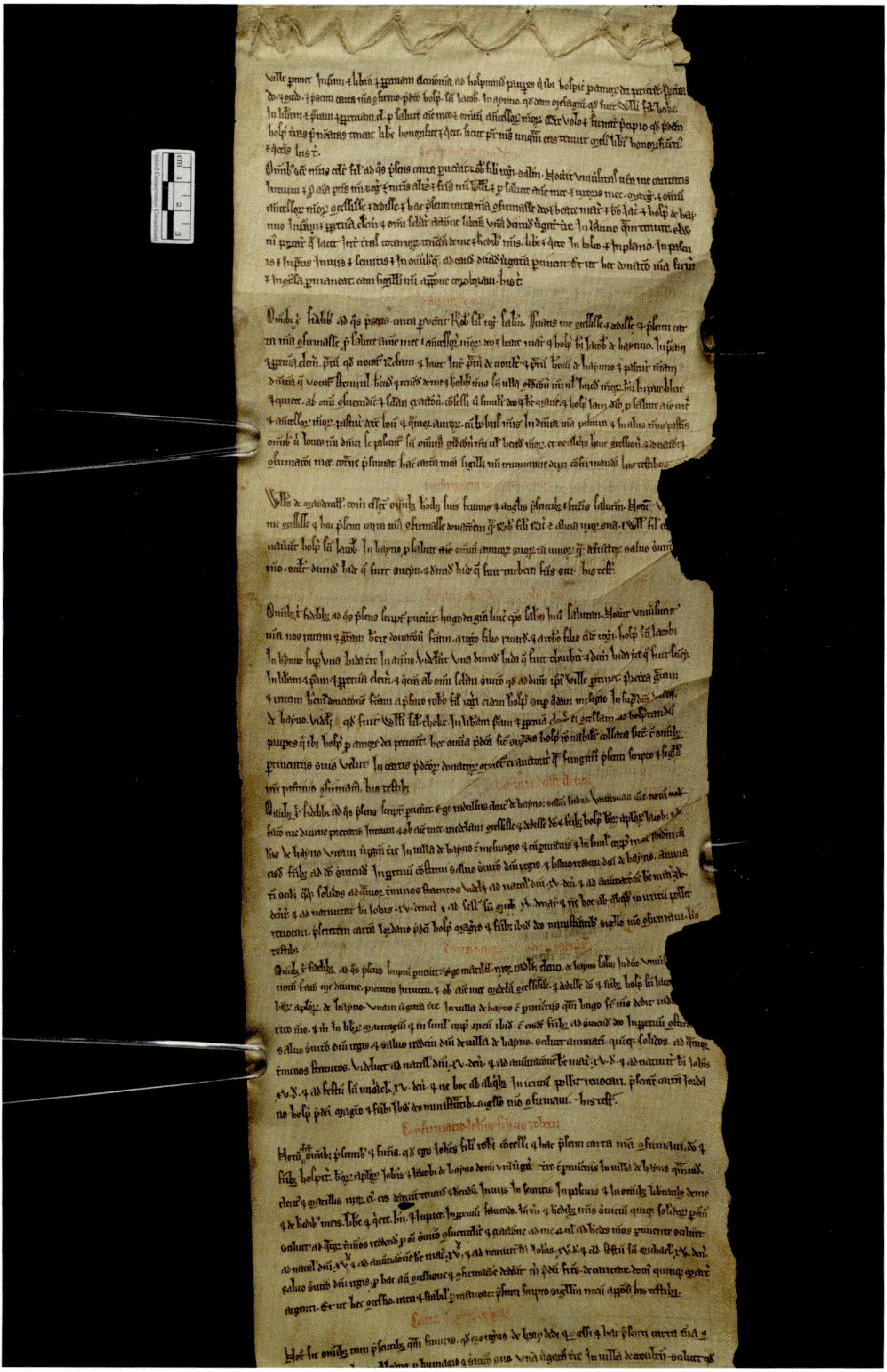

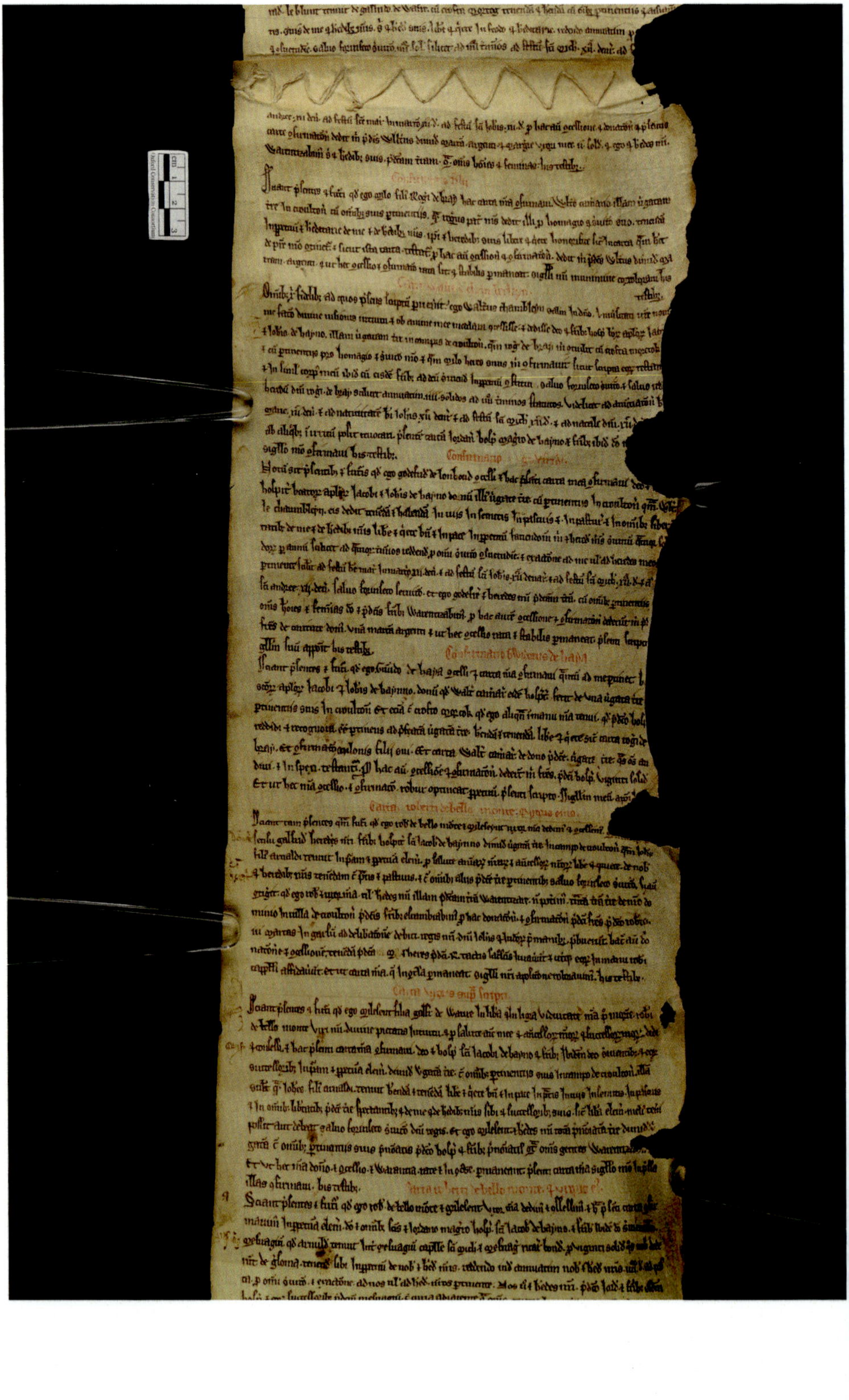

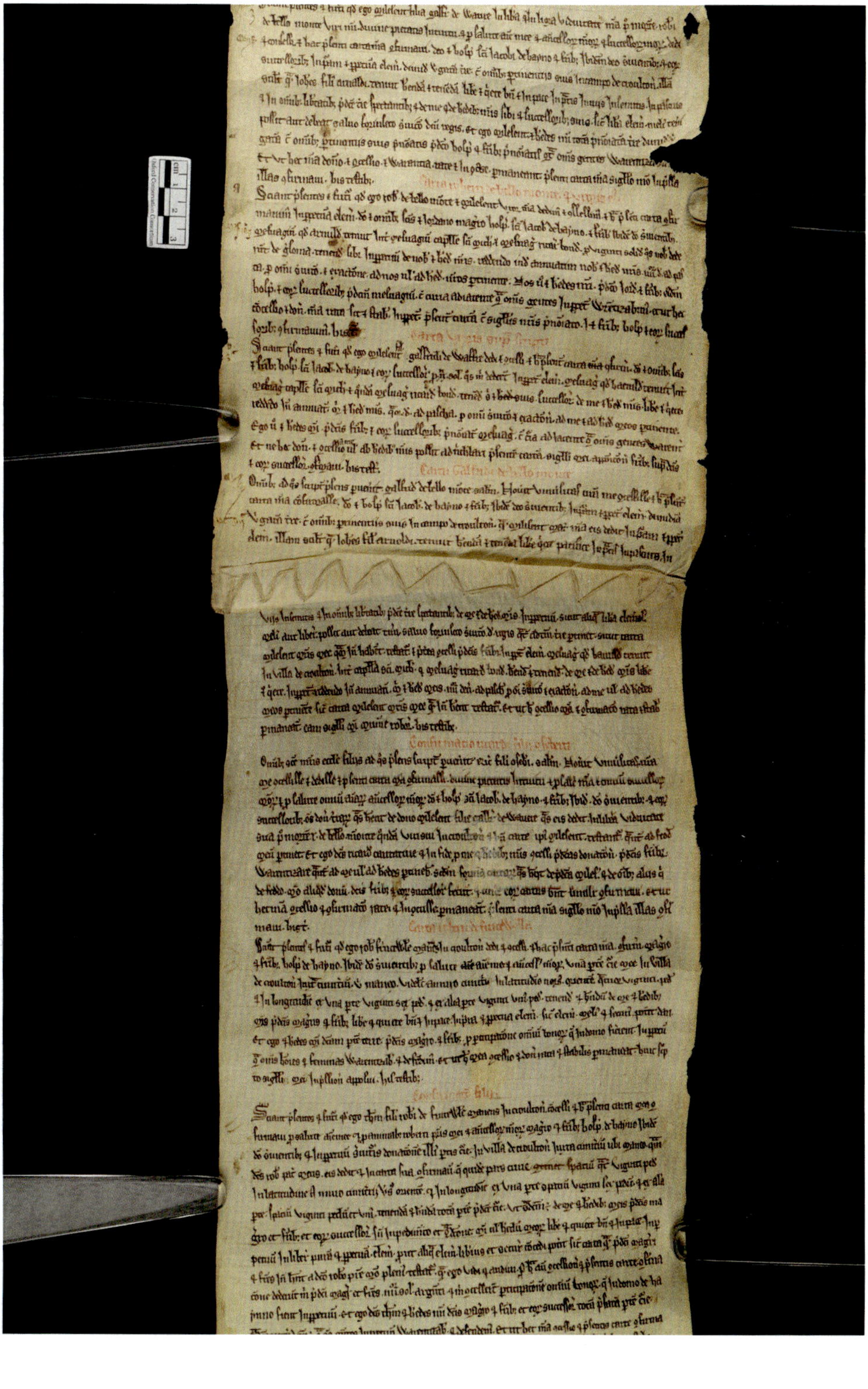

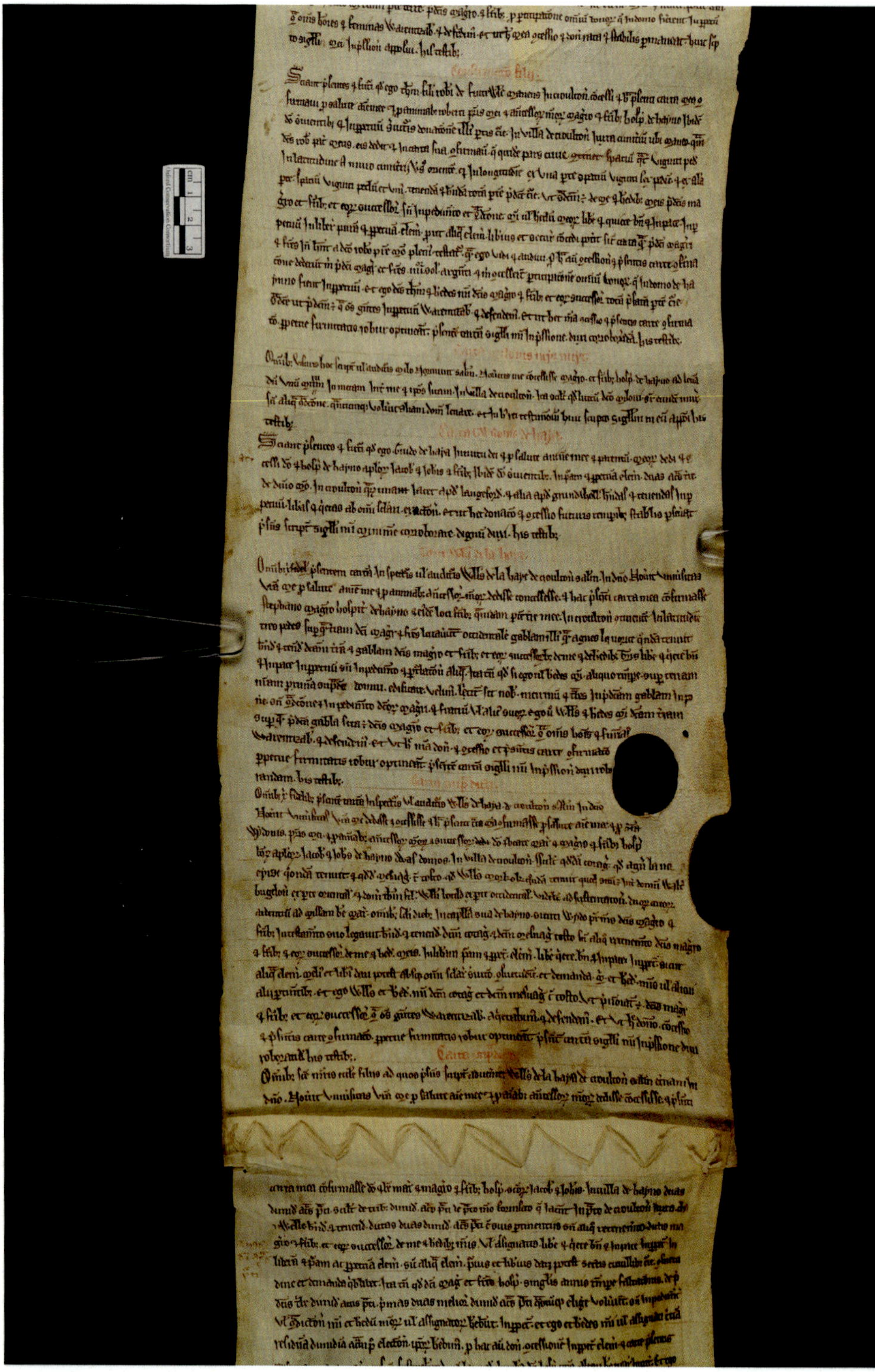
cm 1 2 3
Oxford Conservation Consortium

[illegible] ... pretie firmitatis robur optineat presenti cartam sigilli mei impressione dum
roboravi hiis testibus.

Carta [illegible]

Omnibus sancte matris ecclesie filiis ad quos presens scriptum pervenerit Willelmus de la bayse de Coulton salutem eternam in
domino. Noverit universitas vestra me pro salute anime mee et parentum antecessorum meorum dedisse concessisse et presenti

carta mea confirmasse deo et beate marie et magistro et fratribus hospitalis sanctorum Iacobi et Iohannis in villa de bayno duas
dimidias acras prati scilicet de tribus dimidiis acris prati de prato meo Fouleslaw quod iacent in prato de Coulton iuxta do
... habendas et tenendas dictas duas dimidias acras prati cum omnibus pertinentiis suis ... dicto magistro et fratribus et eorum successoribus de me et heredibus meis vel assignatis libere et quiete bene et in pace imperpetuum in
liberam et puram ac perpetuam elemosinam sicut aliqua elemosina purius et liberius dari potest ... solutam
dine et demandis quibuslibet. Ita tamen quod dicti magister et fratres hospitalis singulis annis tempore falcationis de predictis tribus dimidiis acris prati primas duas meliores dimidias acras prati quascumque eligere voluerint sine impedimento
vel contradictione mei et heredum meorum vel assignatorum habebunt imperpetuum et ego et heredes mei vel assignati tertiam
residuam dimidiam acram post electionem ipsorum habebimus. Pro hac autem donatione concessione imperpetuum elemosina et carte presentis
confirmatione dicti magister et fratres sustinebunt unam lampadem in ecclesia dicti hospitalis coram altari beate marie imperpetuum. Et ego
Willelmus et heredes mei vel assignati duas dictas dimidias acras prati singulis annis ... magistro et fratribus dicti
hospitalis et eorum successoribus ... cum omnibus pertinentiis ... dictis magistro et fratribus hospitalis et eorum successoribus contra omnes
gentes imperpetuum warantizabimus acquietabimus et defendemus et purgabimus sicut puram meram liberam et perpetuam elemosinam.
In cuius rei testimonium presenti carte sigilli mei impressionem duxi roborandam hiis testibus.

Carta [illegible]

Omnibus Christi fidelibus presentem cartam audituris Willelmus de bayse de Coulton salutem. Noveritis me pro salute anime mee et
animabus antecessorum et successorum meorum dedisse concessisse et hac carta mea confirmasse deo et beate marie et magistro
et fratribus hospitalis beatorum apostolorum Iacobi et Iohannis de bayno unam acram terre mee in villa de Coulton scilicet dimidiam
acram in campo [illegible] que iacet [illegible] inter terram ... et terram ... Beamond et dimidiam acram in campo
australi que extendit ... inter terram hospitalis de bayno et terram Galfridi ... pro anima ... ... Wa[illegible]
patris mei et anime matris mee et ... eorum annuatim ... celebrand[a] ... quibus nomina eorum scribantur
in martilogio dicti hospitalis. Habendam et tenendam dictis magistro et fratribus et eorum successoribus libere quiete bene et in pace
absque omni seculari servitio consuetudine demanda et ... aliis pertinentiis scilicet imperpetuum in liberam puram et perpetuam elemosinam sicut aliqua elemosina ... et liberius dari potest. Et ego Willelmus et heredes mei dictam ... dictis magistro et fratribus
et eorum successoribus contra omnes gentes warantizabimus acquietabimus et defendemus. Quod ut ratum sit presenti carte sigilli
mei impressionem roboravi. hiis testibus.

Carta de [illegible]

Universis sancte matris ecclesie filiis ad quos presens scriptum pervenerit magister Reginaldus de ... salutem. Noverit universitas vestra
me dedisse pro salute anime mee et antecessorum meorum deo et beate marie et sancto Iacobo hospitalis de bayno et magistro et fratribus
ibidem deo servientibus domum cum pertinentiis que sita est inter domum que fuit Galfridi ... et inter domum ... de la ...
... quam Iohannes ... tenet ... in ... de eadem domo ... vel heres ... habendam et
tenendam libere et quiete bene et in pace sicut puram et perpetuam elemosinam reddendo inde annuatim domino comiti de Wincestre
... ad ... terminos scilicet ad festum sancti michaelis ... et ... ad ... pro omni ...
... pro omni exactione servitio et demanda. Et ut hec mea donatio et ... rata et inconcussa permaneat presenti scripto
sigillum meum apposui hiis testibus.

Confirmatio [illegible] de [illegible]

Hoc sit omnibus sancte matris ecclesie filiis ad quos presens scriptum pervenerit quod ego ... de ... filius Willelmi ... pro salute
anime mee et ... et heredum meorum et antecessorum meorum dedi et confirmavi imperpetuum in puram et perpetuam elemosinam deo
et beate marie et hospitali apostolorum Iacobi et Iohannis de bayno unam dimidiam summam frumenti annuatim in festo sancti michaelis
... de terra mea de ... ille qui tenuerit vel habuerit. Et ego et heredes mei predictam dimidiam
summam frumenti imperpetuum ... predicto hospitali ... singulis annis ad predictum terminum persolvi-
mus. Et ut hec mea donatio et confirmatio rata et inconcussa permaneat hanc cartam cum sigilli mei munimine roboravi hiis testibus.

Carta Baldewini de [illegible]

Sciant tam presentes quam futuri quod ego Baldewinus de ... dedi et concessi consilio et assensu ... uxoris
mee et Willelmi filii mei heredis mei unam virgatam terre in villa de ... quam ... tenuit reddendo inde
annuatim hospitali sancti Iacobi de bayno ... solidos pro salute anime mee et ... uxoris mee et Willelmi filii mei et patris
Galfridi de ... et ... et parentum omnium antecessorum meorum bene et in pace libere et quiete et honorifice
in villa et extra villam in pratis et pascuis et in ... liberis consuetudinibus et exactionibus in puram et perpetuam
elemosinam. Et ut hec donatio rata et inconcussa permaneat eam sigilli mei appositione corroboravi et
ego ... Baldewinus et heredes mei warantizabimus ... predictam terram predicto hospitali contra omnes gentes
hiis testibus.

Carta uxoris eius super eodem

Sciant tam presentes quam futuri quod ego ... de ... dedi et concessi consilio et assensu Willelmi filii mei heredis mei unam
virgatam terre in villa de ... quam ... filius ... tenuit reddendo inde annuatim hospitali sancti Iacobi de bayno ... solidos pro salute anime mee et Willelmi filii mei et patris mei Galfridi de ... et ... et parentum omnium antecessorum meorum et successorum
bene et in pace libere et quiete et honorifice in villa et extra villam in pratis et pascuis et in omnibus liberis consuetudinibus et exactionibus in puram et perpetuam elemosinam. Et ut hec donatio rata et inconcussa permaneat eam sigillo meo corroboravi.
Et ego predicta ... et heredes mei warantizabimus predicto hospitali hanc predictam donationem contra omnes gentes. hiis testibus.

Confirmatio [illegible]

Sciant presentes et futuri quod ego Willelmus de bayse filius ... de ... concessi et confirmavi donationem quam ... Baldewinus pater et ...
mater mea dederunt hospitali sancti Iacobi de bayno scilicet unam virgatam terre in villa de ... quam ... filius ... tenuit
reddendo inde annuatim hospitali predicto ... sicut carta Baldewini patris mei et ... matris mee testatur. Et ut hec
mea concessio et confirmatio rata et inconcussa permaneat eam sigillo meo corroboravi. hiis testibus.

cm 1 2 3
Oxford Conservation Consortium

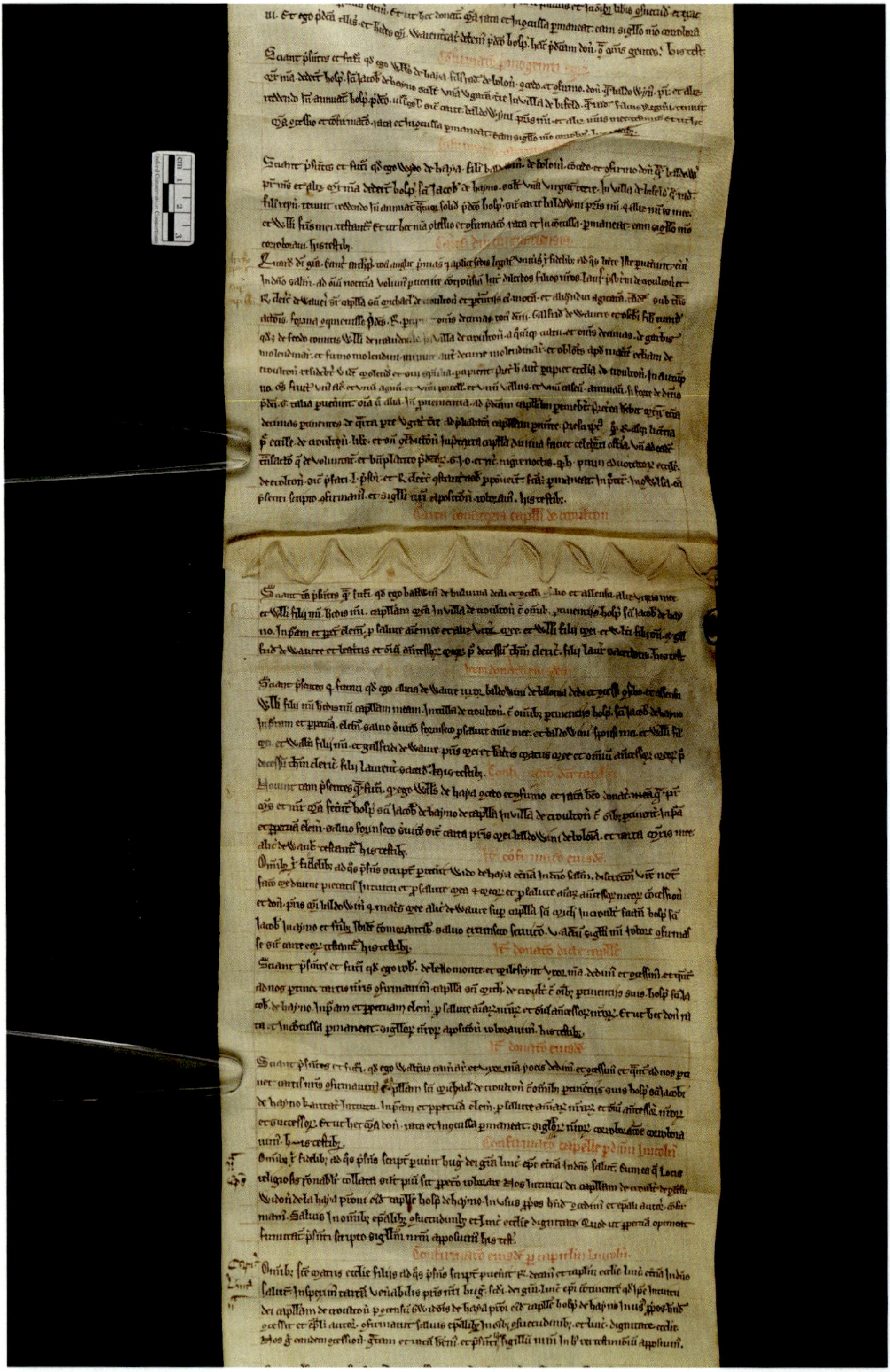

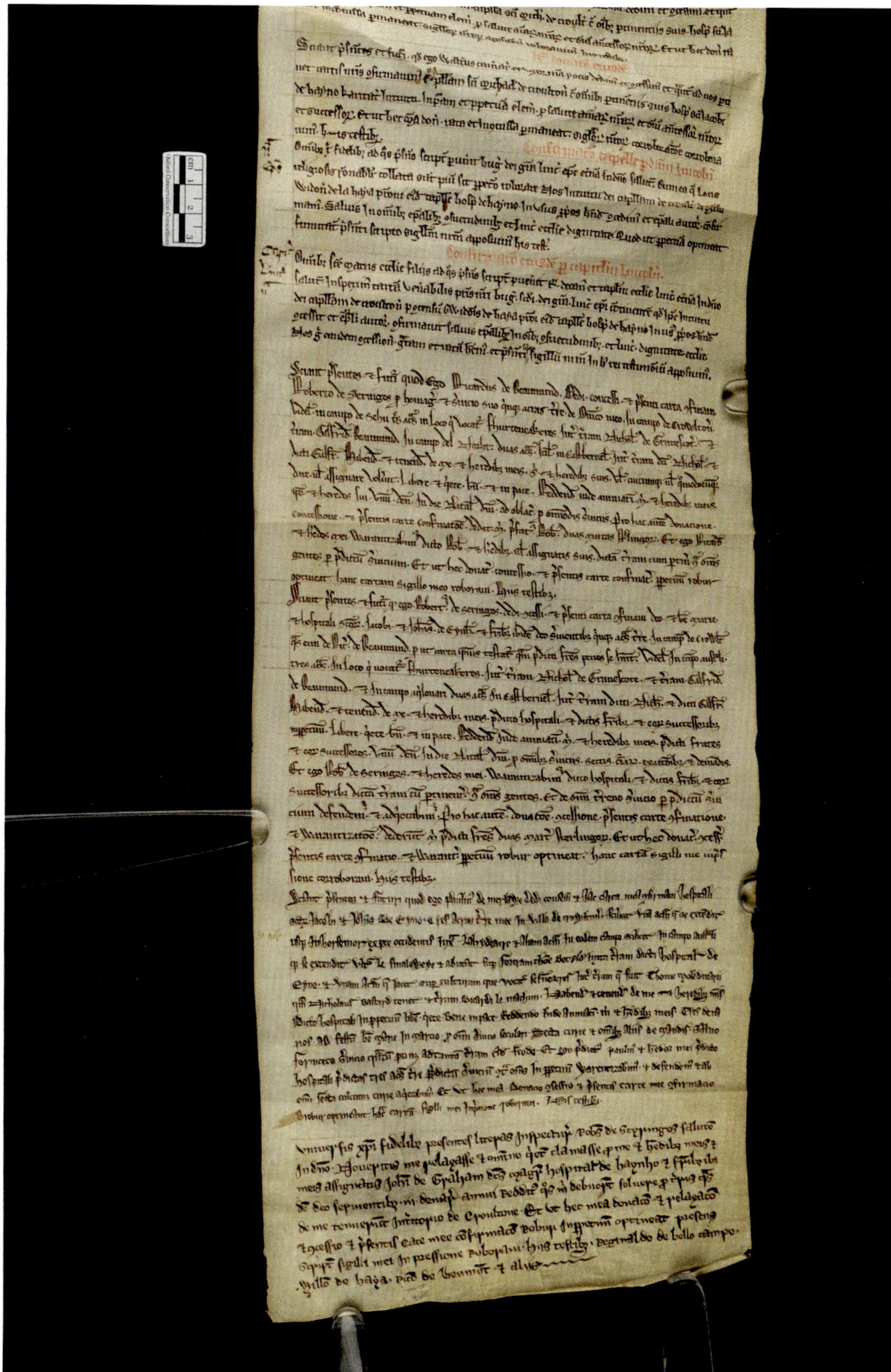

*VERSO*

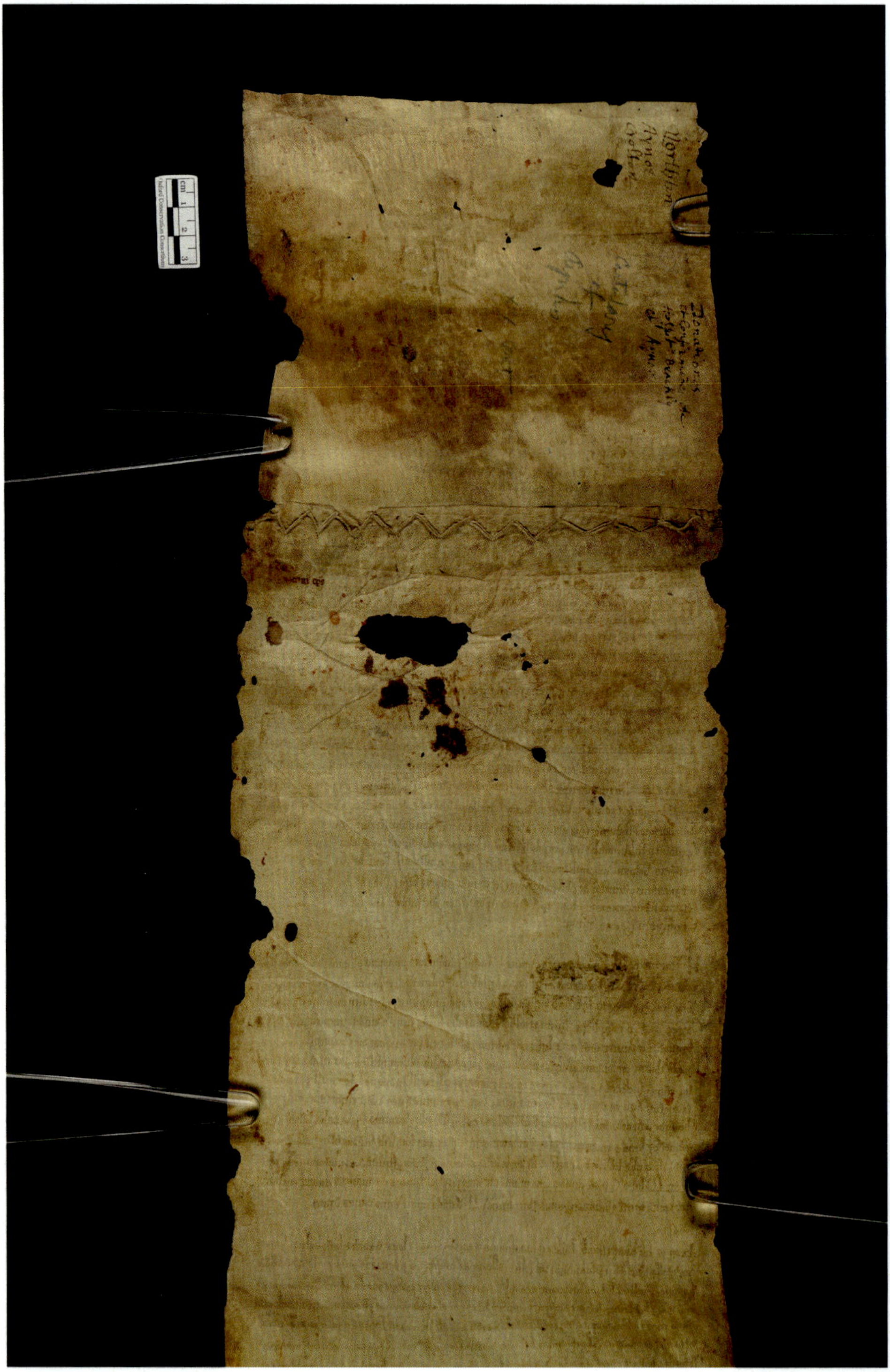

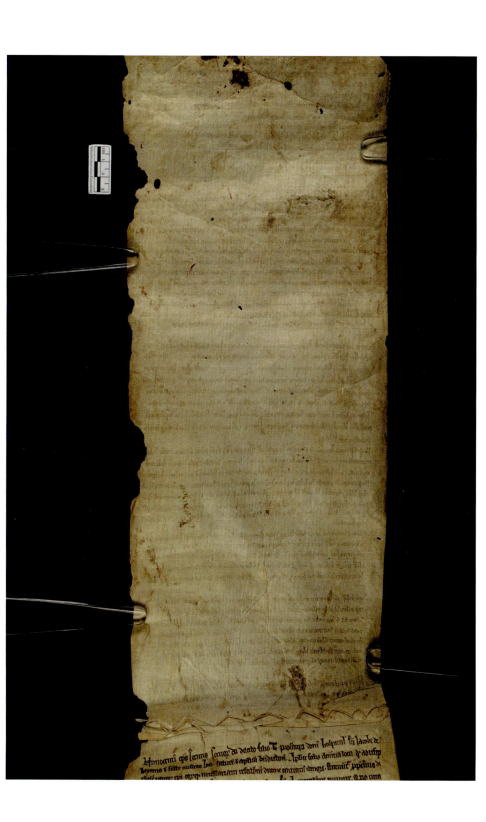
Innocentius eps servus servorum dei dilecto filio T. procuratori domus hospital' sancti Iacobi de

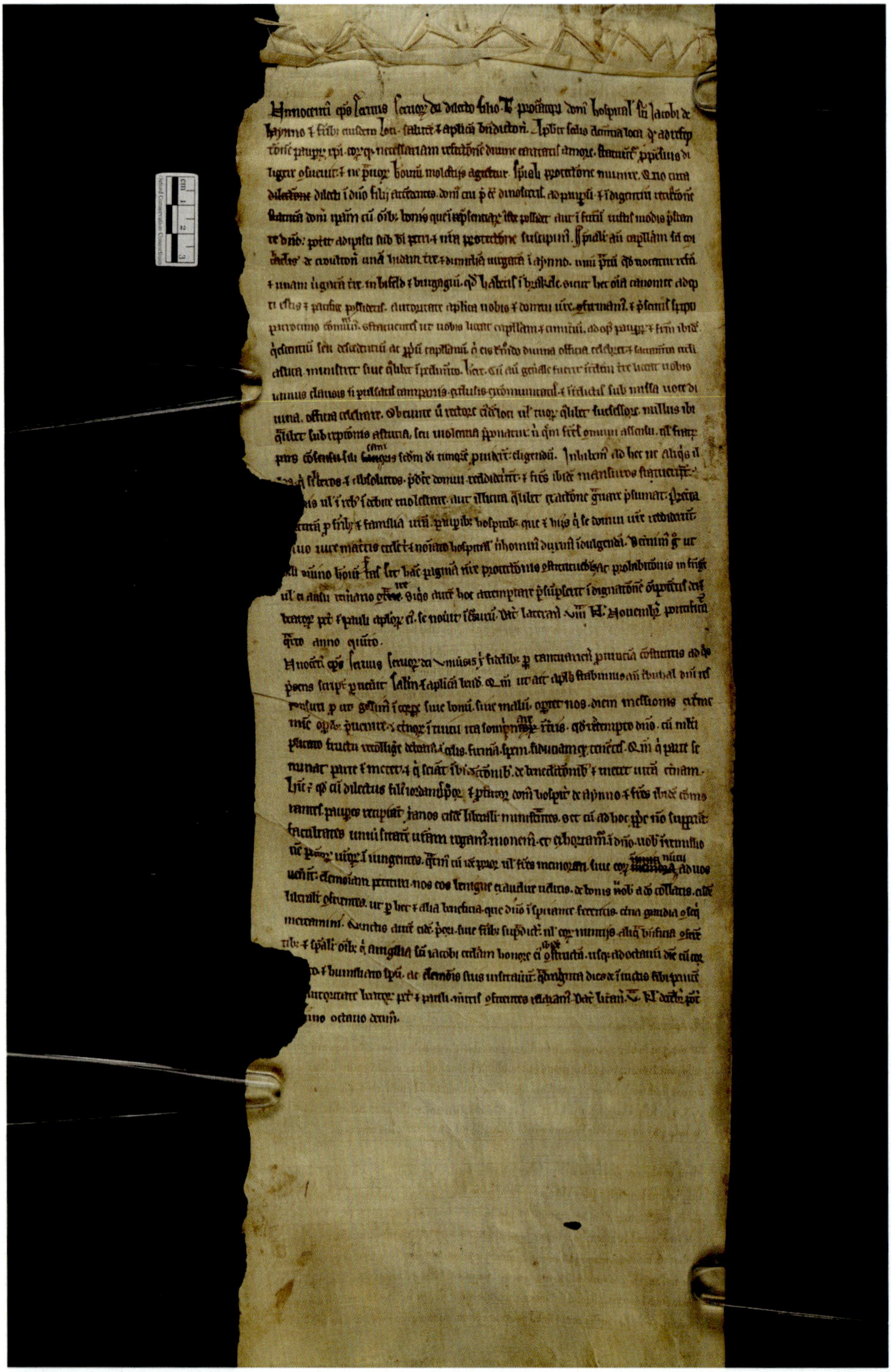
Innocentius episcopus servus servorum dei dilecto filio .. procuratori domus hospitalis sancti Iacobi de
[illegible] et fratribus eiusdem loci salutem et apostolicam benedictionem. [illegible] loci que ad receptionem pauperum Christi eorumque necessariam refectionem divine caritatis amore [illegible] propensius diligere convenit et ne pravorum hominum molestiis agitetur speciali protectione munire. Eapropter
[illegible] dilecti in domino filii [illegible] domum [illegible] ad pauperum et indigentium receptionem
[illegible] domum ipsam cum omnibus bonis que in presentiarum rationabiliter possidet aut in futurum iustis modis prestante
domino poterit adipisci sub beati Petri et nostra protectione suscipimus. Specialiter autem capellam sancti [illegible]
[illegible] unam virgatam terre et dimidiam virgate in [illegible] unum pratum quod vocatur [illegible]
et unam virgatam terre in [illegible] et burgagium quod habetis in [illegible] sicut hec omnia canonice adepti
estis et pacifice possidetis auctoritate apostolica vobis et domui vestre confirmamus et presentis scripti
patrocinio communimus. Statuentes ut vobis liceat capellam et cimiterium ad opus pauperum et fratrum ibidem
commorantium seu decedentium ac proprium capellanum qui eis ibidem divina officia celebret et sacramenta ecclesiastica ministret sine qualibet contradictione habere. Cum autem generale interdictum terre fuerit liceat vobis
clausis ianuis non pulsatis campanis exclusis excommunicatis et interdictis submissa voce divina officia celebrare. Obeunte vero te nunc eiusdem loci procuratore vel tuorum quolibet successorum nullus ibi
qualibet subreptionis astutia seu violentia preponatur nisi quem fratres communi assensu vel fratrum
pars consilii sanioris secundum deum timorem providerint eligendum. Inhibemus ad hec ut aliquis [illegible]
[illegible] quos liberos et absolutos postea domui reddiderint et fratres ibidem mansuros statuerint [illegible]
[illegible] vel in rebus suis [illegible] molestare aut illicita qualibet exactione gravare presumat. Preterea
[illegible] pro fratribus et familia vestra pauperibus hospitibus que et hiis qui se domui vestre reddiderint
[illegible] iure matricis ecclesie [illegible] hospitalis [illegible] indulgendam. Decernimus ergo ut
nulli omnino hominum liceat hanc paginam nostre protectionis confirmationis constitutionis et prohibitionis infringere
vel ei ausu temerario contraire. Si quis autem hoc attemptare presumpserit indignationem omnipotentis dei et
beatorum Petri et Pauli apostolorum eius se noverit incursurum. Datum Laterani viii Kalendas Novembris pontificatus
nostri anno quinto.

Innocentius episcopus servus servorum dei universis Christi fidelibus per Cantuariensem provinciam constitutis ad quos
presens scriptum pervenerit salutem et apostolicam benedictionem. Cum ut ait apostolus stabimus omnes ante tribunal Christi re-
cepturi prout in corpore gessimus sive bonum fuerit sive malum, oportet nos diem messionis extreme
misericordie operibus prevenire ac eternorum intuitu seminare in terris quod reddente domino cum multiplicato fructu recolligere debeamus in celis firmam spem fiduciamque tenentes. Quoniam qui parce seminat parce et metet et qui seminat in benedictionibus de benedictionibus et metet vitam eternam.
Cum igitur ut accepimus dilectus filius .. procurator domus hospitalis de [illegible] et fratres ibidem commorantes pauperes recipiant [illegible] eos caritative liberaliter ministrantes, et cum ad hoc proprie non suppetant
facultates, universitatem vestram rogamus, monemus et exhortamur in domino, vobis in remissionem
vestrorum peccaminum iniungentes quatinus cum [illegible] vel fratres memorati sive eorum nuntii ad vos
venerint elemosinam petituri, vos eos benigne recipiatis [illegible] et de bonis vobis a deo collatis [illegible]
liberaliter conferatis, ut per hec et alia bona que domino inspirante feceritis ad eterna gaudia pervenire
mereamini. [illegible] fratribus supradictis vel eorum nuntiis [illegible]
[illegible] et specialiter omnibus qui [illegible] sancti Iacobi [illegible] usque ad octavam diem [illegible]
[illegible] et humiliter recipiant [illegible] elemosinis suis [illegible]
auctoritate beatorum Petri et Pauli apostolorum [illegible]. Datum Laterani [illegible] Kalendas [illegible] pontificatus nostri
anno octavo decimo.

... facultatem uniuscuiusque usum rigandi monendi et abqueramus dno uob restitutio
... ue pene uiue et ungentis. Ffini ut ue quer ut ftra maneam siue ... nimi
uehit elemosam penitu nos eos tenuqe adaudit uctus. de tomis nob ad collatis ade
... litualt obtineant. ut p hec t alia teneant que dno i tpuamt fecerit etna gaudia e sci
... mereamini. Sancto anime ede peu siue filis supdit n eor nimmis aliū bisinis efut
... ibz t tpali oib3 q tangit tā iacobi eiidam bonere et ostructi usq adoctauū die ... or
... et hunmemo tpi de elemois suis intraiut donquin dico et sctis siū pruer
... aurquatur laterg pot et puelu nims obtinens reclam pax luen T. U actio por
... anno octauo Anū

Sciant presentes et futuri qd Ego Robert de Stiringis dedi t ... ffest i eam cum ostimam coagio
et tribut hospitalis beate stis Iacobi et Iohis de egdo duas acras te in campo de Ostchelme ... jhnia
... aua iacet In campo audruh apd prat cenre eam... Dei se birim ... alia acri iacet in campo brooli apd
... side soli al uupeho me eam oie. Habendu et tenendu de me et heredib3 meis deo congatis et fabr et
... suiseribz. Libere et quiete. Reddedo mi annuatim oib et heredib3 meis unum denariū ad inse
... enimatio seruicu et demandis et ominu captu ... seris Grasti aut donatone concesione et prelatione eai
... te ostinatone uolente mihi pedu ... et hos: Huam. Iohis Steringin. et xpe Robert de
Stiringis et heredes meis... garantizabim erca de demanione ista et ... igese fuerit et teneam duas
... Actis ad he. Cum peruenne sing. die filis et cor successorib3 p Dei seymani toer omus genorg t
... genui. Quis in pnm he. Nomen carti sigili mei inptione ofirmani Hus restibu

Omibz xpi fidelib3 presentem cartam inspectu ut indicie. Tomas de egslied filus Robert in
... eram in Humbille salū. Noueritis me qa salutis sie mee t pie salute aiee Garganice ugone mee
... pro aiab3 antecog et successe meori. Dedisse et hac carta ofirmasse. deo et beate marie
... dngio et stis domus aptor Iacobi t Iohis de erato duas acr tre mee ... unam scilam amboleg
... Croslet sal unam acram in campo albi. Emne dimidia ac iace et pre ocadentali ...
... tim reliraco et tham Fidelin coĭn t alia dimidia ac iace uers oĭentem de Hamuille
... um hospitalis et tham pdca Tome. Et una acra iacet in empo t empo beriah emna
... uia ac et una yast iace in meregris ... et hee priols uene. Ge alia dimidia ac iace sup smale
... bechille ute scim eade hospitale et tham pdci Tome. Hdndes et temendas dco. Gragio et fabr
... et eor successoribz libere t here bene t in pace. Abisqe oim selari seruico t shuernie serus cupti
... temandis in ... Alium penenclio muyenū Saliquam t pupinu t genuin elemoiam hec adei
... enior Melius et liberus tenn dari ut ept pp; lieari qd omibz t singlis anno celebret a mi sainue day
Sugaruer Conuse de hene demnere p hunc ... et in dca hospitali. Qie sta manu ego t ... clesone
... no de omibz t singlis anno fres dci hospitale dednue. de eade eas puannam ad pecositone
... ff. Ego Tomas et heredes mei p nobis duas acr t pediu dco Gragio et fabr et eor
... setpz et omes acenres garantizabim et dendemu et de oim serues agocabuni. Qd in pn
... pntem scripto sigili mei inpresione agefini Hus restibu

Omibz xpi fidelib3 pemenm cartam inspectie ut induruo Robert t Eule edm. Noueritis me
... salute aie mee t pie salute aie monis mee t pe aiab3 antecesso et successog meog ... delicatis anglisse
... ut cora ofirmasse. deo t te marie et stis hospital bonere aptor Iacobi t Iohis... condedit serui...

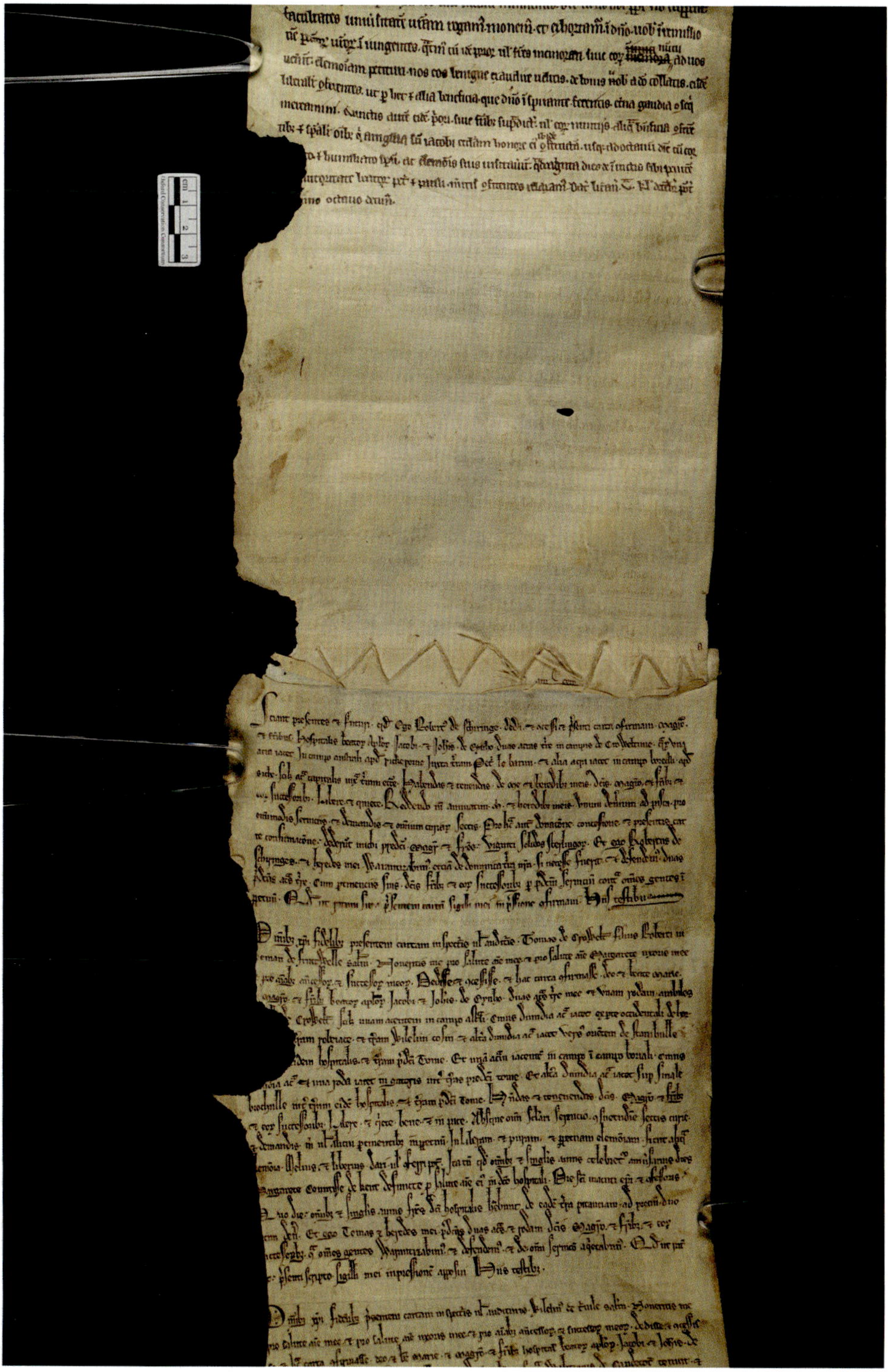

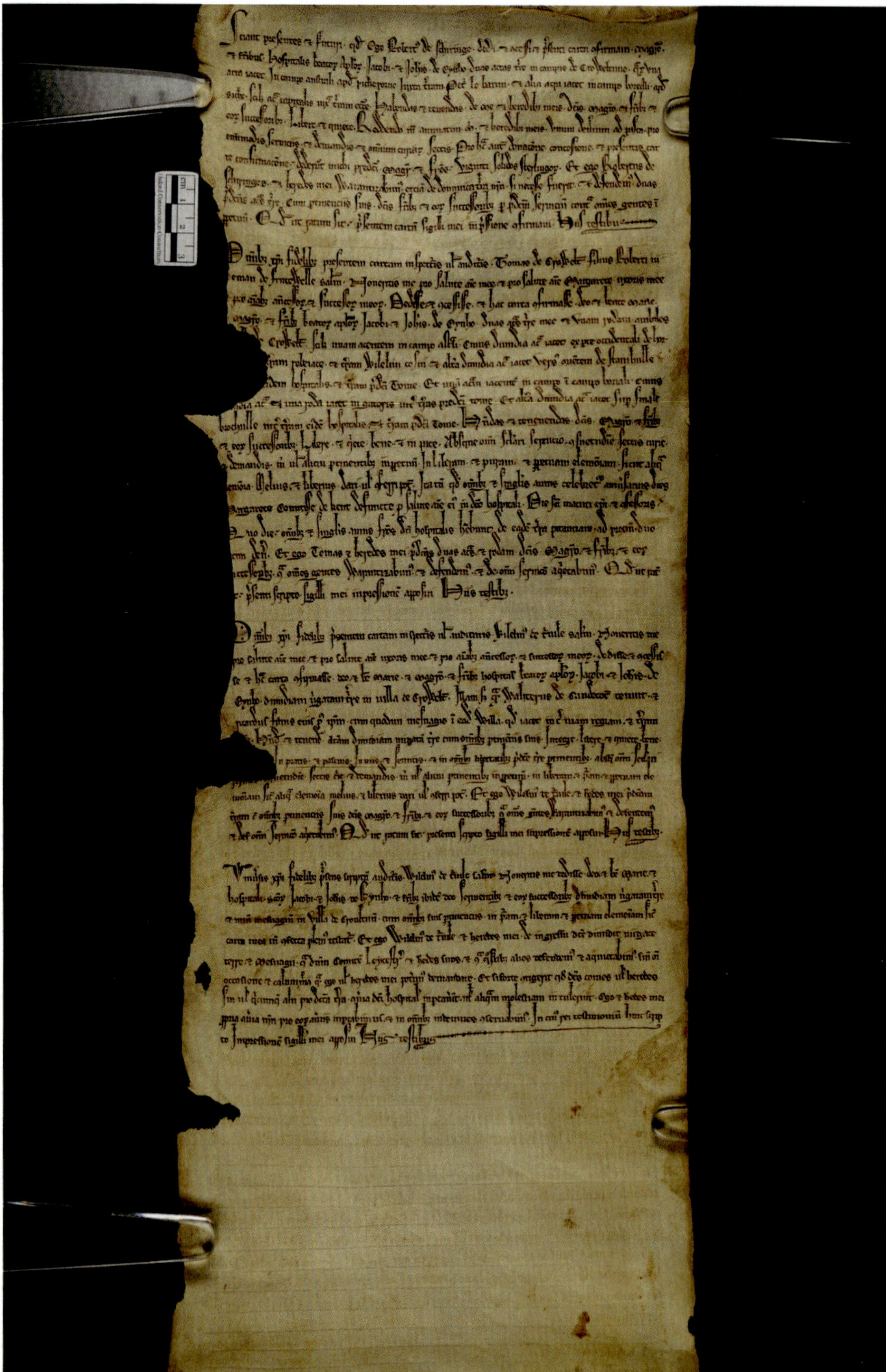

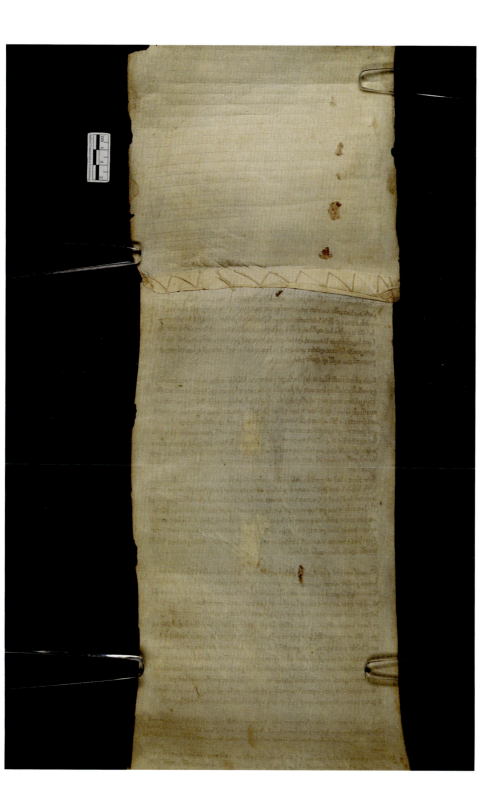

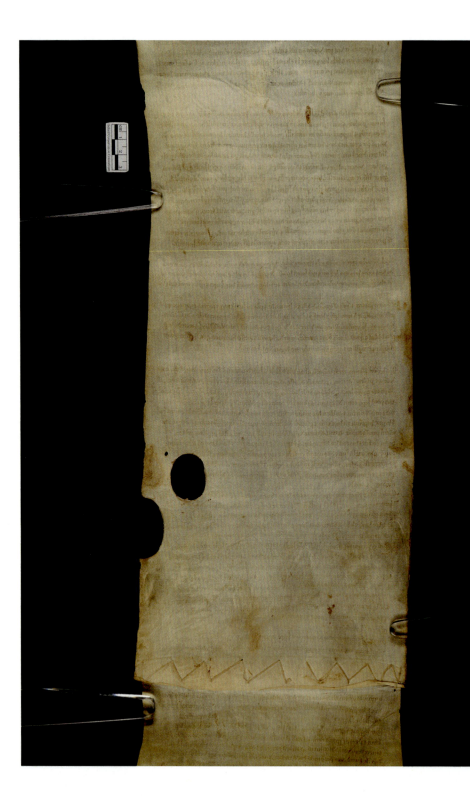

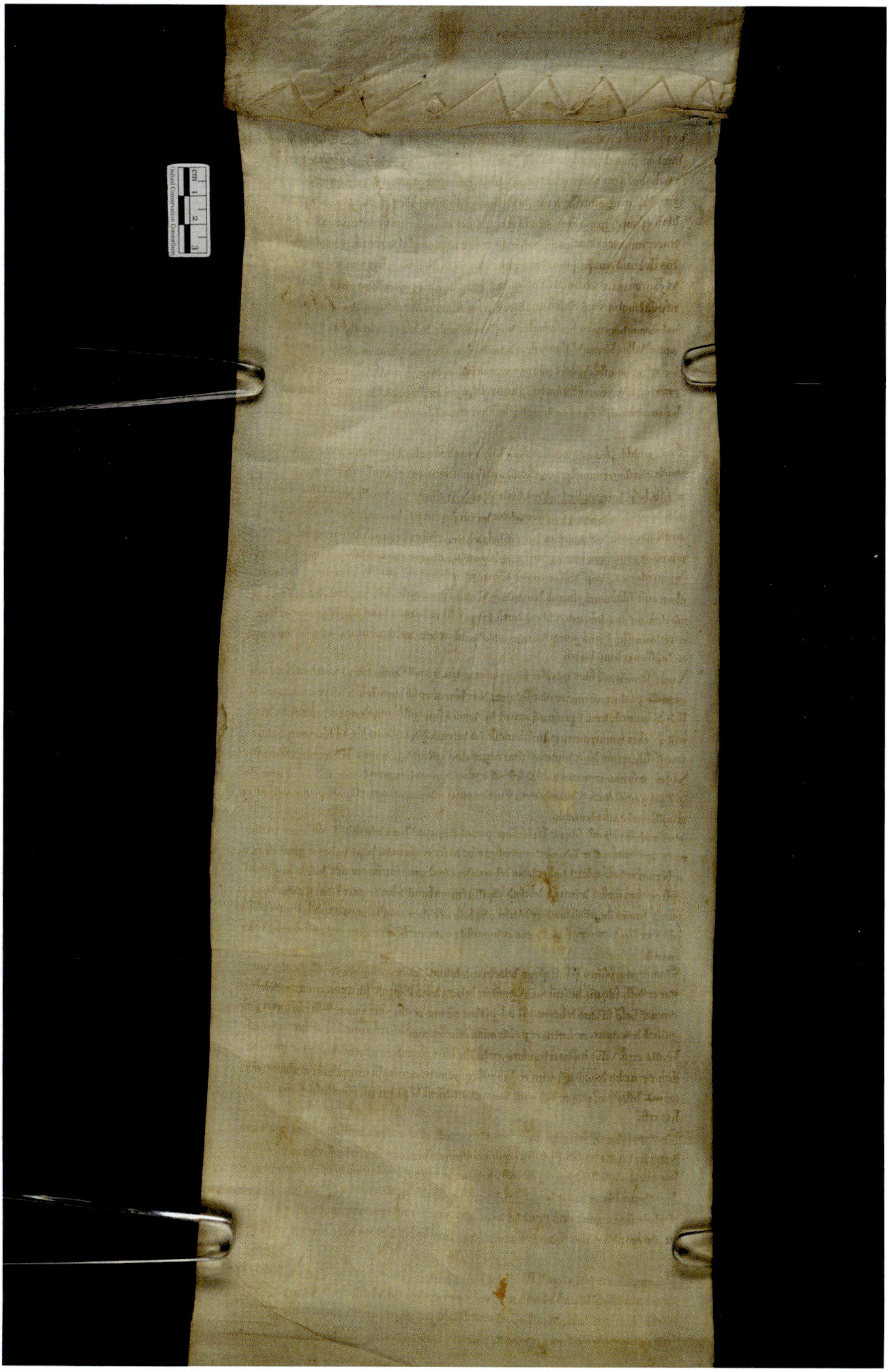

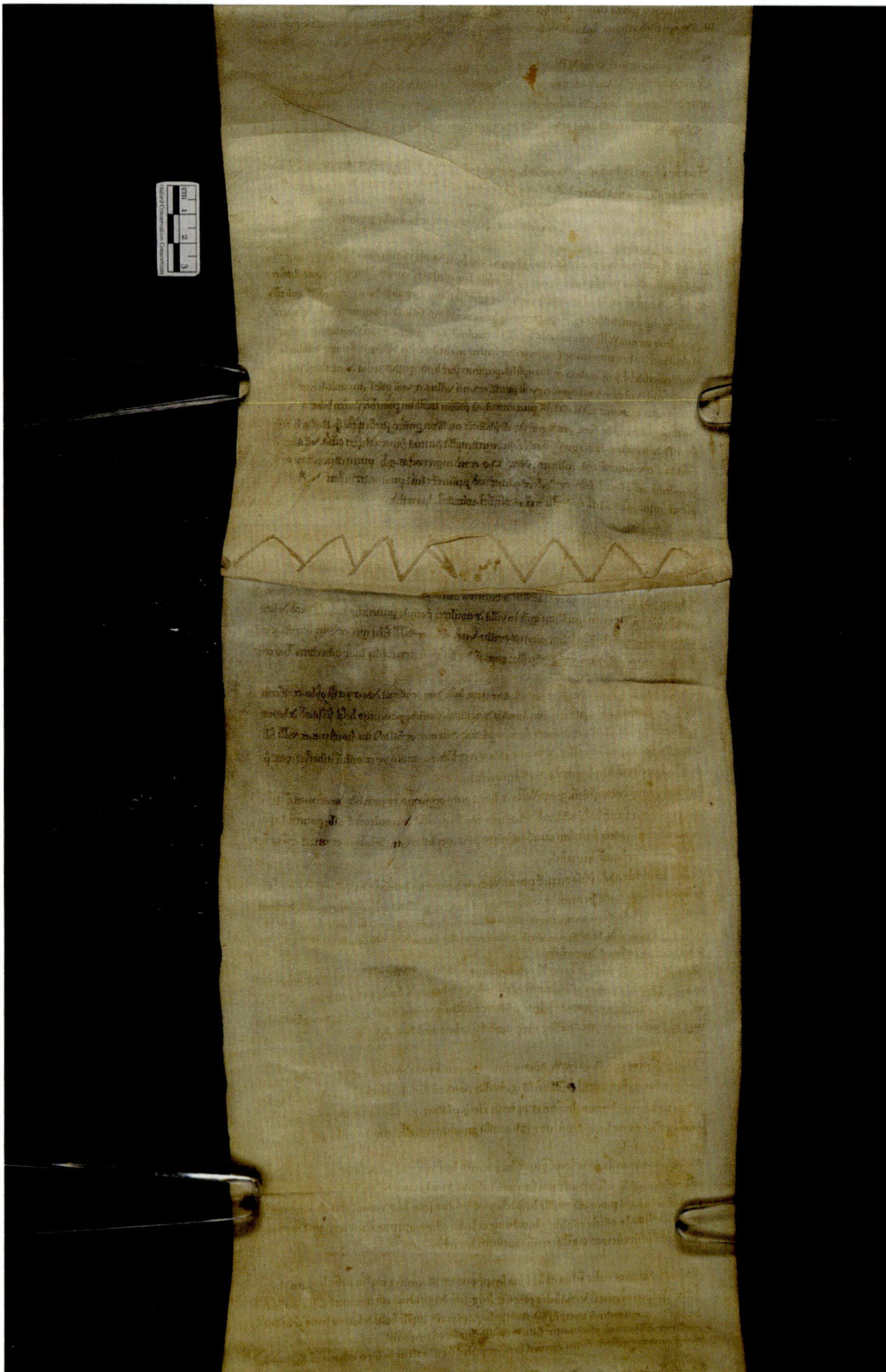

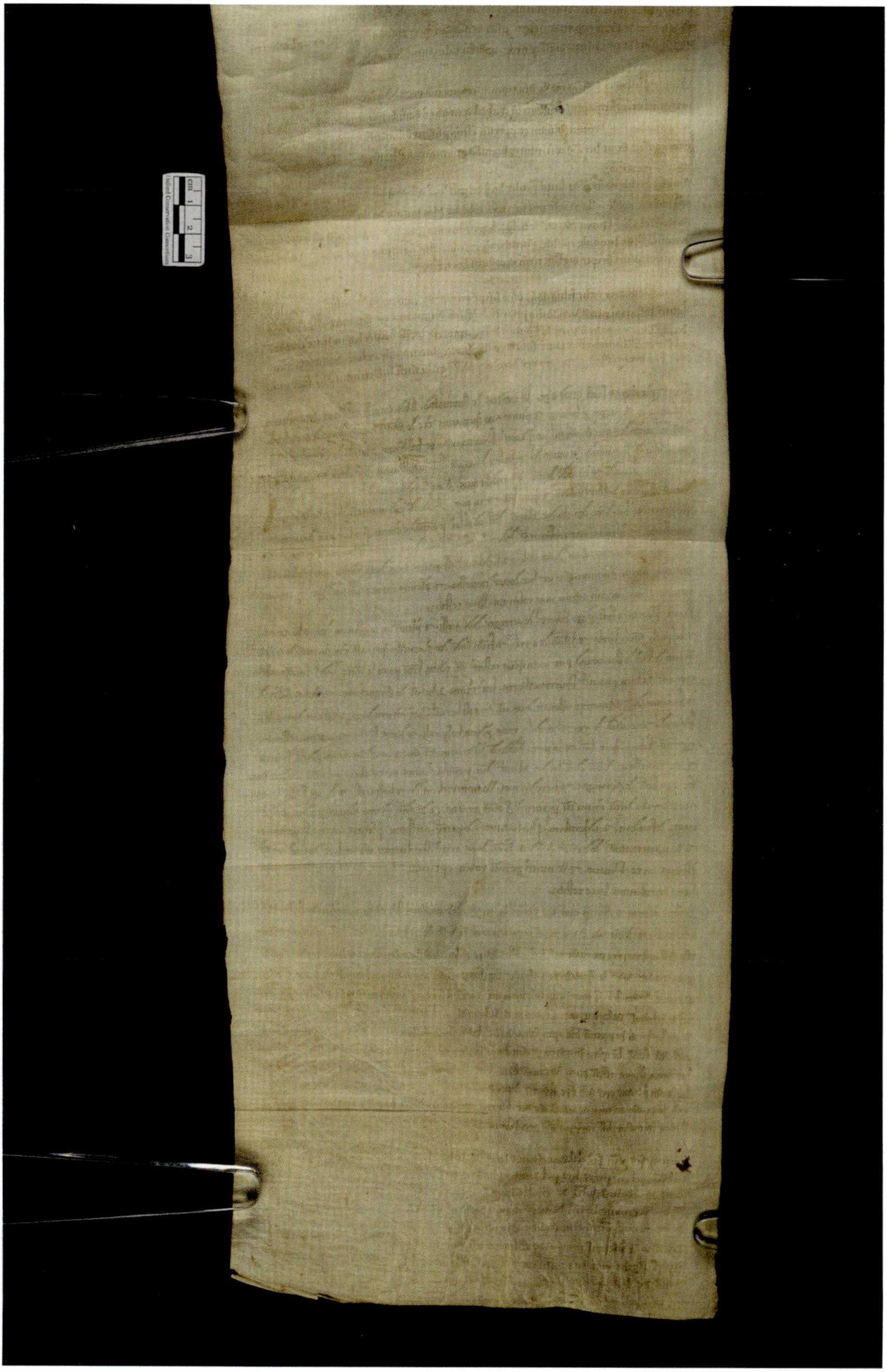

# TEXT AND TRANSLATION

For the present edition, the cartulary serves as the base text (*B*) when it preserves the only copy of a charter. When an original survives (*A*), this becomes the base text, with *B*'s variants noted. *C* is used for the second copy of a charter in the cartulary. When *A* is the base text, line breaks in the original act are noted in superscript numbers between two parallel vertical lines. In terms of orthography, *u*/*v* are kept distinct as vowel and consonant letters, respectively, whereas *i*/*j* are rendered consistently as a vowel and the use of *c*/*t* before *i* plus vowel (*-cio*/*-tio*) has not been standardised. Punctuation has been modernised. Save for occurrences of 'Aenho', 'Ainho', etc., Old English and French words are rendered in italics.

Within the main text, the following symbols are used in the following ways:

( ) = letters supplied by the editors abbreviated by suspension mark (used for all abbreviations that are either unusual or have more than one possible expansion, e.g., qm = quam or quoniam, hospit' = hospitale or hospitalarius, Rog' = Rogerus or Rogerius, Galfr' = Galfridus or Galfredus, etc.)
[ ] = letters missing due to damage in the cartulary/original and supplied from cartulary/original (or by the editors, if missing from both)
{} = letters missing due to damage in cartulary but not in the surviving original
< > = letters supplied by the editors omitted by the scribe (of either cartulary or original)

In the translations, the names of individuals today known by a patronymic indicator are here translated literally (e.g., *Robertus filius Rogeri* = Robert, son of Roger, not Robert Fitz Roger). Likewise, as in the chapters above, surnames/toponymics with multiple forms have been standardised (e.g., Neirenuit/Neirenut/Neirnut/Neyrnut = Neirenuit).

Some minor marginalia were added in what seems to be a single sitting (and certainly no more than two) by a scribe working towards the end of the Middle Ages. These are noted after the translation of the charter next to which they appear.

The reverse of membrane 1 has the following early modern and modern endorsements: Northan'. Aynhoe. Crolton. Donationes et confirmationes, etc, hospit(alium) Brackly et Aynho (? s.xvii); Cartulary of Aynho. XIV cent. (? s.xx). The reverse of membrane 2 has the following early modern endorsement: Aenhoe (? s.xvi).

For ease of reference, the following table lists every act in the cartulary and, where surviving, its corresponding original.

| No. | Act | Original |
|---|---|---|
| **1** | Pope Innocent III | – |
| **2** | Pope Innocent III | – |
| **3** | Roger Fitz Richard | Aynho 21 |
| **4** | Roger Fitz Richard | Aynho 71 |
| **5** | William Fitz Roger | – |
| **6** | William Fitz Roger | Aynho 31 |
| **7** | Robert Fitz Roger | Aynho 19 |
| **8** | Robert Fitz Roger | Aynho 32 |
| **9** | Robert Fitz Roger | – |
| **10** | William de Mandeville, earl of Essex | Aynho 49 |
| **11** | Hugh [of Avalon], bishop of Lincoln | Aynho 22 |
| **12** | Ralph, clerk of Aynho | – |
| **13** | Matilda, wife of Ralph, clerk of Aynho | – |
| **14** | John Fitz Robert | – |
| **15** | Roger de Bray | Aynho 62 |
| **16** | Miles, son of Roger de Bray | Aynho 52 |
| **17** | Walter Chamberlain | Aynho 64 |
| **18** | Geoffrey de Loenhout | – |
| **19** | Guy de la Haye | – |
| **20** | Robert de Beaumont and Melisende, his wife | – |
| **21** | Melisende, daughter of Geoffrey de Wavre, widow of Robert de Beaumont | Aynho 28 |
| **22** | Robert de Beaumont and Melisende, his wife | Aynho 86 |
| **23** | Melisende, daughter of Geoffrey de Wavre | – |
| **24** | Geoffrey de Beaumont | – |
| **25** | Richard, son of Osbert | Aynho 44 |

| No. | Act | Original |
|---|---|---|
| 26 | Robert of Fritwell | Aynho 65 |
| 27 | Thomas, son of Robert of Fritwell | Aynho 63 |
| 28 | Miles Neirenuit | – |
| 29 | Guy de la Haye | Aynho 50 |
| 30 | William (II) de la Haye of Croughton | Aynho 26 |
| 31 | William (II) de la Haye of Croughton | Aynho 53 |
| 32 | William (II) de la Haye of Croughton | Aynho 27 |
| 33 | William (II) de la Haye of Croughton | – |
| 34 | Master Reginald of Halse | – |
| 35 | Richard Hunte of Barford, son of William Hunte | – |
| 36 | Baldwin de Boulogne | Aynho 43 |
| 37 | Alice de Wavre | Aynho 41 |
| 38 | William (I) de la Haye, son of Baldwin de Boulogne | Aynho 42 |
| 39 | Guy de la Haye, son of Baldwin de Boulogne | Aynho 40 |
| 40 | Richard, archbishop of Canterbury | Brackley 76A |
| 41 | Baldwin de Boulogne | Aynho 85 |
| 42 | Alice de Wavre, wife of Baldwin de Boulogne | – |
| 43 | William (I) de la Haye | – |
| 44 | Guy de la Haye | – |
| 45 | Robert de Beaumont and Melisende, his wife | – |
| 46 | Walter Chamberlain and Roeis, his wife | Aynho 30 |
| 47 | Hugh [of Wells], bishop of Lincoln | Aynho 82 |
| 48 | R[oger], dean, and the chapter of Lincoln | Aynho 81 |
| 49 | Richard de Beaumont | – |
| 50 | Robert of Sheering | – |
| 51 | Paulinus of Marlow | Aynho 58 |
| 52 | Robert of Sheering | Aynho 55 |
| 53 | Pope Innocent III | See no. **1** |
| 54 | Pope Innocent III | See no. **2** |
| 55 | Robert of Sheering | – |
| 56 | Thomas of Croughton, son of Robert Newman of Fritwell | Aynho 36 |
| 57 | William de Turville | – |
| 58 | William de Turville | – |

* * *

Confirmaciones
Confirmacio capelle de *Crowltone*
Littera eiusdem
Carta fundatoris
Alia eiusdem
Confirmacio filii
Confirmacio alterius [f]ilii
Confirmacio eiusdem.
Iterum eiu<s>dem
Confirmacio comitis Willelmi
Confirmacio domini Linc'
Carta Radulphi clerici
Carta eiusdem uxoris Radulphi
Confirmacio Iohannis filii Roberti
Carta Rogeri de *Bray*
Confirmacio filii
Carta Walteri *Schamberleyn*
Confirmacio Godefridi
Confirmacio Widonis de Haya
Carta Roberti de Bello Monte et uxoris eius
Carta uxoris supradicti
Carta Roberti de Bello Monte et uxoris eius
Carta uxoris suprascripti
Carta Galfridi de Bello Monte
Confirmacio Ric(ardi) filii Osberti
Carta Roberti de *Frutewelle*
Confirmacio filii
Carta Mylonis *Neyrnut*
Carta Wydonis de Haya
Carta Wydonis de Haya
Carta supradicti
Carta de *Brakekele*
Carta Baldewyni de *Byfeld*
Carta uxoris eius super eodem
Confirmacio primogeniti eorum
Confirmacio alterius filii
Carta domini Cantuariensis
Carta donatoris capelle de *Crowltone*
Item donacio eiusdem
Confirmacio dicte capelle
Item confirmacio eiusdem
Item donacio dicte capelle
Item donacio eiusdem
Confirmacio capelle per dominum Lyncol'
Confirmacio eiusdem per capitulum Lyncol'
Carta Ri[car]di *Beu*[*m*]*unt* de V acris terre
Carta Roberti de *Scyringes* de dictis V acris terre domui de Aynho vendit'
Carta Paulini de *Merlawe* de tribus acris terre

**[Membrane 2]**

## PRIVILEGIA ET CARTE HOSPITALIS DE HAYNO

### 1

25 Oct [1202] – Lateran

### Privilegium Innocentii tertii

Innocentius[(a)] episcopus servus servorum Dei, dilecto filio T. procuratori do(mus) hospit(alis) sancti Iacobi de Hynno[(b)] et fratribus eiusdem loci, salutem et apostolicam benedictionem. Apostolice sedis clementia loca, que ad receptionem[(c)] pauperum Christi eorumque necessariam refectionem divine caritatis amore statuuntur propensius diligere consueuit et, ne pravorum hominum molestiis agitentur, speciali protec[tione munire. Quocirca,[(d)] dilecti] in Domino filii, attendentes domum, cui preesse dinosceris, ad pauperum et indigentium recreationem statut[am], domum ipsam(e) [cum omnibus bonis, que inpresentia]rum(f) iuste possidet aut in futurum iustis modis prestante Domino, poterit adipisci, sub beati Petri et nostra protect[ione suscipimus. Specialiter autem] capellam sancti Michaelis de *C(r)oult'*(g), unam hidam terre et dimidiam virgatam in Aynno, unum pratum quod vocatur *Refam* et unam virgatam terre in *Bifeld* et burgagium quod habetis in *Brakele*,(h) sicut hec omnia canonice adepti estis et pacifice possidetis, auctoritate apostolica vobis et domui vestre confirmamus et presentis scripti patrocinio communimus.(i) Statuentes ut vobis liceat capellam et cimiterium ad opus pauperorum et fratrum ibidem quiescentium seu discedentium(j) ac proprium capellanum, qui eis tantummodo divina officia celebret et sacramenta ecclesiastica ministret, sine(k) quolibet impedimento, habere. Cum autem generale fuerit interdictum terre, liceat vobis ianuis clausis, non pulsatis campanis, exclusis excommunicatis, et interdictis sub missa voce divina officia celebrare. Obeunte vero rectore eiusdem loci, vel tuorum quolibet sucsessorum,(l) nullus ibi qualibet subreptionis astutia seu violentia preponatur, nisi quem fratres communi assensu, vel fratrum pars consilii sanioris,(m) secundum Dei timorem providerint eligendum. Inhibemus ad hec, ne aliquis il[[los]],(n) qui se liberos(o) et absolutos predicte domui reddiderint et fratres ibidem mansuros statuerint, [[in person]]is vel in rebus indebite molestare aut illicita qualibet exactione gravare presumat. Preterea [[sepul]]turam pro fratribus et familia vestra, pauperibus hospitibusque et hiis, qui se domui vestre reddiderint, [[sa]]lvo iure matricis ecclesie, tibi et nominato hospitali nichilominus duximus indulgendam. Decernimus ergo ut [[nu]]lli omnino hominum fas sit hanc paginam nostre protectionis, constitutionis, ac prohibitionis infringere vel ei ausu temerario contraire.(p) Siquis autem hoc attemptare presumseri[t] indignationem omnipotentis Dei et beatorum Petri et Pauli apostolorum eius se noverit incursurum. Dat(um) Lateran(i), VIII(q) k(a)l(endas) novembris, pontificatus nostri(r) anno quinto.

(a) *Rubricated initial* I- *om. C.* — (b) Haynno *C.* — (c) refeptionem *C.* — (d) dilectione *struck through, C.* — (e) ipsam *inserted in interline above* ista, *struck through, B.* — (f) inrepresentiarum *with* re- *struck through, C.* — (g) Croulton' *C.* — (h) in Brak' quod habetis *B.* — (i) -ni- *inserted in interline, C.* — (j) descedentium *C.* — (k) sive *C.* — (l) sucsessore *BC.* — (m) consensusilii *with* -sensu- *struck through and* sanoris *corrected to* sanioris *with* san- *struck through and* sani- *inserted in interline, C.* — (n) *Double square brackets indicate text missing due to damage in C.* — (o) siliberos *BC.* — (p) contrarie *corrected to* contraire *with* -rie *struck through and* -ire *inserted in interline, C.* — (q) VIII[a] *C.* — (r) IIII *B*; quarto *C.*

## Privilege of Innocent III

Bishop Innocent, servant of the servants of God, [sends his] greeting and apostolic blessing to [his] beloved son T., proctor of the house of the hospital of St James of Aynho, and to the brothers of that same place. The mercy of the apostolic see has long been keen to favour places founded for the reception of Christ's poor and their necessary restoration with the love of Divine charity, and to safeguard them with special protection lest they be disturbed by the ingressions of wicked people. Wherefore, beloved sons in the Lord, we, recognising the house over which you are known to preside, established for the reception of the poor and needy, take that house under our and St Peter's protection, with all its goods, which it justly holds at present or that, the Lord being with you, it may in future be able to obtain by just means. Specifically, we confirm with apostolic authority to you and your house, and strengthen with the protection of this present writing, the chapel of St Michael of Croughton, one hide of land and half a virgate in Aynho, one meadow called *Refam* and one virgate of land in Byfield, and a burgage which you have in Brackley, just as you have canonically received and peacefully possess all this. Ordaining that it may be permitted for you to have a chapel and cemetery for the work of the poor and the brothers resting and dying there, and [for them] to have their own chaplain, who will celebrate the divine offices and administer the ecclesiastical sacraments only for them, without any impediment whatsoever. When the land is placed under a general interdict, however, you are permitted to keep the doors shut, not to ring the bells, [and] to exclude the excommunicated and interdicted from the saying of divine Mass. Upon the death of the rector of that place, or any of your successors, let none be promoted there by any kind of subtle contrivance or violence, but only he whom the brothers by common consent, or the wiser part of them, shall decide to elect in the fear of God. To this end, we forbid anyone should presume to harass unduly or burden in any unlawful manner, in persons or in things, those who have handed themselves over to the aforementioned house, free and absolved, and have resolved to stay as brothers there. Moreover, we have likewise decided to grant to you and the [afore]named hospital the [right of] burial for the brothers and your family, for the poor and guests, and for those who hand themselves over to your house, saving the rights of the mother church. We therefore decree that no one has the right to violate this our document of protection, statute, and prohibition or dare recklessly act against it. But if anyone should dare attempt this, let him know that he incurs the wrath of almighty God and of his blessed Apostles Peter and Paul. Given at the Lateran on the eighth kalends of November in the fifth year of our pontificate.

## 2

27 Nov [1215] – Lateran

**Litera eiusdem**

Innocentius[a] episcopus servus servorum Dei, universis Christi fidelibus per Cantuarien' provinciam constitutis ad quos presens scriptum pervenerit, salutem et apostolicam benedictionem. Q(uonia)m, ut ait apostolus, stabimus ante tribunal Domini responsivi prout gessimus in corpore, sive bonum sive malum, oportet nos diem messionis extreme misericordie operibus prevenire, et eter[n]orum intuitu ita seminare[b] in terris quod, reddente[c] Domino, cum multiplicato fructu recolligere debeamus in celis, firmam spem fiduciamque tenentes, q(uonia)m qui parce seminat, parce et metet, et qui seminat in benedictionibus, de benedictionibus et metet[d] <in> vitam eternam. Huic est quod cum dilectus filius Iordanus prior et procurator domus hospitalis de Haynno[e] et fratres ibidem commorantes, pauperes recipiant Christianos[f] eisdem liberaliter ministrantes. Set cum ad hoc proprie non suppetant facultates universitatem vestram[g] rogamus monemus et exhortamus in Domino vobis in remissionem peccatorum vestrorum iniungentes, quatinus cum idem prior vel fratres memorati sive eorum nuntii[h] ad vos venerint elemosinam petituri, vos[i] eos benigne exaudire[j] velitis, de bonis vobis[k] a Deo collatis eisdem liberaliter conferentes, ut per hec et alia beneficia que Domino inspirante feceritis[l] eterna gaudia consequi mereamini. Cunctis autem eidem priori sive fratribus supradictis vel eorum nuntiis aliqua beneficia conferentibus et specialiter omnibus qui a vigilia sancti Iacobi ecclesiam honore eius ibidem[m] constructam, usque ad octavum diem, cum cor[[de contrit]]o[n] et humiliato spiritu, ac elemosinis suis, visitauerint, quadraginta dies d[e] iniunctis sibi peniten[[tiis, a]]utoritate[o] beatorum Petri et Pauli meritis confidentes,[p] relaxamus. Dat(um) Laterani,[q] V[r] k(a)l(endas) decembris, pont[[ificatus <nostri> a]]nno octavo decimo.

(a) *Rubricated initial* I- *om. C.* — (b) sompniorum *corrected to* sominare (sic) *with expunging dot under* -p- *and* -ior' *struck through, and with* -i- *and* -are *inserted in interline, C.* — (c) reddempto *BC, with* -d- *inserted in interline, C.* — (d) et qui seminat … metet *om. B.* — (e) Aynno *C.* — (f) rcipiant *followed by* ibidem *with epxunging dots underneath, B.* — (g) nostram *B.* — (h) nuntii *inserted in interline above* memora *and* i(m)imici, *both struck through and the latter itself inserted in interline, C.* — (i) nos *BC.* — (j) exadire *B.* — (k) nobis *corrected to* vobis *with* n- *struck through and* v- *inserted in interline, C.* — (l) inspirantes *corrected to* inspirante *by* -s *struck through, and* fecerites *corrected to* feceritis *with expunging dot underneath final* -e- *and* -i- *inserted in interline B.* — (m) ibidem *inserted in interline, C.* — (n) *Double square brackets indicate text missing due to damage in C.* — (o) Domini *struck through, B.* — (p) confitentes *BC.* — (q) Lit(er)an(i) *BC.* — (r) V$^{a}$ *C.*

### Letter of the same

Bishop Innocent, servant of the servants of God, [sends his] greeting and apostolic blessing to all the faithful in Christ in the [archiepiscopal] province of Canterbury whom this document may reach. Because, as the apostle says, we will stand before the tribunal of the Lord to answer for what we have done in this [earthly] body, whether good or bad [2 Corinthians 5:10], it is proper that we prepare for the day of harvest [i.e., Judgement] with works of the utmost mercy, and to sow on earth, with a view to eternity, that which, with God repaying [it] with multiplied fruit, we ought to reap in heaven, keeping a firm hope and trust, since he who sows sparingly reaps sparingly, and he who sows bountifully will reap bountifully in [2 Corinthians 9:6] eternal life. This is why [our] beloved son Jordan, prior and proctor of the house of the hospital of Aynho, and the brothers dwelling there receive poor Christians, ministering liberally to them. But since the[ir] resources are not sufficient for this purpose, we beseech, admonish, and encourage you all in the [name of the] Lord [and] in remission of your sins, that whenever the same prior and the [afore]mentioned brothers or their envoys come to you requesting alms, you should listen to them kindly, giving to them liberally from the goods bestowed on you by God, so that you may merit joy everlasting through this and other benefits done through God's inspiration. Now, to all those conferring any benefits to the same prior or the aforementioned brothers or their envoys, and especially to all who, from the vigil of St James until the octave day, should visit the church built there in his honour, with a contrite heart and humble spirit, and with his alms, trusting in the authority and merits of blessed Peter and Paul, we remit forty days of penance enjoined to them. Given at the Lateran on the fifth kalends of December in the eighteenth year of our pontificate.

*Note*. This indulgence was issued three days before the closure of the Lateran Council. The use of the form *Quoniam ut ait* with regards to indulgences is discussed in Sayers, *Papal Government*, pp. 114–15 and Vincent, 'Pardoners' Tales', p. 53.

### 3

[*c*.1170]

### [Cart]a fundatoris

Rogerus filius Ricardi omnibus hominibus et amicis suis[(a)] francis et anglis, clericis et |[1]| laicis, presentibus et futuris, salutes. Sciatis me dedisse et concessisse et presenti carta mea |[2]| confirmasse Azuro servienti meo, pro servitio suo, unam virgatam terre in villa de |3| Aenho,(b) quam Robertus *le Brankere* tenuit cum omnibus eiusdem terre pertinentiis, et cum |4| masagio suo illi scilicet et heredibus suis tenendam de me et heredibus meis, in feo-|5|-do et hereditate, honorifice libere et quiete ab omnibus serviciis, et consuetudinibus, |6| et exactionibus, salvo servicio regis et comitis, reddendo(c) inde singulis annis V(d) |7| solidos ad IIII[or] terminos: ad festum sancti Michaelis XV(e) denarios, ad Natale(f) XV |8| denarios, ad Pasca XV denar(ios), ad festum sancti Iohannis XV den(arios). Quare volo et fir-|9|-miter precipio, quod Azurus prememoratus et heredes sui habeant et teneant terram iamdictam |10| cum omnibus pertinentiis suis in terra lucrabili, in pratis, in pasturis, et in omnibus aliis |11| libertatibus, et liberis consuetudinibus, bene et in pace, libere et quiete ab omnibus servitiis [de] |12| me et heredibus meis, per servicium prenominatum.(g) Testibus istis:(h) *Aeliz* de Esexa uxore |13| mea, Roberto filio meo, Waltero decano, Willelmo de Asinis, Roberto de Sancto Claro, |14| Rog(er)o filio Iohannis constab(ulario) Cestr(ie), *Albot*(i) *Pucin*, Michaele *Pucin*, Rad(ulfo) *Guer*, |15| Roberto de *Wigemor*, Gaufrido *Pucin*, Roberto *Wrange*, Ric(ardo) fratre eius, Turberno |16| persona de Aenho, Willelmo filio *Suain*, Philippo clerico, et multis aliis.

(a) suis *om. B.* — (b) Haynno *B.* — (c) redendo *B.* — (d) V[e] *B.* — (e) XV[cim] *B.* — (f) Domini *add. B.* — (g) *Corrected from* prenominatim *with expunging dot under* -i- *and* -u- *in superscript, B.* — (h) *B ends here.* — (i) *This reading is uncertain.*

### The founder's charter

Roger, son of Richard, [sends his] greetings to all his men and friends, [both] French and English, clerks and laypeople, present and future. Know that I have given, conceded, and confirmed with this my present charter to my servant Azurus, for his service, one virgate of land in the vill of Aynho, which Robert le Brankere held, with everything pertaining to that same land, and with its messuage, to be held by him and his heirs from me and my heirs, in fief and inheritance, fittingly, free and quit from all services, customs, and exactions, saving the king's and earl's service, thence rendering 5s each year on four occasions: 15d at the feast of St Michael, 15d at Christmas, 15d at Easter, [and] 15d at the feast of St John. I therefore wish and firmly instruct that the aforementioned Azurus and his heirs have and hold the said land with everything pertaining to it in profitable land, in meadows, in pastures, and in all other freedoms and free customs, well and in peace, free and quit from all services, from me and my heirs on account of the aforementioned service. With these witnesses: my wife Alice of Essex; my son Robert; Walter the dean; William de *Asinis*; Robert de St Clere; Roger, son of John the constable of Chester; Albot Pucin; Michael Pucin; Ralph Guer; Robert of Wigmoor; Geoffrey Pucin; Robert Wrange [and] his brother, Richard; Turbern, parson of Aynho; William, son of Svein; Philip the clerk; and many others.

*Original.* MCA, Aynho 21. Endorsed: Rog(erus) filius Ric(ardi). Auzur(us). Aynho (s.xv); Eynno (s.xv). Dimensions: 146 × 192 + 30 mm. Sealed *sur double queue*, parchment tag through three slits, seal impression missing.

*Note.* It is unclear what connection this charter has to Aynho Hospital, save for the fact that it concerns land in that vill. Macray dated this act *c.*1170 × 1180, but it presumably predates no. **4**. Robert de St Clere is among the witnesses of Earl William's acts of 1170 granting Aynho to Roger Fitz Richard.

## 4

[1170 × 20 Feb 1171]

### [Alia] eiusdem

Rog(erus) filius Ric(ardi), Linco[lniens]i episcopo et universis sancte matris ecclesie filiis, presentibus et futuris, salutem. |[1]| Sciatis me dedisse i[n hos]pitalitatem Deo et sancte Marie et sancto Iacobo dimidiam hidam terre in |[2]| Ainho,[a] illam scilicet[b] dimi[di]am hidam quam *Turbern*[c] tenuit, et aliam dimidiam hidam terre quam *Suein*[d] |[3]| tenuit in puram et perpetu[am] elemosinam, ad hospitandum pauperes fratres qui hospitium ibi pro amore |[4]| Dei petierint, in bosco, [in] plano, in pratis, in pasturis, in viis, in semitis, in molendinis, et in omnibus al[iis] |[5]| liberis consuetudinibus et libertatibus, liberas[e] et quietas ab omnibus secularibus servi[ciis] ad me et heredes meos |[6]| pertinentibus. Et hanc do[n]ationem feci concessu[f] Willelmi filii mei et Roberti, pro salute anime mee et pro anima |[7]| com(itis) Gaufr(idi), et pro salut[e] anime com(itis) Willelmi, et pro salute anime *Alize*[g] sponse mee, et pro salute anime |[8]| Willelmi filii mei et Roberti [filii] mei et *Alize* filie mee, et pro animabus omnium antecessorum meorum. His t(estibus):[h] |[9]| Iohanne constab(ularii) Cestrie, [Turber]to persona, Waltero capellano, Willelmo de *Adles*, Roberto de *Seint Cler*, |[10]| Stephano fratre comite de *[Rich]emu(n)d*, Adam de *Duttun'*, Willelmo *Patric*, Roberto filio Rog(er)i, Willelmo |[11]| de *Ca(n)vile*, Rog(er)o *Bur[du]n*, Willelmo *Legat*, Hugone filio Rad(ulfi), Ada(m) de *Roing'*, Osberto maresc(allo).

(a) Haynno *B.* — (b) silicet *B.* — (c) Thurbern, *with first* -r- *inserted in interline B.* — (d) Sueyn *B.* — (e) libera *B.* — (f) consessu B. — (g) Alicie B. — (h) *B ends here.*

## Another of the same

Roger, son of Richard, [sends his] greeting to the bishop of Lincoln and all children of the holy mother Church, present and future. Know that I have given in hospitality to God, St Mary, and St James half a hide of land in Aynho, namely that half a hide which Turbern held, and another half a hide of land that Svein held, in pure and perpetual alms, for sheltering poor brothers seeking to be received there for the love of God, in woodland, open land, meadows, pastures, roads, paths, mills, and in all other free customs and freedoms, free and quit of all secular services pertaining to me and my heirs. And I have made this donation with the consent of my son[s] William and Robert, for the salvation of my soul and the souls of Earl Geoffrey, Earl William, my betrothed Alice, my sons William and Robert and my daughter Alice, and all my ancestors. With these witnesses: John, constable of Chester; Turbern the parson; Walter the chaplain; William de *Adles*; Robert de St Clere; Stephen, brother of the earl of Richmond; Adam of Dutton; William Patric; Robert, son of Roger; William de Canville; Roger Burdun; William Legat; Hugh, son of Ralph; Adam of Roding; Osbert the marshal.

*Original.* MCA, Aynho 71. Endorsed: Rog(erus) filius Ric(ardi). Aynho (s.xv). Dimensions: 140 × 78 + 10 mm. Sealed *sur double queue*, tag and seal impression missing.

*Note.* Dated *c.*1180 × 1190 by Macray, but it is much earlier. The *terminus a quo* is determined by the grant of Aynho to Roger Fitz Richard in that year by the earl of Essex. The witness Stephen, brother of the earl of Richmond, is a little-known illegitimate son of Alan, 1st Earl of Richmond. His brother, Conan IV, duke of Brittany and earl of Richmond, died on 20 February 1171, providing the *terminus ad quem*. For Adam of Dutton, who witnesses this act as a member of the retinue of John, constable of Chester, see *Early Ches. Charts.*, pp. 21–2. Other witnesses of the act above were also part of John's entourage, including, perhaps, the aforementioned Stephen, since he appears alongside William Patric, William de Canville, Roger Burdun, and William Legat in a charter by which the constable grants land to Adam of Dutton (ibid., no. 6, p. 14), although it is possible that this act and the one above were issued at the same time.[1] William Legat was a scribe of the constable's charters (Hodson, 'Last Witness', pp. 73–4), but this act is not in his hand.

1 John's charter is also witnessed by a Robert, son of Roger, whom Geoffrey Barraclough identifies as a son of Roger, son of Alured de Cumbray: *Early Ches. Charts.*, p. 15. It seems more likely, however, that this individual is John's brother-in-law, Robert Fitz Roger, and that his act, which Barraclough dates 1172 × 1181, was issued around the same time as Roger Fitz Richard's act for Aynho.

## 5

[1170/1 × *c*.1180, perhaps *c*.1170/1]

### Confirmatio filii

Sciant presentes et futuri quod ego Willelmus filius Rog(er)i concedo et confirmo et ratam habeo donationem quam pater meus fecit hospitali sancti Ia(cobi) in Haynno de dimidia hida terre que fuit *Thurbern* et dimidiam hidam terre que fuit *Sueyn*, in Haynno, sicut confirma<vi>t ei[a] pater meus per cartam suam, liberas et quietas ab omni seculari servicio quod ad dominium ipsius ville pertinet, ut de exitu illius terre habeant necessario pauperes hospitari querentes propter Deum, et ut nichil in alios[b] usus transferatur, nisi tamen in usus pauperorum. Hoc feci pro salute anime com(itis) Gaufr(idi) domini fundi et anime patris mei et matris et omnium vivorum et defunctorum parentum meorum. His t(estibus).

(a) eis *with expunging dot under* -s, *B.* — (b) alienos B.

### The son's confirmation

May all present and future know that I, William, son of Roger, concede and confirm and consider valid the donation my father has made to the hospital of St James in Aynho of half a hide of land that was Turbern's and half a hide of land that was Svein's, [both] in Aynho, as my father has confirmed by his charter, free and quit from all secular service pertaining to the demesne of that vill, so that from the revenue of that land the poor seeking hospitality with God may have what is necessary, and so that nothing is transferred to other uses except for the use of the poor. This I did for the salvation of the soul of Earl Geoffrey, lord of the fee, and the soul of my father, and [those] of my mother and all my relations alive and dead. With these witnesses.

*Note*. This act is difficult to date precisely without a witness list. However, the statement that William confirmed his father's donation for the soul of Geoffrey (III) de Mandeville, earl of Essex and 'lord of the fee', who died in 1166, echoes the sentiment of his father's act above (no. **4**). It is possible that Geoffrey's name appears in error, with the Aynho cartularist misreading an abbreviated form of William de Mandeville's name, which in the Latin could also begin with the letter 'G' ('Guillelmus'). If this were so, then this charter would have been issued before the earl of Essex's death in 1189. If the reference to Geoffrey is taken as correct, which seems more likely, then it would suggest William Fitz Roger issued this act shortly after Aynho Hospital's foundation and thus closer, chronologically, to Geoffrey de Mandeville's death a few years earlier. As discussed in Chapter 1, it is likely that William Fitz Roger issued this confirmation as heir to his mother's inheritance, giving his consent to the hospital's foundation within a manor that would one day pass to him.

## 6

[*c*.1180 × 14 Nov 1189, likely *c*.1180 × 25 May 1186]

### Confirmatio alterius filii

Venerabilibus dominis et amicis episcopo Lincolniensi, comiti Willelmo, et omnibus amicis et hominibus suis francis et anglis, Willelmus filius Rog(er)i, salutem. Notum sit vobis me |1| dedisse et hac[a] presenti carta mea[b] confirmasse Deo et hospitali sancti Iacobi in Haino[c] dim(idiam)[d] hidam terre que fuit Turberni,[e] quam pater meus et mater mea dederunt eidem |2| hospitali, et in incrementum donationis eorum ego do eidem hospitali dimidiam hidam que fuit Sueini.[f] Et has omnes terras do ei[g] liberas ab omni seculari |3| servicio, cum omnibus sibi pertinentiis, sicut aliquis plenius tenuit illud tenementum ante eos. Quare volo quod predictum hospitale in usum pauperum qui illuc |4| devenient hospitaturi, teneant predictas terras liberas et quietas ab omni seculari servicio, pro salute anime patris et matris mee, et domini mei comitis[h] |5| Willelmi et omnium amicorum meorum tam vivorum quam mortuorum. Testibus his:[i] Willelmo de *Ver*, Willelmo filio Nicholai de *Writle*, Rog(er)o filio Iohannis |6| constabularii de *Cestre*, Roberto de *Sencler*, Ada(m) de *Roinges*, Hugone filio Rad(ulfi), Willelmo camerario Willelmi de *V(er)*, Gileberto pincerna Willelmi de *V(er)*, |7| Roberto de *Burgate*, Teobaldo, Ric(ardo) f[i]lio Nicholai de *Writle*.

(a) ac *B*. — (b) mea *om. B*. — (c) Haynno B. — (d) dim(idiam) *inserted in interline, A*. — (e) Turbern *B*. — (f) Sueyn *B*. — (g) eis *corrected with expunging dot beneath* -s *A*; eis *B*. — (h) com<i>tis *B*. — (i) *B has* His testibus *and ends here.*

### The other son's confirmation

William, son of Roger, [sends his] greeting to [his] venerable lords and friends, the bishop of Lincoln, Earl William, and all [his] men and friends [both] French and English. May it be known to you that I have given and confirmed with this my present charter to God and the hospital of St James in Aynho half a hide of land that was Turbern's, which my father and mother gave to the same hospital, and increasing their donation I give to the same hospital half a hide of land that was Svein's. And all these lands I give to them free from all secular service, with all their appurtenances, just as all others have clearly held this tenement before them. I therefore wish that the aforementioned hospital holds the aforementioned lands free and quit from all secular service for use by the poor who seek hospitality there, for the salvation of my father's soul, and [those] of my mother, my lord Earl William, and all my friends alive and dead. With these witnesses:

William de Vere; William, son of Nicholas of Writtle; Roger, son of John the constable of Chester; Robert de St Clere; Adam of Roding; Hugh, son of Ralph; William, chamberlain of William de V[ere]; Gilbert, cupbearer of William de V[ere]; Robert of Burgate; Theobald; Richard, son of Nicholas of Writtle.

*Original.* MCA, Aynho 31. Endorsed: W. filius Rog(eri). Aynho. Comiti Willelmo (s.xv). Dimensions: 261 × 63/40 mm. Sealed *sur simple queue*; tongue 236 mm, seal impression missing. Wrapping tie fragment.

*Note.* Dated by Macray *c.*1180 × 1190, but the reference to William de Mandeville, earl of Essex, means it must have been issued before his death on 14 November 1189. If the first witness in the list is William Fitz Roger's uncle, William de Vere, later bishop of Hereford, as seems likely, then it would appear the charter was issued before his election to that post on 25 May 1186. As bishop, William is known to have had a chamberlain called William, although it seems unlikely that this is the chamberlain by that name among the witnesses here, as the William who served his episcopal namesake also served William de Vere's predecessor, Robert Foliot (1174–86) (*EEA*, vol. 7, pp. lviii–lix). Robert of Burgate is a member of that family who held the manor of Burgate, Suffolk, from the earls of Oxford (V. Brown (ed.), *Eye Priory Cartulary and Charters* (2 vols, Woodbridge, 1992–4), vol. 2, p. 47). He is likely the individual by that name whose seal is affixed to two charters in the British Library (W. de G. Birch, *Catalogue of Seals in the Department of Manuscripts in the British Museum* (6 vols, London, 1887–1900), vol. 2, nos. 7606–7, p. 529).

## 7

[1190 × *c.*1192, perhaps 1190]

### Confirmatio filii

Noverint tam presentes quam futuri, quod ego Robertus filius Rog(er)i concedo |1| et confirmo et ratam habeo donationem quam pater meus fecit hos-|2|-pitali sancti Iacobi in Ainho[a] de una[b] hida terre cum omnibus perti-|3|-nentiis suis, scilicet de dimidia hyda[c] terre que[d] fuit Thurberni et de |4| dimidia hyda[e] terre que fuit Sweini,[f] in Ainho,[g] sicut carta patris |5| mei testatur, liberam et quietam ab omni seculari servicio quod ad dominium |6| ipsius **[Membrane 3]** ville pertinet, in puram et liberam et perpetuam elemosinam, ad hospi-|7|-tandum pauperes qui ibi hospitium pro amore Dei petierint. Preterea do |8| et concedo et presenti carta mea confirmo predicto hospitali sancti Iacobi in |9| Ainho[h] quoddam mesagium, quod fuit Willelmi filii *Thoke*,[i] in liberam et |10| puram[j] et perpetuam elemosinam, pro[k] salute anime mee et omnium antecessorum |11| meorum. Quare volo et firmiter precipio quod predictum hospitale terras prenominatas |12|

teneat libere, honorifice et quiete, sicut pater meus unquam eas tenuit |[13]| melius liberius honorificentius et quietius.[l] Hiis[m] testibus:[n] Willelmo de *Pirhowe*, Ro-|[14]]-berto de Sancto Claro, Waltero Guntardo, Olivero monacho, Rog(er)o de Creissi, |[15]| Galfr(ido) filio Iohannis const(abularii) Cestrie, Willelmo de Marisni, Galfr(ido) *Puci*(*n*), Iohanne de Furn(ingho).

(a) Aynno *B.* — (b) hida *with expunging dots underneath, B.* — (c) hida *B.* — (d) que *inserted in interline, B.* — (e) hida *B.* — (f) Sueyn *B.* — (g) Haynno *B.* — (h) Aynno *B.* — (i) Hoke *B.* — (j) purram *B.* — (k) p<ro> *B.* — (l) *Corrected from* quietis *with* -u- *inserted in interline, B.* — (m) His *B.* — (n) *B ends here.*

### The son's confirmation

May all present and future know that I, Robert, son of Roger, concede, confirm, and consider valid the donation my father has made to the hospital of St James in Aynho of one hide of land with everything pertaining to it, namely of half a hide of land that was Turbern's and half a hide of land that was Svein's, [both] in Aynho, as my father's charter testifies, free and quit from all secular service pertaining to the demesne of that vill, in pure, free, and perpetual alms for sheltering the poor who seek hospitality there for the love of God. I also give, concede, and confirm with my present charter to the aforementioned hospital of St James in Aynho a certain messuage that was William's, son of Hoke, in free and pure and perpetual alms, for the salvation of my soul and the souls of all my ancestors. I therefore wish and firmly instruct that the aforementioned hospital should hold the aforementioned lands freely, fittingly, and peacefully, just as my father once held them right freely, fittingly, and peacefully. With these witnesses: William of Perio; Robert de St Clere; Walter Guntard; Oliver the monk; Roger de Cressy; Geoffrey, son of John the constable of Chester; William de *Marisni*; Geoffrey Pucin; John of Farthinghoe.

*Original.* MCA, Aynho 19. Endorsed: Confirmatio Rob(erti) f(ilii) Rog(eri) (s.xv); Ayno (s.xvii). Dimensions: 143 × 119 + 13 mm. Sealed *sur double queue*, parchment tag through three slits. Seal: round, fragmentary, white wax painted brown: 54 mm. A knight on horseback (head and hands destroyed). Legend: destroyed. Counterseal: oval, 24 mm. Indistinct, perhaps the Flight into Egypt or St Martin Dividing His Cloak. Legend: ✠ [S]IG[I]LLVM S[ECRETVM].

*Note.* Dated by Macray *c.*1190 × 1200, but must have been issued before *c.*1192, as the donation of the messuage formerly belonging to William, son of Hoke, was confirmed by Hugh, bishop of Lincoln, around 1192 (and certainly no later than March 1195, no. **11**). The presence of Robert's stepson, Roger de Cressy, among the witnesses suggests Robert was already married to Roger's mother, Margaret de Chesney. They were betrothed before Michaelmas 1190. The presence of his nephew, Geoffrey, whose father died on crusade in 1190, also suggests a date close to this year. Perio (also sometimes referred to in the literature as Pirho) was later home to a medieval hospital (VCH, *Northampton*, vol. 2, p. 163).

## 8

[*c*.1191 × 1200/7]

### Confirmatio eiusdem

Omnibus sancte matris ecclesie filiis ad quos presens carta pervenerit, Robertus filius Rog(eri), salutem. Noverit |[1]| universitas vestra me caritatis intuitu et pro anima patris mei Rog(eri) et matris *Aliz* et fratris mei Willelmi, |[2]| et pro salute anime mee et uxoris mee, Marg(arite), et omnium antecessorum meorum, concessisse et dedisse et |[3]| hac presenti carta mea confirmasse Deo et beate Marie et beato Iacobo et hospitali de Aino,[(a)] |[4]| in puram et perpetuam elemosinam et omni seculari actione liberam, unam dimidiam virgatam terre |[5]| in Aino[(b)] quam tenuit Elwinus porcarius, que iacet inter terras cotariorum, tenendam de me et heredibus |[6]| meis, libere et quiete, in bosco et in plano, in pascuis et in pratis, in viis et semitis, et in omnibus |[7]| que ad eandem dimidiam virgatam pertinent. Et ut hec donatio mea firma et inconcussa permaneat, eam sigilli mei appositione coroboravi. His t(estibus):[(c)] Willelmo filio Rocelini, Roberto de Sancto *Cler*, Wal-|[8]|-tero *Guttard'*, Olivero monaco, Ad(am) Daco, magister Simone, Rog(ero) de C(re)ssi, Iohanne filio Roberti, et multis aliis.

(a) Haymno *B*. — (b) Hainno, *with* -a- *inserted in interline B*. — (c) *B ends here.*

### Confirmation of the same

Robert, son of Roger, [sends his] greeting to all children of the holy mother Church whom this present charter may reach. May you all know that I have conceded, given, and confirmed with this my present charter, for charity's sake and for the salvation of the souls of my father Roger, my mother Alice, and my brother William, and for my own soul and [those] of my wife Margaret, and of all my ancestors, to God, blessed Mary, blessed James, and the hospital of Aynho, in pure and perpetual alms, and free from all secular service, half a virgate of land in Aynho that Elwin the swineherd held, which lies between the lands of the cottagers, to be held from me and my heirs, free and quit, in woodland and open land, in pastures and meadows, in roads and paths, and in all else that pertains to that half a virgate. And so that this my donation remains valid and intact, I have corroborated it with the affixing of my seal. With these witnesses: William, son of Rocelin;

Robert de St Clere; Walter Guttard'; Oliver the monk; Adam Daco; Master Simon; Roger de Cressy; John, son of Robert; and many others.

*Original.* MCA, Aynho 32. Endorsed: Robertus filius Rog(eri). Aynho (s.xv). Dimensions: 190 × 87/79 + 10 mm. Sealed *sur double queue*, parchment tag through one slit, seal impression missing.

*Note.* Dated by Macray *c.*1180 × 1190, but must be from around 1190, since the charter mention's Robert's wife, Margaret, to whom he was married by Michaelmas that year, her first husband having died in 1188/9. The final two witnesses are Robert's stepson and his son by Margaret, the latter of whom was likely born around 1191, which provides the *terminus a quo*. The *terminus ad quem* is harder to determine, although Roger de Cressy came of age in 1207 and cannot be found in his stepfather's retinue after that date.

## 9

[*c.*1185 × 22 Nov 1214, perhaps *c.*1185/6 × 1190]

### Iterum eiusdem

Omnibus Christi fidelibus ad quos presens carta pervenerit, Robertus filius Rog(eri), salutem. Sciatis me concessisse et dedisse et presenti carta mea confirmasse, pro salute anime mee et antecessorum meorum, Deo et beate Marie et hosp(itali) beati Iacobi de Haynno, in puram et perpetuam elem(osinam), pratum quod vocatur *Refam*, que iacet inter pratum de *Croult'* et pratum hominium de Haynno et pasturam meam dominicam que vocatur *Stenirul*, habendum et tenendum de me et heredibus meis, sine ulla contradictione mei vel heredum meorum, bene <et> in pace, libere et quiete ab omni consuetudine et seculari exactione. Consessi vero similiter Deo et beate Marie et hosp(itali) iamdicto, pro salute anime mee et antecessorum meorum, pasturam decem bovum et quatuor affrorum,[a] cum bobus meis in dominica mea pastura et in aliis meis pasturis omnibus ubi boves mei dominici se pascentur, sine omnia[b] contradictione mei vel heredum meorum. Et ne aliquis huic concessioni et donationi et confirmationi mee contraire presumat, hanc cartam meam sigilli mei munimine duxi confirmandam. His testibus.

(a) aurorum *B.* – (b) omnim *with* -a *inserted in interline above* -m, *not erased, B.*

### Another of the same

Robert, son of Roger, [sends his] greeting to all the faithful in Christ whom this present charter may reach. Know that I have conceded, given, and confirmed with this my present charter, for the salvation of my soul and [those] of my ancestors, to God, blessed Mary, and the hospital of St James of Aynho, in pure and perpetual alms, the meadow known as *Refam*, which lies between the meadow of Croughton and that of the people of Aynho, and my demesne pasture called *Stenirul*, to have and to hold from me and my heirs, without any objection from me or my heirs, well and in peace, free and quit of all custom and secular exaction. I have likewise conceded to God, blessed Mary, and the aforementioned hospital, for the salvation of my soul and [those] of my ancestors, the pasture of ten oxen and four draught horses, together with my oxen in my demesne pasture and in all my other pastures, wherever my demesne oxen graze, without any objection from me or my heirs. And to ensure that nobody presumes to contradict this my concession, donation, and confirmation, I have thought fit that this charter be fortified with the protection of my seal. With these witnesses.

*Note*. This act is difficult to date precisely without a witness list. The broad parameters are therefore the date by which Robert's father was dead and Robert's own death. However, the fact that this charter makes no mention of Robert's wife, nor his son, as is the case in no. **8**, may suggest that it dates from before his marriage to Margaret de Chesney.

## 10

[*c*.1180 × 14 Nov 1189, perhaps *c*.1185/6]

### Confirmatio co[m]itis [W]illelmi

Willelmus de *Mandevill'*, comes *Essex'*, omnibus hominibus suis francis et anglis, presentibus et futuris, salutem. Notum v{obis sit} me conces-|1|-sisse et hac presenti mea carta[a] confirmasse donationem quam Rog(erus)[b] filius Ri(cardi) et Aelicia[c] uxor sua et Willelmus filius e{orum do}naverunt hospi-|2|-tali sancti Iacobi in Haino,[d] pro salute[e] omnium amicorum suorum tam vivorum quam defunctorum, salvo serviti{o} meo, scilicet dimidiam hide |3| que fuit *Swein*[f] et dim(idiam) hide que fuit T(ur)b(er)ti[g] fratris sui. Testibus istis:[h] Iohanne de *Rokell'*, Hasculfo capell(ano), Roberto filio Rog(eri), Iohanne de *La*(*m*)*born*(*e*), |4| Hugone capell(ano), Willelmo de *Hairon*, Silvestro filio Sim(onis), Ric(ardo) de *P*(*er*)*tenhal'*, et multis aliis.

(a) carta mea *B*. — (b) Robertus *B*. — (c) Alicia *B*. — (d) Hayno *B*. — (e) anime *struck through, B*. — (f) Sueyn *B*. — (g) Turbern *B*. — (h) *B has* His test(ibus) *and ends here.*

### Earl William's confirmation

William de Mandeville, earl of Essex, [sends his] greeting to all his men, [both] French and English, present and future. May it be known to you that I have conceded and confirmed with this my present charter the donation that Roger, son of Richard, his wife Alice, and their son William have given to the hospital of St James in Aynho for the salvation of all their friends alive and dead, saving the service due me, namely half a hide that was Svein's and half a hide that was Turbert's, his brother's. With these witnesses: John de Rochella; Hasculph the chaplain; Robert, son of Roger; John of Lambourne; Hugh the chaplain; William de Hairon; Sylvester, son of Simon; Richard of Pertenhall; and many others.

*Original.* MCA, Aynho 49. Endorsed: Confirmatio Willelmi Mandevill'. Comes. Aynho (s.xv). Dimensions: 220 × 64 + 23 mm. Sealed *sur double queue* on green cords through three holes. Seal: round, fragmentary, white wax painted brown: approx. 78 mm. A knight on horseback, sword in right hand and shield in left, the rear legs of the horse thrust out behind it. Legend: [...] [COME]S ESSE[X]I/E.

*Note.* Dated by Macray *c.*1180 × 1190 but must have been issued before the earl's death on 14 November 1189. Since it identifies William Fitz Roger as a donor to the hospital, it must have been issued after no. **6**. Also cf. the discussion above (Chapter 2). Hasculph the chaplain is presumably to be identified with the chaplain by that name who attempted to divert the funeral of William's father to Chicksands (Greenway and Watkiss (eds), *Walden Monastery*, p. 40). The seal is William's second, being closely modelled on that of his friend, Philip I, count of Flanders (1168–91), with whom he went on crusade in 1177/8. John of Lambourne died at the siege of Acre in 1190 (Bennett, *Elite Participation*, p. 333).

## 11

[*c.*1192 × ? Mar 1195]

### Confirmatio domini Lincoln[ie]ns'

Omnibus Christi fidelibus ad quos presens scriptum pervenerit, Hugo Dei gratia Linc(olniensis) episcopus, salutem in vero salutari. Noverit universitas |1| vestra nos ratam et gratam habere donationem f[acta]m a Rog(er)o filio Ricardi et a Roberto filio eiusdem Rog(er)i, hospitali sancti Iacobi in |2| Ainho[(a)] super una hida terre in Ainho,[(b)] v[idelicet] una dim(idia) hida que fuit Turberni[(c)] et dim(idia) hida[(d)] que fuit Sweini,[(e)] in liberam, et puram, |3| et perpetuam elemosinam, et quietam ab [omn]i seculari servitio quod ad dominium ipsius ville pertinet. Preterea gratam et ratam habemus

|4| donationem factam a prefato Roberto filio Rog(er)i eidem hospitali super quodam mesagio in supradicta villa de Ainho,[f] videlicet quod fuit |5| Willelmi filii *Toke*,[g] in liberam, puram, et perp[etu]am elemosinam, ei concessam, ad hospitandum pauperes qui ibi hospicium pro amore Dei petierint. |6| Hec omnia predicta sicut supradicto hospitali [rationa]biliter collata sunt cum omnibus pertinentiis suis velud[h] in cartis predictorum donatorum continentur, |7| ei auctoritate qua fungimur presenti scrip[to et] sigilli nostri patrocinio confirmamus. Hiis[i] testibus:[j] Haim(one) decano Linc(olniensis) ecclesie, Roberto *Hu*(*n*)-|8|-*tedon*' et magistro Rog(er)o Leircestren', archidiaconis, magistro Ric(ardo) de Swalewecliva, Ingelramo capellano, Roberto de Capella, |9| Hugone de Sancto Edwardo, Willelmo cl[erico d]ecani, Hugone de *Rolveston*', Eustachio de *Wilton*', et aliis multis.

(a) Haynno, *with* -a- *inserted in interline B.* — (b) Aynno *B.* — (c) Thurber' *B.* — (d) terre *add B.* — (e) Suey' *B.* — (f) Hayno *B.* — (g) Thoke *B.* — (h) velut *B.* — (i) His *B.* — (j) *B ends here.*

## The lord [bishop] of Lincoln's confirmation

Hugh, by God's grace bishop of Lincoln, [sends his] greeting in true salvation to all the faithful in Christ whom this present document may reach. May you all know that we consider valid and pleasing the donation made by Roger, son of Richard, and by Robert, son of the same Roger, to the hospital of St James in Aynho of one hide of land in Aynho, namely half a hide that was Turbern's and half a hide that was Svein's, in free, pure, and perpetual alms, and free from all secular service that pertains to the demesne of that vill. We also consider pleasing and valid the donation made by the aforementioned Robert, son of Roger, to the same hospital of a certain messuage in the aforementioned vill of Aynho, namely that which was William's, son of Toke, in free, pure, and perpetual alms, [which was] granted to it for sheltering the poor seeking hospitality there for the love of God. All the above were granted to the aforementioned hospital in accordance with reason, and with everything pertaining to them, as is contained in the charters of the aforementioned donors, and we confirm them with the authority of the present document and the protection of our seal. With these witnesses: Haimo, dean of the church of Lincoln; Robert of Huntingdon and Master Roger of Leicester, archdeacons; Master Richard of Swalecliffe; Ingelram the chaplain; Robert de Capella; Hugh de St Edward; William, the dean's clerk; Hugh of Rolleston; Eustache of Wilton; and many others.

*Original.* MCA, Aynho 22. Endorsed: Facta est collatio per I. Cyrencestr' (s.xiii, preceded and followed by notary's signs?). Dimensions: 185 × 102 + 15 mm. Sealed *sur double queue*, tag and seal impression missing. Pd from A in *EEA*, vol. 4, no. 8, pp. 5–6.

*Note.* The dates are those of Roger [of Rolleston], archdeacon of Leicester (see *EEA*, vol. 4, no. 11, pp. 8–9 for discussion).

## 12

[Nov 1214 × 1232, perhaps Nov 1214 × *c.*1220]

### Carta Radulfi clerici

Omnibus Christi fidelibus ad quos presens scriptum pervenerit, ego Radulfus, clericus de Hayno, salutem in Domino. Universitati vestre notum[(a)] facio me, divine pietatis intuitu, et ob anime mee medelam, concessisse et dedissse Deo et fratribus hosp(italis) beatorum apostolorum Iacobi et Iohannis de Hayno unam virgatam terre in villa de Hayno, cum mesuagio et cum pertinenciis, et insimul corpus meum ibidem cum eisdem fratribus ad Deo serviendum in perpetuum constitui, salvo servitio domini regis, et salvo redditu domini de Hayno, annuatim scilicet quinque solidos ad quatuor terminos statutos, videlicet ad Natale Domini XV den(arios), et ad annunciationem beate Marie XV den(a)r(ios), et ad nativitate beati Iohannis XV denar(ios), et ad festum sancti Michaelis XV denar(ios). Et ne hoc ab aliquibus[(b)] in irritum possit revocari, presentem cartam Iordano predicti hosp(italis) magistro et fratribus ididem Deo ministrantibus, sigillo meo confirmavi. His testibus.

(a) vobis *struck through, B.* — (b) *Corrected from* aliq(uo)s *with expunging dot under* -s, *and* -ibus *inserted in interline B.*

### Ralph the clerk's charter

I, Ralph, clerk of Aynho, [send my] greeting in the Lord to all the faithful in Christ whom this present document may reach. I make it known to you all that, for the sake of holy piety and for the cure of my soul, I have conceded and given to God and the brothers of the hospital of the blessed Apostles James and John of Aynho one virgate of land in the vill of Aynho, with a messuage and what pertains to it, and I have established my body in company with the same brothers in that place to serve God in perpetuity, saving the king's service and the lord of Aynho's rent, namely 5s payable each year on four occasions, namely 15d at Christmas, 15d at the Annunciation of the blessed Mary, 15d at the nativity of blessed John, and 15d at the feast of St Michael. And lest this be recalled or rendered invalid by anyone, I have confirmed the present charter to Jordan, master of the aforementioned hospital, and the brothers who serve God there, with my seal. With these witnesses.

*Note*. This donation was confirmed by John (I) Fitz Robert (no. **14**), who succeeded his father in November 1214. The *terminus ad quem* of the broader date range is the presentation of Peter of Maldon as master of Aynho Hospital. Ralph does not appear in the record beyond *c.*1220 (no. **29**), which provides the *terminus ad quem* of the narrower dates.

## 13

[Nov 1214 × 1232, perhaps Nov 1214 × *c.*1220]

### Carta uxoris [eius]dem Radulfi

Omnibus Christi fidelibus ad quos presens scriptum pervenerit, ego Matildis, uxor Radulfi, clerici de Hayno, salutem in Domino. Univer[sitati vestre] notum facio me, divine pietatis intuitu, et ob anime mee medelam, concessisse et dedissse Deo et fratribus hosp(italis) sancti Iaco[bi et sancti Iohannis] beatorum apostolorum de Hayno, unam virgatam terre in villa de Hayno, cum pertinenciis, quam Hugo, frater meus, dedit Rad[ulfo ma]rito meo et mihi in liberum maritagium, et insimul corpus meum ibidem cum eisdem fratribus ad serviendum Deo in perpetuum constit[ui], salvo servitio domini regis, et salvo redditu domini de villa de Hayno, scilicet annuatim quinque solidos ad quatuor terminos statutos, videlicet ad Natale Domini XV den(arios), et ad annunciationem beate Mar(ie) XV d(enarios), et ad nativitate beati Iohannis XV d(enarios), et ad festum sancti Michaelis[(a)] XV den(arios). Et ne hoc ab aliquibus in irritum possit revocari, presentem cartam Iordano hosp(italis) predicti magistro et fratribus ibidem Deo ministrantibus, sigillo meo confirmavi. His test(ibus).

(a) -h- *of* Michaelis *inserted in interline, B.*

### Charter of the same Ralph's wife

I, Matilda, wife of Ralph, clerk of Aynho, [send my] greeting in the Lord to all the faithful in Christ whom this present document may reach. I make it known to you all that, for the sake of holy piety and for the cure of my soul, I have conceded and given to God and the brothers of the hospital of the blessed Apostles St James and St John of Aynho one virgate of land in the vill of Aynho, with its appurtenances, which Hugh, my brother, gave to my husband Ralph and to me in frank-marriage, and I have established my body in company with the same brothers in that place to serve God in perpetuity, saving the king's service and the lord of the vill of Aynho's rent, namely 5s payable each year on four occasions, namely 15d at Christmas,

15d at the Annunciation of the blessed Mary, 15d at the nativity of blessed John, and 15d at the feast of St Michael. And lest this be recalled or rendered invalid by anyone, I have confirmed the present charter to Jordan, master of the aforementioned hospital, and the brothers who serve God there, with my seal. With these witnesses.

*Note*. For the date, see above, no. **12**.

## 14

[Nov 1214 × 1232, perhaps Nov 1214 × *c*.1220]

### Confirmatio Iohannis filius Roberti

Notum sit[a] omnibus presentibus et futuris quod ego Iohannes filius Roberti concessi et hac presenti carta mea confirmavi, Deo et fratribus hospit(alis) beatorum apostolorum Iohannis et Iacobi de Hayno, donum unius virgate terre, cum pertinenciis, in villa de Hayno, quam Rad(ulfus) clericus et Matillis uxor eius eis dederunt, tenendum et habendum in viis, in semitis, in pascuis, et in omnibus libertatibus de me et de heredibus meis, libere et quiete, bene et in pace, in perpetuum faciendo, inde mihi et heredibus meis servicium q<u>inque solidorum per an(num), scilicet ad quatuor terminos reddend(is), pro omni servitio, consuetudine et exactione ad me[b] vel ad heredes meos pertinente, scilicet ad Natale Domini XV d(enarios),[c] et ad annunciationem beate Marie XV d(enarios),[c] et ad nativitate beati Iohannis XV d(enarios), et ad festum sancti Michaelis XV den(arios), salvo servitio domini regis. Pro hac autem concessione et confirmatione dederunt[d] mihi predicti fratres, de caritate domus, quinque marc(as) argenti. Et ut hec concessio rata et stabilis permaneat, presenti scripto sigillum meum apposui. His testibus.

(a) sit *inserted in interline, B.* — (b) a *struck through, B.* — (c) d(enarios) *inserted in interline, B.* — (d) -r- of dederunt *inserted in interline, B.*

### John, son of Robert's confirmation

May it be known to all present and future that I, John, son of Robert, have conceded and confirmed with this my present charter to God and the brothers of the hospital of the blessed Apostles John and James of Aynho the gift of one virgate of land, with its appurtenances, in the vill of Aynho, which Ralph the clerk and Matilda, his wife, gave to them, to hold and to have in roads, paths, pastures, and in all other freedoms from me and my heirs, free and quit, well and in peace, in perpetual fashion, thence rendering to me and my heirs service of 5s per year for all the service, custom, and exaction pertaining to me and my heirs, [to be paid] on four occasions, namely 15d at Christmas, 15d at the Annunciation of blessed Mary, 15d at the nativity of blessed John, and 15d at the feast of St Michael, saving the king's service. For this concession and confirmation, the aforementioned brothers gave me five marks of silver from the charity of the[ir] house. And so that this concession remains valid and stable, I have attached my seal to this present document. With these witnesses.

*Note.* For the date, see above, no. **12**.

## 15

[*c.*1200 × 1205]

### Carta [Rog]eri de *Bray*

Notum sit omnibus tam presentibus quam futuris, quod ego Rog(erus) de *Brai*[a] dedi et consessi[b] et hac presenti carta mea confirmavi, Waltero *le Chamberleng*,[c] pro hu-|1|-magio et servicio suo, unam virgatam terre in villa de Croultone,[d] scilicet quam[e] Rad(ulfus) *le Blunt* tenuit de Gaufrido[f] de *Wafre*, cum crofta *Mortog*, tenendam et habendam, cum |2| omnibus pertinentiis et aisiamentis suis de me et de[g] heredibus meis sibi et heredibus suis libere et quiete in feudo[h] et hereditarie reddendo[i] annuatim pro {omni servicio} et consuetudine, |3| salvo forinseco servicio, .IIII.$^{\text{or}}$ sol(idos), scilicet ad IIII$^{\text{or}}$ terminos: ad festum sancti Michaelis XII[j] d(enarios), ad {festum sancti} **[Membrane 4]** Andree XII d(enarios), ad festum sancte Marie in Martio XII d(enarios), ad festum |4| sancti Iohannis XII d(enarios). Pro hac autem concessione et donatione et presentis carte confirmatione, dedit mihi predictus Walt(e)rius[k] dimidiam marcam argenti et Margerie uxori mee II sol(idos). |5| Et ego et heredes mei warantizabimus[l] sibi et heredibus suis predictam terram contra omnes homines[m] et feminas. His testibus:[n] Laurencio persona de *Croultone*, Ric(ardo) filio Osb(erti), Ric(ardo) de |6| *Hi(n)tone*, Roberto de *Toreville*, Ric(ardo) de *Leuns*, Bald(wino) de *Boloine*, Roberto de *Beumunt*, Willelmo filio Osb(erti), Rad(ulfo) *Neirnut*, Simone de *Torevile*, Rogero de *Leons*, et multis aliis.

(a) Bray *B.* — (b) concessi *B.* — (c) Gambleyng *B.* — (d) Croultn' *B.* — (e) quod *B.* — (f) Galfrido *B.* — (g) de *om. B.* — (h) feodo *B.* — (i) redendo *B.* — (j) XII$^{\text{ci(m)}}$ *B.* — (k) Walterus *B.* — (l) warentizabimus *B.* — (m) homines *om. A.* — (n) *B ends here.*

### Roger de Bray's charter

May it be known to all present and future that I, Roger de Bray, have given, conceded, and confirmed with this my present charter to Walter Chamberlain, for his homage and service, one virgate of land in the vill of Croughton, namely that which Ralph Blunt held from Geoffrey de Wavre, with the croft of *Mortog*, with all its appurtenances and easements, to hold and to have by him and his heirs from me and my heirs free and quit in fief and inheritance, rendering an annual payment for all service and custom, save foreign service, of 4s [payable] on four occasions, [namely] 12d at the feast of St Michael, 12d at the feast of St Andrew, 12d at the feast of St Mary in March, and 12d at the feast of St John. For this concession, donation, and present charter's confirmation, the aforementioned Walter gave me half a mark of silver and 2s to my wife, Margaret. And my heirs and I will warrant to him and his heirs the aforementioned land against all men and women. With these witnesses: Lawrence, parson of Croughton; Richard, son of Osbert; Richard of Hinton [in the Hedges]; Robert de Turville; Richard de Lyons; Baldwin de Boulogne; Robert de Beaumont; William, son of Osbert; Ralph Neirenuit; Simon de Turville; Roger de Lyons; and many others.

*Original.* MCA, Aynho 62. Endorsed: B(r)ay (? s.xvi). Dimensions: 335 × 79 + 18 mm. Sealed *sur double queue*, parchment tag. Seal: round, fragmentary, white wax painted brown: 50 mm. A knight on horseback, sword in right hand and shield in left. Legend: destroyed.

*Note.* Dated *c.*1200 × 1210 by Macray, but the witness Richard de Lyons, who held land at Warkworth, just outside Banbury (J.J. Howard (ed.), *Miscellanea genealogica et heraldica*, 2nd ser [5 vols, London, 1884–94], vol. 1, p. 50), was dead by 1205, when his son, Roger, levied a fine on his father's lands at Warkworth (*Wavercurt*) to his widow, Juliana, in dower (Baker, *Antiquities*, vol. 1, p. 738).

## 16

[*c.*1200 × 1205]

### Confirmatio filii

Sciant presentes et futuri quod ego Milo filius Rog(er)i de *Brai*(a) hac carta mea confirmavi Waltero |1| camerario illam virgatam terre in *Creulton'*,(b) cum omnibus suis pertinentiis, quam Rog(er)us pater meus dedit illi pro |2| homagio et servicio suo, tenendam in perpetuum et hereditarie de me et de heredibus meis ipsi et |3| heredibus suis, libere et quiete honorifice, sicut in carta quam habet de patre meo continetur, et sicut ipsa[(c)] carta testatur. Pro hac autem concessione et confirmatione dedit mihi predictus Walterus dimidiam |[4]| marcam argenti. Et ut hec concessio et confirmatio rata sit et stabilis permaneat, sigilli mei muni-|[5]|-mine ipsam[(d)] corroboravi. His testibus:[(e)] Laurentio persona *Cruelton'*, Ric(ardo) filio Osberti, Ric(ardo) de *Hin-*|[6]|*-ton'*, Roberto de *T(ur)evill'*, Ric(ardo) de *Leuns*, Balduino de *Bulon'*, Roberto de Bellomonte, Willelmo f(ilio) Osb(erti), |[7]| Rad(ulfo) *Neirenuit*, Sym(one) de *T(ur)evill'*, Rog(er)o de *Leuns*, Thoma scri[ptor]e huius carte.

(a) Bray *B.* — (b) Croulton' *B.* — (c) ista *B.* — (d) ipsam *om. B.* — (e) *B ends here.*

### The son's confirmation

May those present and future know that I, Miles, son of Roger de Bray, have confirmed with this my charter to Walter Chamberlain that virgate of land in Croughton, with all its appurtenances, which my father Roger gave him for his homage and service, to hold in perpetuity and inheritance by him and his heirs from me and my heirs free and quit, fittingly, as is contained in the charter he has from my father, and as this present charter testifies. For this concession and confirmation, the aforementioned Walter gave me half a mark of silver. And so that this concession and confirmation remains valid and stable, I have corroborated it with the protection of my seal. With these witnesses: Lawrence, parson of Croughton; Richard, son of Osbert; Richard of Hinton [in the Hedges]; Robert de Turville; Richard de Lyons; Baldwin de Boulogne; Robert de Beaumont; William, son of Osbert; Ralph Neirenuit; Simon de Turville; Roger de Lyons; Thomas, the scribe of this charter.

*Original.* MCA, Aynho 52. Endorsed: no endorsements. Dimensions: 160 × 85 + 26 mm. Sealed *sur double queue*, parchment tag through one slit. Seal: round, white wax painted brown: 46 mm. A fleur-de-lis, surmounting a crescent. Legend: ✠ S[I]GILL[VM MI]LONIS D[E BR]AI.

*Note.* Dated *c.*1200 × 1210 by Macray, but since the witness list is almost identical to no. **15**, it was likely issued at the same time. A charter for Brackley Hospital shows that Miles' daughter, Mabel, was the wife of Geoffrey de Loenhout (MCA, Astwick and Evenley 64A), who was also a hospital benefactor (no. **18**).

## 17

[*c*.1210]

### Ca[rta] Walt[eri] *Chamberlayn*

Omnibus Christi fidelibus ad quos presens scriptum pervenerit, ego Walt(e)r(us) *Cha(m)belein*,[a] salutem in Domino. Universitati[b] vestre notum facio me[c] divine |1| pietatis[d] intuitu et ob anime mee medelam concessisse et dedisse Deo et fratribus hospitalis beatorum apostolorum Iac{obi} et Iohannis de Heyno[e] |2| illam virgatam terre in campis de *Creulet'*[f] quam Rog(erus)[g] de *Bray* mihi contulit cum croefta[h] *Moretok{e}* et cum pertinentiis pro homa-|3|-gio et servicio meo et quam Milo heres suus mihi confirmavit, sicut scripta eorum testan{tur}, et insimul corpus meum ibidem |4| cum eisdem fratribus ad Deum serviendum inperpetuum constitui, salvo forinseco servicio et salvo red{itu} heredum domini |5| R(o)-g(er)i de *Bray*, scilicet annuatim IIII[or][i] sol(idos) ad quatuor[j] terminos statutos, videlicet ad annunciationem be{ate} Marie duode-|6|-cim[k] den(arios), et ad nativitate beati Iohannis duodecim den(arios), et ad festum sancti Michaelis duodecim d(enarios), et ad Natale[l] duodecim {d(enarios). |7| Et ne hoc} ab aliquibus in irritum possit[m] revocari, presentem cartam Iordano hospitali magistro de |8| Heyno[n] et fratribus ibidem Deo {ministrantibus}, sigillo meo confirmavi. Hiis[o] test(ibus):[p] Roberto de *Turvill'*, |9| Symone de *Turvill'*, Hamu(n)d(o) *Pyr(un)*, Willelmo *Bast(ard)*, Roberto de Bello Monte, Ricardo filio Maze, Radul-|10|-fo *Len Veise*, et multis aliis.

(a) Chamb(e)leyn *B*. — (b) Universsitati *A*. — (c) me facio *B*. — (d) visionis *B*. — (e) Hayno *B*. — (f) Croulton' *B*. — (g) Rog(er)i *A*. — (h) crofta *B*. — (i) IIII *B*. — (j) IIII[o<r>] *B*. — (k) XII[c] *here and at each subsequent occurrence B*. — (l) Domini *add. B*. — (m) posit *B*. — (n) Hayno *B*. — (o) His *B*. — (p) *B ends here.*

### Walter Chamberlain's charter

I, Walter Chamberlain, [send my] greeting in the Lord to all the faithful in Christ whom this present document may reach. I make it known to you all that, for the sake of holy piety and for the cure of my soul, I have conceded and given to God and the brothers of the hospital of the blessed Apostles James and John of Aynho that virgate of land in the fields of Croughton, which Roger de Bray conferred upon me with the croft of *Moretoke* and its appurtenances, for my homage and service, and which his heir Miles confirmed to me, as their documents testify, and I have established my body in company with the same brothers in that place to serve God in perpetuity, saving foreign service and the rent of lord Roger de Bray's heirs, namely 4s payable each year on four occasions, namely 12d at the Annunciation of blessed Mary, 12d at the feast of the birth of blessed John, 12d at the feast of St Michael, and 12d at Christmas. And lest this be recalled or rendered invalid by anyone, I have confirmed the present charter to Jordan, master of Aynho, and the brothers who serve God there, with my seal. With these witnesses: Robert de Turville; Simon de Turville; Haymond Pirun; William Bastard; Robert de Beaumont; Richard, son of Maze; Ralph Len Veise; and many others.

*Original.* MCA, Aynho 64. Endorsed: B(r)ay (? s.xvi). Dimensions: 174 × 87 + 30 mm. Sealed *sur double queue*, parchment tag through three slits, seal impression missing.

*Cartulary marginalia.* Croult' [?] virgat(am) [?] (very indistinct).

## 18

[*c*.1210]

### Confirmatio Godefridi

Notum sit presentibus et futuris quod ego Godefridus de *Lonhoud* concessi et hac presenti carta mea confirmavi Deo et hospit(ali) beatorum apostolorum Iacobi et Ioh(ann)is de Hayno donum illius virgate terre cum pertinentiis in *Croulton'* quam W(a)lt(erus) *le Chaumbleyn* eis dedit, tenendam et habendam in viis, in semitis, in pascuis, et in pasturis, et in omnibus libertatibus de me et de heredibus meis, libere et quiete, bene et in pace, in perpetuum faciendo, inde mihi et heredibus meis servicium quatuor so[li]dorum per annum, scilicet ad quatuor terminos reddend(is), pro omni servitio, consuetudine et exactione ad me vel ad heredes meos pertinente, scilicet ad festum beate Mar(ie) in Martio(a) XII den(arios), et ad festum sancti Ioh(ann)is XII$^{cim}$ denar(ios), et ad festum sancti Michaelis XII$^{cim}$ d(enarios), et ad [festum] sancti Andree XII den(arios), salvo forinseco servitio. Et ego Godefre(dus) et heredes mei predictam terram cum omnibus pertinentiis [contra] omnes homines et feminas Deo et predictis fratribus warentizabimus. Pro hac autem concessione et confirmatione dederunt mihi pred[ictus] fratres de caritate domus unam marcam argenti. Et ut hec concessio rata et stabilis permaneat, presenti script[o si]gillum suum apposuit. His testibus.

(a) -i- of Martio *inserted in interline, B.*

### Geoffrey's confirmation

May it be known to those present and future that I, Geoffrey de Loenhout, have conceded and confirmed with this my present charter to God and the hospital of the blessed Apostles James and John of Aynho the gift of that virgate of land, with its appurtenances, in Croughton, which Walter Chamberlain gave them, to hold and to have from me and my heirs in roads, paths, pastures, common grazing, and all freedoms, free and quit, well and in peace, in perpetual fashion, thence rendering to me and my heirs service of 4s per year for all the service, custom, and exaction pertaining to me and my heirs, [to be paid] on four occasions, namely 12d at the feast of blessed Mary in March, 12d at the feast of St John, 12d at the feast of St Michael, and 12d at the feast of St Andrew. And I, Geoffrey, and my heirs will warrant to God and the aforementioned brothers the aforementioned land, with all its appurtenances, against all men and women. For this concession and confirmation, the aforementioned brothers gave me one mark of silver from the charity of the[ir] house. And to ensure that this concession remains valid and stable, he attached his seal. With these witnesses.

*Note*. This act is difficult to date precisely without a witness list. But it was perhaps issued at the same time as no. **17**, whose grant it confirms. Geoffrey was a benefactor of Brackley Hospital, issuing deeds in its favour between 1218 and 27 January 1238 (MCA, Astwick and Evenley 86A, 91A, 95A, 101A, 102A, 108A, and 129A). Like Geoffrey de Wavre and his son-in-law, Baldwin de Boulogne, Geoffrey de Loenhout seems to have had some connection to the Low Countries (see Chapter 1). His wife was the daughter of Miles de Bray, who was also a hospital benefactor (no. **16**).

## 19

[*c*.1210]

### Confirmatio Gwidonis de Haya

Sciant presentes et futuri quod ego Guuido de Haya concessi et carta mea confirmavi quantum ad me pertinet h[ospitali] sanctorum apostolorum Iacobi et Iohannis de Haynno donum quod Walt(erus) cam(er)ar(ius) eidem hosp(i)t(ali) fecit de una virgata terre [cum] pertinentiis suis in *Croulton'*, et etiam cum crofto *Morcok*, quod ego in aliquando in manu mea tenui, quod predicto hos[pitali] reddidi et recognovi esse pertinens ad prefatam[a] virgatam terre, habendam et tenendam, libere et quiete, sicut carta Rog(er)i de *Bray*, et confirmatio Milonis filii sui, et carta Walt(eri) cam(er)ar(ii) de dono predicte virgate terre, quas omnes audivi et inspexi, testantur.[b] Pro hac autem concessione et confirmatione dederunt mihi fratres predicti hosp(italis) viginti solid(os). Et ut hec mea concessio et confirmatio robur optineat perpetuum presenti scripto sigillum meum apposui. H[is testibus].

(a) *Corrected from* prefeatam, *with expunging dot under* -e-, *B.* — (b) testantiur *B.*

**Guy de la Haye's confirmation**

May those present and future know that I, Guy de la Haye, have conceded and confirmed with my charter to the hospital of the saintly Apostles James and John of Aynho what pertains to me of the gift that Walter Chamberlain made to the same hospital of one virgate of land, with its appurtenances, in Croughton, with the croft of *Morcok*; whatever I have held in my hand at any time that pertains to the aforementioned virgate of land I have surrendered to the aforementioned hospital and recognised [to be theirs], to have and to hold, free and quit, as testify the charter of Roger de Bray, the confirmation of his son Miles, and the charter of Walter Chamberlain concerning the donation of the aforementioned virgate of land, all of which I have heard and seen. For this concession and confirmation, the brothers of the aforementioned hospital gave me 20s. And to ensure that this my concession and confirmation obtains perpetual strength, I have attached my seal to the present document. With these witnesses.

*Note.* For the date, see above, no. **18**.

## 20

[1199 × 1216]

**Carta Roberti de Bello Monte et uxoris eius**

Sciant tam presentes quam futuri quod ego Robertus de Bello Monte et *Mileseynt* uxor mea dedimus et concessimus, [consilio et as]sensu Galfridi, heredis[a] nostri, fratribus hospit(alis) sancti Iacobi de Haynno dimidiam virgatam terre in campo de *Croulton'*, quam Iohannes filius Arnaldi tenuit, in puram et perpetuam elem(osinam), pro salute animarum nostrarum et antecessorum nostrorum, libere et quiete, de nobis et heredibus nostris tenendam, cum pratis et pasturis et cum omnibus aliis predicte terre pertinentibus, salvo forinseco servitio. Si autem contigerit quod ego Robertus et uxor mea vel heredes nostri[b] illam predictam terram warentizare non poterimus, tantam terram terre de nostro dominio in villa de *Croulton'* predictis fratribus escambiabimus. Pro hac donatione et confirmatione predicti fratres predicto Roberto III marcas in garsum ad deliberationem debiti regis nostri domini Iohannis et Iudeorum premanibus prebuerunt. Hanc autem donationem et concessionem tenendam predicta M.[c] et heres predicti R. tactis sacrosanctis iuraverunt et utrique eorum in manu Roberti cappellani affidaverunt. Et ut carta nostra,[d] que [?] inconcussa permaneat, sigilli nostri apositione roboravimus. His testibus.

(a) *Corrected from* heredes, *with expunging dot under* -e- *and* -i- *superscript, B.* — (b) mei *B.* — (c) *Corrected from* predictam Ma- *by erasure of* -m *and* -a, *B.* — (d) mea *B.*

## Charter of Robert de Beaumont and his wife

May those present and future know that I, Robert de Beaumont, and Melisende, my wife, have given and conceded, with the counsel and consent of Geoffrey, our heir, to the brothers of the hospital of St James of Aynho, half a virgate of land in the field of Croughton, which John, son of Arnald, held, in pure and perpetual alms, for the salvation of our souls and [those] of our ancestors, free and quit, to be held from us and our heirs, with meadows and pastures, and with everything else pertaining to the aforementioned land, saving foreign service. Should it transpire, however, that I, Robert, and my wife or our heirs cannot warrant the aforementioned land, we will give the aforementioned brothers the same amount of land from our demesne in the vill of Croughton in exchange. For this donation and confirmation, the aforementioned brothers offered by their hands to the aforementioned Robert three marks as payment in kind, in consideration of the debt of our lord King John and the Jews. Holding this donation and concession, the aforementioned M[elisende] and the heirs of the aforementioned R[obert] have taken an oath by touching the holy Gospels and have each pledged faith in the hands of Robert the chaplain. And to ensure that our charter remains firm, we have corroborated it by attaching our seal. With these witnesses.

*Date*. The mention of King John gives us the broad date of this act.

*Cartulary marginalia*. Donat(io) di(midiam) virgat(am).

## 21

[*c*.1220 × 1230]

### Carta uxoris suprascripti

Sciant presentes et f[utur]i quod ego *Milesent* filia Galfr(idi) de *Wavre* in libera et in ligia viduitate mea, post mortem |1| Roberti d[e] Bello Monte, [viri mei], divine pietatis intuitu, et pro salute anime mee et antecessorum meorum et [succes]sorum meorum, |2| dedi et con[sessi] et hac presenti carta mea confirmavi Deo et [hos]pitali sancti Iacobi de Ayno[(a)] et fratribus ibidem Deo servi-|3|-entibus [et eorum] s[ucce]ssoribus, in puram et perpetuam elemosinam, dimidiam virgatam terre cum omnibus pertinentiis suis in campo |4| de *Crow[el]ton'*,[(b)] illam scilicet quam Iohannes filius Arnaldi tenuit, habendam et tenendam libere et quiete pacifice,[(c)] in p[r]atis, in pascuis, |5| [in v]iis, in semitis,[(d)] et in omnibus libertatibus predicte terre spectantibus,[(e)] de me et de heredibus meis s[ibi et] successoribus |6| s[ui]s, [sicut libera ele]mosina melius teneri possit aut debeat, salvo f[ori]nseco servitio domini regi[s. Et ego] *Mile*-|7|-[*sent* et heredes mei totam] prenominatam dimdiam virgatam terre[(f)] cum omnibus pertinentiis suis prenominatis predicto [h]ospitali et fratri-|8|-[bus prenominatis contra omnes] gentes warantiza{bimus}.[(g)] Et ut hec mea donatio et con[ce]ssio et warantia r[a]te et inconcusse |9| perman[eant, presenti] carta mea sigillo meo inpressa illas confirmavi. Hiis[(h)] testibus:[(i)] domino Nicholao, decano de Grettewr-|10|-dia, A[de capellano] de *Stutesbir'*, Ric(ardo) filio Oseb(erti), Simone de *Turevill'*, Henrico de *Hinton'*, Widone de *la Haye*, |11| W[i]llelmo *B*[*as*]*tard*, [H]enrico *le Gras*, Iohanne de *Grettewrd'*, Willelmo *Foliot*, Iohanne de *Creton'*, et pluribus aliis.

(a) Hayno *B.* — (b) *Croulton' B.* — (c) pacifice *om. and* bene et in pace *add. B.* (d) in viis, in semitis, in pascuis *B.* — (e) et *add. B.* — (f) terre dimdiam virgatam *B.* — (g) warentizabimus *B.* — (h) His *B.* — (i) *B ends here.*

### Charter of the aforementioned's wife

May those present and future know that I, Melisende, daughter of Geoffrey de Wavre, in free and liege widowhood, following the death of my husband, Robert de Beaumont, have given, conceded, and confirmed with this my present charter, for the sake of holy piety and the salvation of my soul, and [those] of my ancestors and successors, to God, the hospital of St James of Aynho and the brothers who serve God there and their successors, in pure and perpetual alms, half a virgate of land, with all its appurtenances, in the field of Croughton, which John, son of Arnald, held, to be held free and quit, peacefully, by them and their heirs from me and my heirs in meadows, pastures, roads, paths, and in all other freedoms observed in the aforementioned land, just as free alms can and should best be held, saving the king's foreign service. And I, Melisende, and my heirs will warrant the entire aforementioned half virgate of land, with all its appurtenances, to the aforementioned hospital and its brothers against all people. And to ensure that this my donation, concession, and warranty will remain valid and intact, I have confirmed this my present charter with the impression of my seal. With these witnesses: lord Nicholas, dean of Greatworth; Adam, chaplain of Stuchbury; Richard, son of Osbert; Simon de Turville; Henry of Hinton [in the Hedges]; Guy de la Haye; William Bastard; Henry le Gras; John of Greatworth; William Foliot; John of Creaton; and many others.

*Original.* MCA, Aynho 28. Endorsed: no endorsements. Dimensions: 194 × 94 + 25 mm. Sealed *sur double queue*, parchment tag through one slit, seal impression missing. Badly damaged by damp.

*Note.* The Adam of Stuchbury among the witnesses is presumably the future master of Aynho Hospital by that name. Many of the witnesses to this act also appear in no. **25**. Henry le Gras appears among the witnesses of charters for Brackley Hospital issued in 1222 × 1224 (MCA, Astwick and Evenley 108A) and *c.*1220 (MCA, Astwick and Evenley 4 and 77A), the last two of which specifically identify him as 'Henry le Gras of Astwick'. He was therefore likely a relative of Rannulf le Gras of this vill who appears in Aynho acts. John of Creaton also appears as a witness to Brackley acts issued *c.*1220 × 1230 (MCA, Astwick and Evenley 13, 83A–86A, Westbury 34A–35A).

*Cartulary marginalia.* Conf(irmatio).

## 22

[after 25 Oct 1202 × 1210]

### Carta Roberti de Bello Monte et uxoris eius

Sciant presentes et futuri quod ego Robertus de Bello Monte et *Milesent* uxor mea[(a)] dedimus et concessimus[(b)] et hac presenti carta confirmavimus, in perpetuam elemosinam, Deo et omnibus sanctis |[1]| et Iordano magistro hospitalis sancti Iacobi de Heyno[(c)] et fratribus ibidem Deo servientibus, mesuagium quod *Haenild*[(d)] tenuit inter mesuagium capelle sancti Michaelis et mesuagium |[2]| Ricardi *Bond'*, pro viginti sol(idos) quos nobis dederunt de garsoma, tenendum sibi inperpetuum de nobis et heredibus nostris, reddendo inde annuatim nobis et heredibus nostris quatuor[(e)] |[3]| denarios ad Pascha,[(f)] pro omni servicio et exactione ad nos vel ad heredes nostros pertinente. Nos vero et heredes nostri predicto Iordano et fratribus eiusdem hospitalis et eorum suc-|4|-cessoribus predictum mesuagium cum curia adiacente contra omnes gentes inperpetuum warantizabimus.(g) Et ut hec concessio et donatio nostra rata sit et stabilis |5| inperpetuum, presentem cartam cum sigillis nostris prenominato Iord(ano)(h) et fratribus hospitalis et eorum successoribus confirmavimus. Hiis(i) testibus:(j) Roberto de T(ur)-villa, |6| Simone filio eius, Hugone *Russel*, Ham(undo) [*Pi*]*run*, Willelmo *Bastard*, Helya de *Faucot*, Ernaldo capellano carte scriptore, et multis aliis ibidem presentibus.

(a) mei *A*. — (b) conssessimus *B*. — (c) Hayno *B*. — (d) Arnuld(us) *B*. — (e) IIIIor *B*. — (f) Pasca *B*. — (g) warentizabimus *B*. — (h) I. *B*. — (i) His *B*. — (j) *B ends here.*

**Charter of Robert de Beaumont and his wife**

May those present and future know that I, Robert de Beaumont, and Melisende, my wife, have given, conceded, and confirmed with this present charter, in perpetual alms, to God and all the saints, and to Jordan, master of the hospital of St James of Aynho, and the brothers who serve God there, the messuage that Haenild held between the messuage of the chapel of St Michael and the messuage of Richard Bond', for 20s, which they gave to us as payment in kind, to be held by them from us and our heirs in perpetuity, thence returning to us and our heirs 4d each year at Easter for all service and custom pertaining to us and our heirs. We and our heirs will warrant the aforementioned messuage, with the adjacent courtyard, to Jordan and the brothers of the same hospital and their successors against all people in perpetuity. And to ensure that this our concession and donation remains valid and stable in perpetuity, we have confirmed the present charter to the aforementioned Jordan and the brothers of the hospital and their successors with our seals. With these witnesses: Robert de Turville; Simon, his son; Hugh Russel; Haymond Pirun; William Bastard; Helya of Falcutt; Ernald the chaplain [and] the charter's scribe; and many others there present.

*Original.* MCA, Aynho 86. Endorsed: Capella de Creuton' (? s.xvii). Dimensions: 231 × 65 + 15 mm. Sealed *sur double queue*, on two parchment tags each through one slit, seal impressions missing.

*Note.* Dated *c.*1200 × 1210 by Macray, but must be after 25 October 1202, date at which no. **1** is addressed to Turbert, proctor of the hospital, whose successor, Jordan, is mentioned in this act.

*Cartulary marginalia*. Mesuag(ium).

## 23

[*c*.1220 × 1230]

### Carta uxoris suprascripti

Sciant presentes et futuri quod ego *Milesent* filia[a] Galfredi de *Waffre* dedi et concessi et hac presenti carta[b] confirm(avi) Deo et omnibus sanctis et fratribus hosp(italis) sancti Iacobi de Hayno et eorum successor(ibus), pro XX[ti] sol(idos) quos mihi dederunt, in perpet(uam) elem(osinam), mesuag(ium) quod Haenildus tenuit inter mesuag(ium) capelle sancti Michaelis et quondam mesuag(ium) Ricardi *Bond'*, tenendum sibi et[c] suis successor(ibus) de me et h(er)ed(ibus) meis, libere et quiete, reddendo inde annuatim mihi et h(er)ed(ibus) meis quatuor d(enarios) ad Pascha, pro omni servitio et exactione ad me et ad h(er)ed(es) meos pertinente. Ego vero et heredes mei predictis fratribus et eorum successoribus prenominatum mesuag(ium) cum curia adiacente contra omnes gentes warent(izabimus). Et ne hec don(atio) et concessio a me[d] vel ab heredibus meis possit ad nichilari, presentem cartam sigilli mei appositione fratribus supradictis et eorum successor(ibus) confirmavi. His test(ibus).

(a) filia *inserted in interline, B.* — (b) mea *struck through, B.* — (c) h(er)ed(ibus) *struck through, B.* — (d) a me *inserted in interline, B.*

### Charter of the aforementioned's wife

May those present and future know that I, Melisende, daughter of Geoffrey de Wavre, have given, conceded, and confirmed with this present charter to God and all the saints, and to the brothers of the hospital of St James of Aynho and their successors in perpetual alms, for the 20s they gave me, the messuage that Haenildus held between the messuage of the chapel of St Michael and the former messuage of Richard Bond', to be held by them and their successors from me and my heirs in perpetuity, free and quit, thence returning to me and my heirs 4d each year at Easter for all service and custom pertaining to me and my heirs. My heirs and I will warrant the aforementioned messuage, with the adjacent courtyard, to the aforementioned brothers and their successors against all people in perpetuity. And to ensure that this donation and concession cannot be rendered void by myself or my heirs, I have confirmed the present charter to the aforementioned brothers and their successors with my seal. With these witnesses.

*Note.* Since this act does not mention Melisende as being in her widowhood (unlike no. **21**), it may have been issued around the same time as no. **22**, whose grant it confirms.

However, Melisende styles herself here in relation to her father, rather than her husband, suggesting Robert was dead. It is also unclear why Melisende would have issued an act in her own name at the same time as no. **22**, which concerns the same property, and which is issued in both her husband's name and her own. Moreover, no. **24** below, issued by her son, Geoffrey, confirms the grant as laid out in no. **23** rather than in no. **22**, while it also confirms the grant of no. **21**, which was certainly issued after Robert de Beaumont's death.

*Cartulary marginalia.* Ut supra [?].

## 24

[*c.*1220 × 1230]

### Carta Galfridi de Bello Monte

Omnibus ad quos scriptum presens pervenerit, Galfridus de Bello Monte, salutem. Noverit universitas vestra me concessisse et hac presenti carta mea confirmasse Deo et hosp(itali) sancti Iacobi de Hayno et fratribus ibidem Deo servientibus, in puram et perpet(uam) elem(osinam), dimidiam virgatam terre cum omnibus pertinentiis suis in campo de *Croulton'* quam *Milisent*, mater mea, eis dedit in puram et perpet(uam) elem(osinam), illam scilicet quam Iohannes filius Arnoldi tenuit, habendam et tenendam libere, quiete, pacifice, in pratis, in pascuis, in **[Membrane 5]** viis, in semitis, et in omnibus libertatibus predicte terre spectantibus de me et de h(er)ed(ibus) meis, inperpetuum, sicut aliqua libera elemosina melius aut liberius possit aut debeat teneri, salvo forinseco servitio d(omini) regis quantum ad tantam terram(a) pertinet, sicut carta *Milesent* matris mee, quam inde habent, testatur. Et preterea concessi predictis fratribus inperpet(uam) elem(osinam) mesuag(ium) quod Hainildus tenuit in villa de *Croulton'* inter capella sancti Michaelis et mesuag(ium) Ricardi *Bond'*, habendum et tenendum de me et de h(er)ed(ibus) meis libere et quiete, inperpet(uum), reddendo inde annuatim mihi et h(er)ed(ibus) meis IIII$^{or}$ den(arios) ad Pascha, pro omni servitio et exactione ad me vel ad heredes meos pertinente, sicut carta *Milesent* matris mee, quam inde habent, testatur. Et ut hec concessio mea et confirmatio rata et stabilis permaneant, eam sigilli mei munimine roboravi. His testibus.

(a) terre *B*.

### Geoffrey de Beaumont's charter

Geoffrey de Beaumont [sends his] greeting to all whom this present document may reach. May you all know that I have conceded and confirmed with this my present charter to God and the hospital of St James of Aynho, and to the brothers who serve God there, in pure and perpetual alms, half a virgate of land, with all its appurtenances, in the field of Croughton, which my mother Melisende gave them in pure and perpetual alms, namely the one that John, son of Arnold, held, to have and to hold free [and] quit, peacefully, in meadows, pastures, roads, paths, and in all other freedoms observed in the aforementioned land from me and my heirs, in perpetuity, just as free alms can and should best be held, saving the king's foreign service, inasmuch as pertains to this land, just as my mother Melisende's charter, which they have, testifies. And I have also conceded to the aforementioned brothers, in perpetual alms, the messuage which Hainildus held in the vill of Croughton between the chapel of St Michael and the messuage of Richard Bond', to have and to hold from me and my heirs free and quit, in perpetuity, returning to me and my heirs 4d each year at Easter for all service and exaction pertaining to me and my heirs, just as my mother Melisende's charter, which they have, testifies. And to ensure that this my concession and confirmation remains valid and stable, I have reinforced it with my seal. With these witnesses.

*Note.* For the date, see no. **23**.

*Cartulary marginalia.* Ut supra, *with manicule pointing to no. 23.*

## 25

[*c.*1220 × 1230]

### Confirmatio Ricardi filii Oseberti

Omnibus sancte matris ecclesie filiis ad quos presens carta[(a)] pervenerit, Ric(ardus) filius Oseb(ert)i, salutem. Noverit universitas vestra |[1]| me concessisse[(b)] et presenti carta mea confirmasse, divine pietatis intuitu, et pro salute mea et omnium successorum |[2]| meorum, et pro salute omnium animarum antecessorum meorum, Deo et hospitali sancti Iacobi de Einho[(c)] et fratribus ibidem Deo ser-|[3]|-vientibus et eorum successoribus, omnes donationes terrarum quas habent de dono *Milicent'*[(d)], filie Galfr(idi) de *Wavere*, quas eis de-|[4]|-dit in libera[(e)] viduitate sua, post mortem Roberti[(f)] de Bello Monte,(g) quondam viri sui, in *Croulton'*, et unde cartas |5| ipsius *Milicent'* habent et sicud carte quas habent de dicta *Milicent'* testantur,(h) quantum ad feodum(i) meum pertinet. Et ego |6| dictus Ric(ardus) caritative et in fide pro me et pro(j) heredibus meis concessi predictas donationes predictis fratribus warantizare(k) quantum |7| ad me vel ad heredes pertinebit, secundum formam cartarum quas habent de predicta *Milicent'*,(l) et de omnibus aliis qui de feodo(m) |8| meo aliquod donum dictis fratribus et eorum successoribus fecerunt, et unde eorum cartas habent similiter confirmavi. Et ut hec mea |9| concessio et confirmatio rate et inconcusse permaneant, presenti carta mea sigillo meo impressa(n) illas confirmavi. Hiis(o) testi-|10|-bus:(p) Simone de *Turevill'*, Henrico de *Hinton'*, Ydone de *la Haye*, Willelmo *Bastard*, Henrico *le Gras*, Iohanne de *Grettewrd'*, |11| *Wilekin Foliot*, Iohanne de *Creton'*, et pluribus aliis.

(a) scriptum *B.* — (b) et dedisse *add. B.* — (c) Hayno *B.* — (d) Milesent *B.* — (e) -r- *of* libera *inserted in interline, B.* — (f) R. *B.* — (g) *Superfluous tilde above* M-, *B.* — (h) et bene carte ipsius Milesent testantur *B.* — (i) foedum *A.* — (j) pro *om. B.* — (k) warentizare *B.* — (l) Miles(ent) *B.* — (m) foedo *A*; feddo *B.* — (n) inpressa *B.* — (o) His *B.* — (p) *B ends here.*

### Richard son of Osbert's confirmation

Richard, son of Osbert, [sends his] greeting to all children of the holy mother Church whom this present charter may reach. May you all know that I have conceded and confirmed with this my present charter, for the sake of holy piety and the salvation of my soul and [those] of all my successors, to God and the hospital of St James of Aynho, and to the brothers who serve God there and their successors, all donations of lands in Croughton, inasmuch as it pertains to my fief, which they have from the gift of Melisende, daughter of Geoffrey de Wavre, which she gave them in her free widowhood following the death of Robert de Beaumont, her former husband, and in respect of which they have Melisende's charters, and as the charters they have of her testify. And I, the said Richard, have conceded charitably and in [good] faith for myself and my heirs to warrant to the aforementioned brothers the aforementioned donations, inasmuch as they concern me and my successors, according to the charters they have from the aforementioned Melisende and from anyone else who gave the said brothers and their successors any gift from my fief, and whereof they have their charters, I have likewise confirmed. And so that this my concession and confirmation remain valid and intact, I have confirmed them by impressing the present charter with my seal. With these witnesses: Simon de Turville; Henry of Hinton [in the Hedges]; Guy de la Haye; William Bastard; Henry le Gras; John of Greatworth; Wilekin Foliot; John of Creaton; and many others.

*Original*. MCA, Aynho 44. Endorsed: no endorsements. Dimensions: 182 × 98 + 19 mm. Sealed *sur double queue*, on parchment tag through one slit, seal impression missing.

*Note*. Many of the witnesses to this act also appear in no. **21**.

## 26

[*c*.1250 × 1260]

### Carta Roberti de *Frutewelle*

Sciant presentes et futuri quod ego Robertus de[a] *Frutewell'*,[b] manens in *Croulton'*, dedi et concessi et hac presenti carta mea confirmavi |1| magistro et fratribus hospitalis de Eyno[c] ibidem Deo servientibus, pro salute[d] anime mee et antecessorum meorum, unam partem curie mee in |2| villa de *Croulton'* iuxta cimiterium, ubi maneo, videlicet a muro cimiterii in latitudine versus[e] orientem quatuor viginti pedum et in |3| longitudine ex una parte viginti sex pedum et ex alia parte viginti unius pedum, tenendam et habendam[f] de me et heredibus meis predictis magistro[g] |4| et fratribus libere,[h] quiete, bene et in pace, in pura et perpetua elemosina, sicut elemosina melius et securius poterit dari. Et ego et heredes |5| mei dictam parte terre predictis magistro et fratribus pro participatione omnium bonorum que in domo fierent[i] in perpetuum contra omnes homines et feminas warantiza-|6|-bimus[j] et defendemus.[k] Et ut hec mea donatio et concessio[l] rata et stabilis permaneat huic scripto sigilli mei inpressione apposui. Hiis[m] |7| t(estibus):[n] Willelmo de Haye in *Croulton'*, Nicholao *Bastard*, Galfr(ido) *Baumund*, Ricardo *Beumund*, Nicholao clerico de Eyno, Huberto de Ey-|8|-n(o), Waltero *Westt'* de *Walton'*, Iohanne clerico de *Finem(er)e*, et aliis.

(a) de *om. B.* — (b) Friutew(el)le *B.* — (c) Hayno *B.* — (d) anime *struck through, B.* — (e) norsus *B.* — (f) habendum *B.* — (g) magistris *B.* — (h) et *add. B.* — (i) fierent *with superfluous tilde above* -e-, *B.* — (j) warentizabimus *B.* — (k) defendimus *B.* — (l) concessio et donatio *B.* — (m) His *B.* — (n) *B ends here.*

### Robert of Fritwell's charter

May those present and future know that I, Robert of Fritwell, dwelling in Croughton, have given, conceded, and confirmed with this my charter, for the salvation of my soul and [those] of my ancestors, to the master and brothers of the hospital of Aynho who serve God there, a part of my courtyard in the vill of Croughton next to the cemetery, where I dwell, namely eighty feet in width from the cemetery wall to the east and twenty-six feet in length on one side and twenty-one feet in length on the other side, to hold and to have by the aforementioned master and brothers from me and my heirs, free, quit, well and in peace, in pure and perpetual alms, just as alms should be best and securely given. And my heirs and I will warrant the said part of land, in perpetuity, to the aforementioned master and brothers, for participation in all the good things that might happen in the[ir] house, and we will defend it against all men and women. And so that this my donation and concession remain valid and stable, I have attached to this document the impression of my seal. With these witnesses: William de la Haye in Croughton; Nicholas Bastard; Geoffrey Beaumont; Richard Beaumont; Nicholas, clerk of Aynho; Hubert of Aynho; Walter Westt' of Walton [Grounds]; John, clerk of Finmere; and others.

*Original.* MCA, Aynho 65. Endorsed: Fretwele. Crowlton (s.xv); Pars cur' gardin iuxta cimiterium (? s.xvi). Dimensions: 220 × 52 + 14 mm. Seal: oval, white wax painted brown: 30 mm. A fleur-de-lis. Legend: SIGILL(*vm*) ROB(*ert*)I D(*e*) FRVTEW[...].

*Note.* This Robert appears elsewhere as Robert Newman (no. **56**).

## 27

[*c*.1260 × 1270, perhaps *c*.1250 × 1260]

### Confirmatio filii

Sciant presentes et futuri quod ego Thomas filius Roberti de *Frutewelle*, manens in *Croultun*',[a] concessi et hac presenti carta |[1]| mea confirmavi pro salute anime mee et pro animabus Roberti patris mei et antecessorum meorum magistro et fratribus hospitalis |[2]| de Eyneho[b] ibidem Deo servientibus et inperpetuum servituris donationem illius partis curie in villa de *Croultun*'[c] iuxta cimiterium, ubi ma-|[3]|-neo, quantum dictus Robertus pater meus eis dedit et in carta sua confirmavit, que quidem pars curie continet spatium quatuor viginti |[4]| pedum in latitudine a muro cimiterii versus orientem, et in longitudine ex una parte spatium viginti sex pedum et ex alia par-|[5]|-te spatium viginti pedum et unius, tenendam et habendam totam partem predicte curie, ut supradictum est, de me et here-|[6]|-dibus meis predictis magistro et fratribus et eorum successoribus sine inpedimento et contradictione mei vel heredum meorum, libere,[d] quiete, bene |[7]| et in pace, inperpetuum, in liberam, puram et perpetuam elemosinam, prout aliqua elemosina liberius et securius concedi poterit, sicut carta quam pre-|[8]|-dicti magister et fratres inde habent a dicto Rob(er)to patre meo plenius testatur, quam ego vidi et audivi. Pro hac autem concessione et presentis carte con-|9|-firmatione dederunt michi[(e)] predicti magister et fratres quatuor[(f)] solid(os) argenti et michi[(g)] concesserunt participationem omnium bonorum que in domo de Eyneho[(h)] |10| fient inperpetuum. Et ego dictus Thomas et heredes mei dictis magistro et fratribus et eorum successoribus totam prefatam partem curie supradicte, ut pre-|11|-dictum est, contra omnes gentes inperpetuum warantizabimus[(i)] et defendemus. Et ut hec mea concessio et presentis carte confirmatio perpetue firmitatis |12| robur optineant, presentem cartam sigilli mei inpressione duxi roborandam[(j)]. Hiis[(k)] testibus:[(l)] Willelmo de *Haye* in *Croultun'*, Nicholao *Bastard*, Gal-|13|-frido *Beumund*, Ricardo *Beumund*, Nicholao clerico de Eyneho, Huberto de eadem villa, Waltero *West* de *Walton'*, Roberto *Fraunceis* |14| clerico, et aliis.

(a) Croulton' *B.* — (b) Hayno *B.* — (c) Croulton' *B.* — (d) et *add. B.* — (e) mihi *B.* — (f) IIII[or] *B.* — (g) mihi *B.* — (h) Haynno *B.* — (i) warentizabimus *B.* — (j) corroborandam *B.* — (k) His *B.* — (l) *B ends here.*

### The son's confirmation

May those present and future know that I, Thomas, son of Robert of Fritwell, dwelling in Croughton, have conceded and confirmed with this my present charter, for the salvation of my soul and the souls of my father, Robert, and my ancestors, to the master and brothers of the hospital of Aynho, who serve and forever will serve God there, the donation of that part of the courtyard in the vill of Croughton next to the cemetery, where I dwell, inasmuch as my father, the said Robert, gave them and confirmed with his charter, namely the part of the courtyard consisting of eighty feet in width from the cemetery wall to the east and twenty-six feet in length on one side and twenty-one feet in length on the other side, for the aforementioned master and brothers and their successors to hold and to have the entire part of the aforementioned courtyard, as said above, from me and my heirs without impediment or objection from me and my heirs, free, quit, well and in peace, in perpetuity, in free, pure, and perpetual alms, just as all alms may be given freely and securely, as the charter that the aforementioned master and brothers have from my father, the said Robert, clearly testifies, which I have seen and heard. For this concession and present charter's confirmation, the aforementioned master and brothers gave me 4s in silver and relinquished to me, in perpetuity, participation in all the good things that happen in the[ir] house at Aynho. And I, the said Thomas, and my heirs will warrant to the aforementioned master and brothers, and to their successors, all the aforesaid part of the aforesaid courtyard, as already said, in perpetuity, and will defend it against all men and women. And to ensure that this my concession and present charter's confirmation remain firm in perpetuity, I have thought fit that this present charter be corroborated with the impression of my seal. With these witnesses: William de la Haye in Croughton; Nicholas Bastard; Geoffrey Beaumont; Richard Beaumont; Nicholas, clerk of Aynho; Hubert of the same vill; Walter West' of Walton [Grounds]; Robert Fraunceis, clerk; and others.

*Original.* MCA, Aynho 63. Endorsed: T. Fretuel'. Crowlto' (s.xv); De parte curie iuxta cimiterium (? s.xvi). Dimensions: 202 × 101 + 25 mm. Sealed *sur double queue*, parchment tag through one slit, seal impression missing. The charter is in the hand of Robert Fraunceis, who also wrote no. **30**.

*Note.* Dated *c.*1260 × 1270 by Macray, but since the witness list is nearly identical to no. **26**, it is possible that these acts were both issued around the same time. This Thomas is referred to in other Aynho charters as Thomas Newman (nos. **56**, **A12–A13**, **A16–17**, **A19**).

## 28

[*c.*1212 × *c.*1235]

### Carta Milonis *Neyrnuyt*

Omnibus visuris hoc scriptum vel audituris, Milo *Nornuuit*, salutem. Noveritis me concessisse magistro et fratribus hosp(italis) de Hayno ad levandum unum murum[(a)] in metam inter me et ipsos sitam in villa de *Croulton'*, ita scilicet quod licitum dicto Miloni super eundem murum sine aliqua contradictione quantumque voluerit aliam domum levare. Et in huius rei testimonium huic scripto sigillum meum apposui. His testibus.

(a) -ru- *of* murum *inserted in interline, B.*

### Miles Neirenuit's charter

Miles Neirenuit [sends his] greeting to all those seeing or hearing this document. May you know that I have conceded to the master and brothers of the hospital of Aynho [the right] to erect one wall in the boundary between me and them located in the vill of Croughton, so that the said Miles will have the right to build another house of whatever size he wants beyond that wall without any objection. And I have attached my seal to this document as testimony in this matter. With these witnesses.

*Note.* The dates are given by Miles Neirenuit's appearances in the record (see Keats-Rohan (ed.), *Domesday Descendants*, pp. 1048–9).

## 29

[*c*.1220]

### Carta Gwidonis de Haya

Sciant presentes et futuri quod ego Guido de Haya, intuitu Dei, et pro salute anime mee |[1]| et parentum meorum, dedi et concessi Deo et hospitali sanctorum apostolorum Iacobi et |[2]| Iohannis de Ainho[(a)] et fratribus ibidem Deo servientibus, in puram et perpetuam elemosinam, duas |[3]| acras terre de dominio meo in *Creweltun'*,[(b)] quarum una[(c)] iacet apud *Langeford'* et alia |[4]| apud *Grundhole*,[(d)] habendas et tenendas inperpetuum, liberas et quietas ab omni seculari |[5]| exactione. Et ut hec donatio et concessio futuris temporibus stabilis perseveret, [(e)] pre-|[6]|-sens scriptum sigilli mei munimine corroborare dignum duxi. Hiis[(f)] testibus:[(g)] domino |[7]| Roberto de *Turevill'*, Hamone *Piru(n)*, Willelmo *Bastard*, Roberto de Bello Monte, Ada |[8]| vicario de *Creweltun'*, Rad(ulfo) de *la Hide*, Ric(ardo) de *Duni(n)tun'*, Rad(ulfo) clerico de Ainho, |[9]| Roberto de Colecestra huius carte scriptore, et multis aliis.

(a) de Hayno apostolorum Iacobi et Iohannis *B*. — (b) Croulton' *B*. — (c) *Corrected from* unam *with* -m *struck through, B*. — (d) Grundihell' *B*. — (e) perseverat *B*. — (f) His *B*. — (g) *B ends here.*

### Guy de la Haye's charter

May those present and future know that I, Guy de la Haye, for God's sake and for the salvation of my soul and [those] of my relatives, have given and conceded to God and the hospital of the blessed Apostles James and John of Aynho, and to the brothers who serve God there, in pure and perpetual alms, two acres of land of my demesne in Croughton, one of which lies at *Langeford'* and the other at *Grundhole*, to have and to hold in perpetuity, free and quit from all secular exaction. And to ensure that this donation and concession remains stable in future times, I have thought fit to corroborate the present document with the protection of my seal. With these witnesses: lord Robert de Turville; Haimo Pirun; William Bastard; Robert de Beaumont; Adam, vicar of Croughton; Ralph de la Hide; Richard of Donnington; Ralph, clerk of Aynho; Robert of Colchester, scribe of this charter; and many others.

*Original*. MCA, Aynho 50. Endorsed: Gwydo de la Hay (s. xv). Dimensions: 170 × 88 + 21 mm. Sealed *sur double queue*, parchment tag through three slits. Seal: round, white wax painted brown: 35 mm. Shield, three bars, over them a bandlet, a label of five points. Legend: ✠ S[IG]ILL(*vm*) WIDON(*is*) DE LA HAIE.

## 30

[*c*.1245 × 1250]

### Carta Willelmi de *la Haye*

Omnibus Christi fidelibus presentem cartam inspecturis vel audituris, Willelmus de *la Haye* de *Croultun'*,[a] salutem in Domino. Noverit universitas vestra |1| me, pro salute anime mee et pro animabus antecessorum meorum, dedisse, concessisse[b] et hac presenti carta mea confirmasse, fratri[c] Stephano ma-|2|-gistro hospitalis de Eyneho[d] et eiusdem loci fratribus, quamdam parte terre mee, in *Croultun'*,[e] continentem in latitudine tres pedes, |3| super quam terram dicti magister et fratres levaverunt occidentalem gablam illius domus[f] quam Agnes *la Noreche*[g] quondam tenu-|4|-it, habendam et tenendam dictam terram et gablam dictis magistro et fratribus et eorum successoribus de me et[h] heredibus meis, libere,[i] |5| quiete, bene et in pace, inperpetuum sine inpedimento et perturbatione aliqua, ita tamen quod si ego vel heredes mei aliquo tempore super terram |6| nostram proximam supradicte domui edificare velimus licitum[j] sit nobis meirinum et trabes in predictam gablam inponere sine contra-|7|-dictione et inpedimento dictorum magistri et fratrum vel alicuius suorum. Ego vero Willelmus et heredes mei dictam terram super quam pre-|8|-dicta gabla sita est dictis magistro et fratribus et eorum successoribus contra omnes homines et feminas inperpetuum[k] warantizabimus[l] et |9| defendemus. Et ut hec mea donatio,[m] concessio et presentis carte confirmatio perpetue firmitatis robur optineant, presentem |10| cartam sigilli mei inpressione duxi roborandam. Hiis[n] testibus:[o] Henrico *Pyrun*, Nicholao de *Grimescote*, Galfrido *Beumund*, |11| Ricardo *Beumund*, Thoma *Neyrnut*, et aliis.

(a) Croulton' *B*. — (b) concessesse *B*. (c) fratri *om*. *B*. (d) Hayno *B*. (c) Croulton' *B*. — (f) domus *om*. *B*. — (g) Norice *B*. — (h) de *add*. *B*. — (i) et *add*. *B*. — (j) *Corrected from* lecitum *with expunging dot under* -e- *and* -i- *inserted in interline, B*. — (k) inperpetuum *om*. *B*. — (l) warentizabimus *B*. — (m) et *add*. *B*. — (n) His *B*. — (o) *B ends here.*

### William de la Haye's charter

William de la Haye of Croughton [sends his] greeting in the Lord to all the faithful in Christ who may examine or hear the present charter. May you all know that I have given, conceded, and confirmed with this my present charter, for the salvation of my soul and for the souls of my ancestors, to brother Stephen, master of the hospital of Aynho, and the brothers of the same place, a certain part of my land in Croughton, measuring three feet in width, on which the said master and brothers have erected the western gable of the house once held by Agnes la Noreche, with the said master and brothers and their successors having and holding the said land and gable from me and my successors free, quit, well and in peace, in perpetuity, without any impediment or other disturbance, on the condition that should my heirs or I ever wish to build on our land next to the aforementioned house, it shall be lawful for us to place timberwork and beams in the aforementioned gable without objection or impediment by the said master and brothers or any of their men. And I, William, and my heirs will warrant the said land in which the aforementioned gable is located to the said master and brothers and their successors and defend it against all men and women in perpetuity. And so that this my donation, concession, and present charter's confirmation remain firm in perpetuity, I have thought fit that this present charter be corroborated with the impression of my seal. With these witnesses: Henry Pirun; Nicholas of Grimscote; Geoffrey Beaumont; Richard Beaumont; Thomas Neirenuit; and others.

*Original.* MCA, Aynho 26. Endorsed: Carta duarum dimidiarum acrarum prati (s. xv, scored through). Dimensions: 232 × 109 + 25 mm. Sealed *sur double queue*, parchment tag through one slit, seal impression missing. The charter is in the hand of Robert Fraunceis, who also wrote no. **27**.

## 31

[*c.*1260 × 1270]

### Carta supradicti

Omnibus Christi fidelibus presentem cartam inspecturis vel audituris Willelmus de Haya de *Crowlton'*,[(a)] salutem eternam[(b)] in Domino. Noverit universitas vestra me pro salu-|1|-te anime mee et pro anima Wydonis patris mei et pro animabus antecessorum et successorum meorum dedisse, concessisse et hac presenti carta mea confirmasse[(c)] |2| Deo et beate Marie et magistro et fratribus hospitalis beatorum apostolorum Iacobi et Iohannis de Eynno[(d)] duas[(e)] domos in villa de *Crowlton'*,[(f)] scilicet |3| quoddam cotagium quod Agnes *la Noieyse*[(g)] quondam[(h)] tenuit et quoddam mesuagium cum tofto quod Willelmus *Morcok*[(i)] quondam tenuit, quod situm est inter domum |4| Walteri *Bugeloue*[(j)] ex parte orientali et domum Thome filii Willelmi *Botyld*[(k)] ex parte occidentali, videlicet ad sustentationem duorum cereorum ardentium ad missam beate |5| Marie omnibus diebus seculi[(l)] in capella sua de Eynno,[(m)] sicuti Wydo pater meus dictis magistro et fratribus in testamento suo legavit, habendum et tenendum dictum |6| cotagium et dictum mesuag(ium) cum[(n)] tofto sine aliquo r[eten]emento dictis magistro et fratribus et eorum successoribus de me et heredibus[o] meis, in liberam, puram et perpetuam |7| elemosinam, libere, quiete, bene et in pace, in[perpe]tuum, sicut aliqua elemosina melius et liberius dari potest, absque omni seculari servicio, consuetudine |8| et demanda michi[p] et heredibus meis vel alicui alii pertinentibus. Et ego Willelmus et heredes mei dictum cotagium et dictum mesuagium cum tofto, ut prenominatum est, |9| dictis magistro et fratribus et eorum successoribus contra omnes gentes warantizabimus,[q] aquietabimus, et defendemus. Et ut hec donatio, concessio et presentis |10| carte confirmatio perpetue firmitatis robur optineant presentem cartam sigilli mei inpressione duxi roborandam. Hiis[r] testibus:[s] Ric(ard)o *Neirenut*, |11| tunc tempore rectore ecclesie de *Crowlton'*, Henrico *Pyrun*, Nicholao de *Grimeschot'*, Roberto de *Seringes*, Galfr(ido) de *Beumund'*, Huberto de Eynho, Ric(ard)o |12| de *Beumund'*, et multis aliis.

(a) Croulton' *B.* — (b) eternam *om. B.* — (c) dedisse et concessisse et hac presenti carta mea confirmasse, pro salute anime mee et pro anima Wydonis, patris mei, et pro animabus antecessorum meorum et successorum, *followed by* dedi *struck through, B.* — (d) Hayno *B.* — (e) *Corrected from* doas *with* -u- *written over* -o-, *B.* — (f) Croulton' *B.* — (g) Noeyise *B.* — (h) q(u)oondam *B.* — (i) Morkok *B.* — (j) Bugelou' *B.* — (k) Botild *B.* — (l) seculi diebus *B.* — (m) Hayno *B.* — (n) cum *om. B.* — (o) h<er>ed(ibus) *B.* — (p) mihi *B.* — (q) warentizabimus *B.* — (r) His *B.* — (s) *B ends here.*

## Charter of the aforementioned

William de la Haye of Croughton [sends his] eternal greeting in the Lord to all the faithful in Christ who may examine or hear the present charter. May you all know that I have given, conceded, and confirmed with this my present charter, for the salvation of my soul, the soul of my father, Guy, and the souls of my ancestors and successors, to God and the blessed Mary, and to the master and brothers of the hospital of the blessed Apostles James and John of Aynho two houses in the vill of Croughton, namely the cottage that Agnes la Noieyse once held and a certain messuage with the toft that William Morcok once held, which is situated between the house of Walter Bugeloue on the eastern part and the house of Thomas, son of William Botild, on the western part, for the sustenance of two wax candles to be burned during the daily mass of St Mary in their chapel at Aynho, just as my father Guy bequeathed to the said master and brothers in his will, with the said master and brothers and their successors having and holding the said cottage and messuage, with toft, without any hindrance from my heirs and me in free, pure, and perpetual alms, free, quit, well and in peace, in perpetuity, just as all alms should rightly and freely be given, free from all secular service, custom, and demands pertaining to me, my heirs, or anybody else. And I, William, and my heirs will warrant and release to the said master and brothers and their successors the said cottage and messuage with toft, as named above, and defend it against all people. And to ensure that this my donation, concession, and confirmation with the present charter remain firm in perpetuity, I have thought fit that this present charter be corroborated with the impression of my seal. With these witnesses: Richard Neirenuit, rector at this time of the church of Croughton; Henry Pirun; Nicholas of Grimscote; Robert of Sheering; Geoffrey Beaumont; Hubert of Aynho; Richard Beaumont; and many others.

*Original.* MCA, Aynho 53. Endorsed: Carta Willelmi de la Hay in qua conti(n)e(t)ur Murkokcroft (s.xv); Hay (? s.xvi). Dimensions: 230 × 100 + 19 mm. Sealed *sur double queue*, parchment tag through one slit, seal impression missing.

**32**

[*c*.1260 × 1270]

**Carta supradicti**

Omnibus sancte matris ecclesie[(a)] filiis ad quos presens scriptum pervenerit,[(b)] Willelmus de *la Haye*[(c)] de *Croulton*', salutem eternam in Domino. Noverit universi-|1|-tas vestra me, pro salute anime mee et pro animabus antecessorum meorum, dedisse, concessisse et presenti **[Membrane 6]** carta mea confirmasse Deo et beate Marie |2| et magistro et fratribus hospitalis sanctorum Iacobi et Iohannis in villa de Eynho[(d)] duas dimidias acras prati, scilicet de tribus dimidiis acris prati de |3| prato meo forinseco que iacent in prato de *Croulton*' iuxta *Charewelle*, habendas et tenendas dictas duas dimid(ias) acras prati, cum suis pertinentiis, |4| sine aliquo retenemento, dictis magistro et fratribus et eorum successoribus de me et heredibus meis vel assignatis,[(e)] libere,[(f)] quiete, bene et in pace, inperpetuum, |5| in liberam et puram ac perpetuam elemosinam, sicut aliqua elemosina purius et liberius dari potest, sine[(g)] sectis cuiuslibet[(h)] curie, consuetudine et deman-|6|-da quibuslibet, ita tamen quod dicti magister et fratres dicti[(i)] hospitalis singulis annis tempore falcationis de predictis tribus dimid(iis) acris prati primas duas |7| meliores dimid(ias) acras prati quascumque eligere voluerint,[(j)] sine impedimento[(k)] vel contradictione mei et heredum meorum vel assignatorum, habebunt, inper-|8|-petuum, et ego et heredes mei vel assignati tertiam residuam dimidiam acram prati[(l)] post electionem ipsorum habebimus. Pro hac autem donatione, concessione |9| inperpetuum elemosinata et carte presentis confirmatione dicti magister[(m)] et fratres sustinebunt unum[(n)] lampadem in ecclesia dicti hospitalis coram altari bea-|10|-te Marie inperpetuum. Et ego sepedictus Willelmus et heredes mei vel assignati dictas duas(o) dimid(ias) acras prati singulis annis a predictis magistro et fratri-|11|-bus dicti hospitalis et eorum successoribus eligendas cum suis pertinenciis, ut prenominatum est, dictis magistro(p) et fratribus(q) et eorum successoribus contra omnes |12| gentes inperpetuum warantizabimus,(r) adquietabimus, et defendemus et protegemus, sicut puram, meram, liberam et perpetuam elemosinam nostram. In cuius |13| rei testimonium presentem cartam sigilli mei impressione(s) duxi roborandam. Hiis(t) testibus:(u) domino Roberto de *Pynkeneye*, Henrico de *Hynton'*, Nicholao(v) |14| de *Grimescot'* in *Croulton'*, Roberto de *Schyringe*, Huberto de Eynho, Waltero *West* de *Walton'*, Nicholao de Eynho clerico, Iohanne de eadem clerico, |15| Galfrido *Beumunt*, et aliis.

(a) eccllesie *A.* — (b) advenerit *B.* — (c) Haya *B.* — (d) Hayno *B.* — (e) *First* -s- of assignatis *inserted in interline, B.* — (f) et *add. B.* — (g) sine *om. B.* — (h) cuiullibet *B.* — (i) dicti *om. B.* — (j) voluerunt *B.* — (k) inpedimento *B.* — (l) prati *om. B.* — (m) magistri *B.* — (n) unam *B.* — (o) asignati duas dictas *B.* — (p) magister *B.* — (q) hosp(italis) *add. B.* — (r) warentizabimus *B.* — (s) inpressione *B.* — (t) His *B.* — (u) *B ends here.* — (v) Nochol(ao) *A.*

## Charter of the aforementioned

William de la Haye of Croughton [sends his] eternal greeting in the Lord to all children of the holy mother Church whom this present document may reach. May you all know that I have given, conceded, and confirmed with this my present charter, for the salvation of my soul and the souls of my ancestors, to God and blessed Mary, and to the master and brothers of the hospital of saints James and John in the vill of Aynho, two half acres of meadowland from the three half acres of meadowland of my outlying meadow that lies in the meadow of Croughton near [the] Cherwell [river], with the said master and brothers and their successors having and holding the said two half acres of land and what pertains to them, without any hindrance, from me, my heirs or assignees, free, quit, well and in peace, in perpetuity, in free, pure, and perpetual alms, just like all alms should be purely and freely given, without any court obligations, custom, or demand, on the condition that the said master and brothers of the said hospital may first choose from the aforementioned three half acres of meadowland the two best half acres of meadowland each year at mowing time, without impediment or objection from me, my heirs or assignees, and have them in perpetuity; and my heirs or assignees and I will have the remaining third half acre of meadowland after their selection. For this donation, concession in perpetual alms, and the present charter's confirmation, the said master and brothers will maintain a lamp in the church of the said hospital before the altar of the blessed Mary in perpetuity. And I, the said William, and my heirs or assignees will warrant and release to the master and brothers and their successors the said two half acres of meadowland, as named above, with their appurtenances, selected each year by the aforementioned master and brothers of the said hospital and their successors, and defend and protect them against all people in perpetuity, just like our pure, absolute, free, and perpetual alms. As testimony in this matter, I have thought fit that this present charter be corroborated with the impression of my seal. With these witnesses: lord Robert of [Moreton] Pinkney; Henry of Hinton [in the Hedges]; Nicholas of Grimscote in Croughton; Robert of Sheering; Hubert of Aynho; Walter West of Walton [Grounds]; Nicholas, clerk of Aynho; John, clerk of the same [place]; Geoffrey Beaumont; and others.

*Original.* MCA, Aynho 27. Endorsed: Hay (? s.xvi). Dimensions: 208 × 125 + 20 mm. Sealed *sur double queue*, parchment tag through one slit, seal impression missing. The scribe of this act is the same as one of the cartulary's continuators (Scribe B), who copied nos. **49–50**.

*Cartulary marginalia.* Duas di(midias) acras prati.

## 33

[*c*.1245 × 1260/70]

### Carta supradicti

Omnibus Christi fidelibus presentem cartam audituris Willelmus de Haya de *Croulton*' salutem. Noveritis me, pro salute anime mee et animabus antecessorum et successorum meorum, dedisse, concessisse et hac carta mea confirmasse Deo et beate Marie et magistr<o> et fratribus hosp(italis) beatorum apostolorum Iacobi et Iohannis de Hayno unam acram terre mee in villa de *Croulton*', scilicet dimidiam acram in campo aquilonari que iacet supra *Rowelowe* inter terram persone et terram Roberti *Beumond*, et dimidiam acram in campo australi que extendit ultra *Salt(er)estrete* inter terram hosp(italis) de Hayno et terram Galfr(idi) *Otuer*, videlicet per aniversarium Gwidonis patris mei et Amicie matris mee et puerorum meorum annuatim in ecclesia sua celebrandum in diebus quibus nomina eorum notantur in martilogio dicti hosp(italis), habendam et tenendam dictis magistro et fratribus et eorum successor(ibus) libere et quiete, bene et in pace, absque omni seculari servitio, consuetudine <et> demanda mihi vel alicui pertinentibus, scilicet inperpetuum, in liberam, puram et perpetuam elem(osinam), sicut aliqua elem(osina) melius et liberius dari potest. Et ego Willelmus et heredes mei dictam acram dictis magistro et fratribus et eorum successor(ibus) contra omnes gentes warantizab(imus), adquietabimus et defendemus. Quod ut ratum sit presentem cartam sigilli mei inpressione roboravi. His test(ibus).

**Charter of the aforementioned.**

William de la Haye of Croughton [sends his] greeting to all the faithful in Christ who may hear this present charter. May you know that I have given, conceded, and confirmed with this my present charter, for the salvation of my soul and the souls of my ancestors and successors, to God and blessed Mary, and to the master and brothers of the hospital of the blessed Apostles James and John of Aynho, one acre of my land in the vill of Croughton, namely half an acre in the northern field that lies above *Rowelowe*, between the land of the parson and the land of Robert Beaumont, and half an acre in the southern field that extends beyond *Salterestrete* between the land of the hospital of Aynho and the land of Geoffrey Otuer, for the anniversary of my father Guy, and [those of] my mother Amicia and my boys, to be celebrated annually in their church on the days marked with their names in the hospital's book of obits, to be had and held by the said master and brothers and their successors, free and quit, well and in peace, free from all secular service, custom, and demand pertaining to me or anyone else, in perpetuity and in free, pure, and perpetual alms, just as all alms should best and freely be given. And I, William, and my heirs will warrant and release to the said master and brothers and their successors the said acre and defend it against all people. In order that this is valid, I have strengthened the present charter with the impression of my seal. With these witnesses.

*Note*. This act is difficult to date precisely without a witness list. The *terminus a quo* is given by the earliest mention of William (II) de la Haye and the *terminus ad quem* by the date at which the main cartulary scribe (Scribe A) was working (see Chapter 4). The Robert Beaumont whose land is mentioned here is presumably not the same individual as Robert de Beaumont, who was dead by *c*.1220 × 1230 (no. **21**), assuming, of course, the land is not here being referred to by a previous association with this individual.

**34**

[1207 × 1219]

**Carta de *Brakele***

Universis sancte matris ecclesie filiis ad quos presens scriptum pervenerit, magister Reginaldus de Also, salutem. Noverit universitas vestra me[(a)] pro salute anime mee et antecessorum meorum Deo et beate Marie et sancto

Iacobo hosp(itali) de Hayno et magistro et fratribus ibidem Deo servientibus, domum cum pertinentiis, que sita est inter domum que fuit Galfr(idi) *Tanewomb'* et inter domum Ade de *la Quarere*, quam Iohannes *Franceys* tenet, quietam clamasse cum omni iuramento quam de eadem domo habui vel habere potui, habendam et tenendam libere et quiete, bene et in pace, sicut puram et perpet(uam) elem(osinam), reddendo inde annuatim domino comiti de *Wincestre* VI den(arios) ad tres anni terminos, scilicet ad festum sancti Michaelis II d(enarios), et ad purificationem beate Marie II d(enarios), et ad Pentecostem II d(enarios), pro omni exactione, servitio et demanda. Et ut hec mea donatio et quieta clamatio rata et inconcussa permaneat, presenti scripto sigillum meum apposui. His testibus.

(a) dedisse *struck through, B.*

### Charter of Brackley

Master Reginald of Halse [sends his] greeting to all children of the holy mother Church whom this present document may reach. May you all know that, for the salvation of my soul and [those] of my ancestors, I have quit-claimed to God and blessed Mary, and to the hospital of Aynho, and the master and brothers who serve God there, the house, with its appurtenances, situated between the house that was Geoffrey Tanewomb's and the house of Adam de la Quarere, which John Fraunceis holds, with all rights I have had and have been able to have to that house, to be had and held free and quit, well and in peace, as pure and perpetual alms, thence rendering 6d each year to the lord earl of Winchester on three occasions, namely 2d on the feast of St Michael, 2d on the Purification of the blessed Mary, and 2d at Whitsun, for all exaction, service, and demand. And so that this my donation and quit-claim remain valid and intact, I have affixed my seal to the present charter. With these witnesses.

*Note.* The reference to the earl of Winchester means this act must have been issued after Brackley passed to Saer de Quincy through his marriage to Margaret de Beaumont, daughter of Robert de Beaumont, earl of Leicester (†1190), following the death without issue of Margaret's brother, Robert, in 1204. Sear de Quincy was made 1st Earl of Winchester in 1207 and died in 1219. Sear was succeeded by his second son, Roger de Quincy. He took possession of his father's lands in 1221 but did not receive the title of earl of Winchester until after Margaret's death in 1235 (R. Oram, 'Quincy, Roger de, earl of Winchester (c. 1195–1264)', *ODNB* 2004). Master Reginald of Halse appears in numerous Brackley charters in the period 1210 × 1230, often alongside Geoffrey Tanewomb (MCA, Brackley 184, 2A, 52A, 132A, B178, B182, C33, D21), who was his brother (MCA, Astwick and Evenley 108A), but he seems to have been dead by the mid-1230s, when the land which he formerly held in Brackley was given to its hospital by Earl Roger, i.e., after 1235 (MCA, Brackley D90). Geoffrey Tanewomb is identified as being the father of a certain Richard Fraunceis, who became a brother at Brackley Hospital around 1260 (MCA, Astwick and Evenley 8), and certainly before 6 February 1261, when he is specifically identified as being among the brethren (MCA, Brackley 70A). Richard was perhaps a relative of the clerk Robert Fraunceis, a scribe of Aynho acts (see Chapter 3).

## 35

[bef. 1260/70]

### Carta Ricardi de *Bereford*

Notum sit omnibus sancte matris ecclesie filiis ad quos presens scriptum pervenerit quod ego Ricardus *Hunte* de *Bereford*, filius Willelmi *Hunte*, pro salute mea et Agn(er)t(ae) uxoris mee et heredum meorum et antecessorum meorum, dedi et[(a)] confirmavi inperpet(uum), in puram et perpetuam elem(osinam), Deo et beate Marie et hosp(itali) apostolorum Iacobi et Iohannis de Hayno unam dimidiam summam frumenti annuatim in festo sancti Michaelis omni occasione post posita de terra mea de *B(er)eford* quicumque illam terram tenebit vel habebit. Et ego et heredes mei predictam dimidiam summam frumenti inperpet(uum) sine fraude et dilatione predicto hosp(itali) nomine elem(osine) singulis annis ad predictum terminum persolvemus. Et ut hec mea don(atio) et confirmatio rata et inconcussa permaneat, hanc cartam meam sigilli mei munimine roboravi. His test(ibus).

(a) et *repeated in error, B.*

### Richard of Barford's charter

May it be known to all children of the holy mother Church whom this present document may reach that I, Richard Hunte of Barford, son of William Hunte, have given and confirmed in perpetuity, for the salvation of my soul and [those] of my wife, Agnerta, and my ancestors and heirs, in pure and perpetual alms, to God and blessed Mary, and to the hospital of the blessed Apostles James and John of Aynho, a half measure of grain from my land at Barford each year at the feast of St Michael, reserved under all circumstances, for as long as I shall have and hold it. And my heirs and I will pay the aforementioned half measure of grain to the aforementioned hospital as alms every year at the said time, in perpetuity, without deceit or delay. And so that this my donation and confirmation remain valid and intact, I have strengthened this my charter with the protection of my seal. With these witnesses.

*Note.* Richard Hunte of Barford is seemingly known only by this act, which, shorn of its witness list, is impossible to date precisely. It must have been issued, however, before the date at which the main cartulary scribe (Scribe A) is known to have worked (see Chapter 4).

## 36

[bef. 25 Oct 1202]

### Carta Baldowini de *Bifeld*

Sciant tam presentes quam futuri quod ego Baldewinus[(a)] de Bolunia dedi et concessi, consilio et assesnu *Aeliz*[(b)] uxoris mee et Willelmi filii mei, |1| heredis mei, unam virgatam terre in villa de *Bifeld'* quam Rad(ulfus) filius Regineri tenuit, reddendo inde annuatim hospitali sancti Iacobi |2| de Aenho quatuor[(c)] solid(os), pro salute anime mee et *Aeliz*[(d)] uxoris mee et Willelmi filii mei, et pro anima Gaufr(idi) de *Waffre*[(e)] et Beatricis et pro |3| animabus omnium antecessorum meorum, bene et in pace, libere et quiete et honorifice, in villa et extra villam, in pratis et in pascuis et in |4| omnibus liberis consuetudinibus et exactionibus, in puram et perpetuam elemosinam. Et ut hec donatio mea rata et inconcussa permaneat, |5| eam sigilli mei appositione corroboravi.[(f)] Et ego[(g)] Baldwinus[(h)] predictus et heredes mei warantizare[(i)] debemus hanc predictam terram prefato hospi-|6|-tali contra omnes homines. Hiis[(j)] testibus:[(k)] Turberto et Iordano, capellanis, Ric(ardo) de *Hinton'*, Roberto de *Turvill'*, Osb(erto) filio Ric(ardi) de *Hint'*, Waltero |7| camerario, Roberto de Bellomonte, Rog(er)o de *Costenti(n)*, Warino de Verineto, Rad(ulfo) clerico de Aenho, Willelmo de *Bifed'*, et multis aliis.

(a) Baldowynus *B.* — (b) Aliz *B.* — (c) Hayno IIII[or] *B.* — (d) Aliz *B.* — (e) Galfridi de Wavere *B.* — (f) apositione coroboravi *B.* — (g) Rad' *struck through, B.* — (h) Baldowynus *B.* — (i) warentizare *B.* — (j) gentes. His *B.* — (k) *B ends here.*

### Baldwin's charter concerning Byfield

May those present and future know that I, Baldwin de Boulogne, have given and conceded, in pure and perpetual alms, with the counsel and consent of Alice, my wife, and my son William, my heir, one virgate of land in the vill of Byfield, which Ralph, son of Reginer, held, thence rendering 4s each year to the hospital of St James of Aynho, for the salvation of my soul and [those] of Alice, my wife, and William, my son, and for the soul of Geoffrey de Wavre and [that of his wife,] Beatrice, and for the souls of all my ancestors, well and in peace, free and quit and fittingly, inside and outside the vill, in meadows and pastures, and in all free customs and exactions. And so that this my donation remains valid and intact, I have corroborated it with the affixing of my seal. And I, the aforementioned Baldwin, and my heirs shall warrant this aforementioned land to the said hospital against all people. With these witnesses: Turbert and Jordan, chaplains; Richard of Hinton [in the Hedges]; Robert de Turville; Osbert, son of Richard of Hinton [in the Hedges]; Walter Chamberlain; Robert de Beaumont; Roger of the Cotentin; Warin de *Verineto*; Ralph, clerk of Aynho; William of Byfield; and many others.

*Original.* MCA, Aynho 43. Endorsed: pro Bifeld' (s.xiii). Dimensions: 234 × 70 + 24 mm. Sealed *sur double queue*, parchment tag through three slits, seal impression missing. This act is in the hand of the same scribe as nos. **37–38**.

*Note.* Dated *c.*1200 × 1210 by Macray, but this donation must have been made before 25 October 1202, when Innocent III confirmed the hospital's possessions, including one virgate of land at Byfield (**no. 1**). Roger of the Cotentin is listed as landholder at Hargrave in a twelfth-century survey of Northamptonshire (Keats-Rohan (ed.), *Domesday People*, p. 104). On the translation of 'de Bifeld' as 'concerning Byfield' rather than 'of Byfield', see Chapter 1 (p. 40, n. 148).

## 37

[bef. 25 Oct 1202]

### Carta uxoris eius super eodem

Sciant tam presentes quam futuri quod ego *Aeliz* de *Waffre*[(a)] dedi et concessi, consilio et assensu Willelmi filii mei, |1| heredis mei, unam virgatam terre in villa de *Bifeld'*, quam Rad(ulfus) filius Regineri tenuit, reddendo inde annu atim hos-|2|-pitali sancti Iacobi de Aenho quatuor[(b)] solid(os), pro salute anime mee et Willelmi filii mei, et pro anima Gaufridi |3| de *Waffre*[(c)] et Beatricis et pro animabus omnium antecessorum meorum et successorum, bene et in pace, libere et quiete |4| et honorifice, in villa et extra villam, in pratis et pascuis et in omnibus liberis consuetudinibus et exactionibus, in |5| puram et perpetuam elemosinam. Et ut hec donatio mea rata et inconcussa permaneat, eam sigillo |6| meo corroboravi. Et ego predicta *Aeliz*[(d)] et heredes mei warantizare[(e)] debemus predicto hospitali hanc |7| predictam donationem contra omnes homines. Hiis[(f)] testibus:[(g)] Turberto et Iordano, capell(anis), Ric(ardo) de *Hinton'*, |8| Roberto de *T(ur)vill'*, Osb(erto) filio Ric(ardi) de *Hint'*, Waltero camerario, Roberto de Bello Monte, Rog(er)o de

|9| *Costenti(n)*, Warino de Verineto, Rad(ulfo) clerico de Aenho, Willelmo de *Bifeld'*, et multis aliis.

(a) Aliz de Wavere, *with* -a- *inserted in interline, B.* — (b) Hayno IIII$^{or}$ *B.* — (c) Galfridi de Wavere *B.* — (d) Alis' *B.* — (e) warentizare *B.* — (f) gentes. His *B.* — (g) *B ends here.*

### His wife's charter concerning the same

May those present and future know that I, Alice de Wavre, have given and conceded, in pure and perpetual alms, with the counsel and consent of my son William, my heir, one virgate of land in the vill of Byfield, which Ralph, son of Reginer, held, thence rendering 4s each year to the hospital of St James of Aynho, for the salvation of my soul and [that] of William, my son, and for the soul of Geoffrey de Wavre and [that of his wife,] Beatrice, and for the souls of all my ancestors and successors, well and in peace, free and quit and fittingly, inside and outside the vill, in meadows and pastures, and in all free customs and exactions. And so that this my donation remains valid and intact, I have corroborated it with my seal. And I, the aforementioned Alice, and my heirs shall warrant this aforementioned land to the said hospital against all people. With these witnesses: Turbert and Jordan, chaplains; Richard of Hinton [in the Hedges]; Robert de Turville; Osbert, son of Richard of Hinton [in the Hedges]; Walter Chamberlain; Robert de Beaumont; Roger of the Cotentin; Warin de *Verineto*; Ralph, clerk of Aynho; William of Byfield; and many others.

*Original.* MCA, Aynho 41. Endorsed: Bifeld' (s.xiv/s.xv); Byfeld' (s.xv). Dimensions: 181 × 80 + 26 mm. Sealed *sur double queue*, parchment tag through three slits, seal impression missing. This act is in the hand of the same scribe as nos. **36**, **38**.

*Note.* Dated *c.*1200 × 1210 by Macray, but same as no. **37**.

## 38

[bef. 25 Oct 1202]

### Confirmatio primogeniti eorum

Sciant presentes et futuri quod ego Willelmus de Haia,[a] filius Bald(winus)[b] de Bolon(ia), concedo et confirmo donationem quam Baldwinus[c] |1| pater <meus> et *Aeliz*[d] mater mea dederunt hospitali sancti Iacobi de Aenho,[e] scilicet unam[f] virgatam terre[g] in villa de *Bifeld*, |2| quam Rad(ulfus) filius Regineri tenuit, reddendo inde annuatim hospitali predicto quatuor[h] solid(os) sicut carte Baldwini[(i)] patris |[3]| mei et *Aeliz*[(j)] matris mee testantur. Et ut hec concessio et confirmatio mea[(k)] rata et[(l)] inconcussa permaneat, eam |[4]| sigillo meo corroboravi. Hiis[(m)] testibus:[(n)] Turberto et Iordano, capellanis, Ric(ardo) de *Hinton'*, Roberto de Turville, Osb(erto) filio Ric(ardi) |[5]| de *Hint'*, Waltero camerario, Roberto de Bello Monte, Rog(er)o de *Costenti(n)*, Warino de Verineto, Rad(ulfo) clerico de |[6]| Aenho, Willelmo de *Bifeld'*, et multis aliis.

(a) Haya *B.* — (b) Rad' *B.* — (c) Baldowynus *B.* — (d) Aliz *B.* — (e) Hayno *B.* — (f) *Erasure of letters* vi- *before* unam, *A.* — (g) t(er)rre *A.* — (h) IIII[or] *B.* — (i) Baldowyni *B.* — (j) Aliz *B.* — (k) mea concessio et confirmatio *B.* — (l) in *repeated in error, A.* — (m) His *B.* — (n) *B ends here.*

## Their firstborn's confirmation

May those present and future know that I, William de la Haye, son of Baldwin de Boulogne, concede and confirm the donation that Baldwin, my father, and Alice, my mother, gave to the hospital of St James of Aynho, namely one virgate of land in the vill of Byfield, which Ralph, son of Reginer, held, thence rendering 4s each year to the said hospital, as the charters of Baldwin, my father, and Alice, my mother, testify. And so that this my concession and confirmation remain valid and intact, I have corroborated it with my seal. With these witnesses: Turbert and Jordan, chaplains; Richard of Hinton [in the Hedges]; Robert de Turville; Osbert, son of Richard of Hinton [in the Hedges]; Walter Chamberlain; Robert de Beaumont; Roger of the Cotentin; Warin de *Verineto*; Ralph, clerk of Aynho; William of Byfield; and many others.

*Original.* MCA, Aynho 42. Endorsed: no endorsements. Dimensions: 203 × 66 + 30 mm. Sealed *sur double queue*, parchment tag through three slits. Seal: round, fragmentary, white wax painted brown: 36 mm. A mythical creature or perhaps a lion or a wolf (head missing). Legend: destroyed. This act is in the hand of the same scribe as nos. **36–7**.

*Note.* Dated *c.*1200 × 1210 by Macray, but same as nos. **36–7**, which were written by the same scribe at the same time.

## 39

[bef. 25 Oct 1202]

### Confirmatio alterius filii

Sciant presentes et futuri quod ego Wido[a] de Haya, filius Baldewinus[b] de Boloin(ia), concedo et confirmo donationem quam Baldewinus[b] pater meus et *Aliz* mater mea dederunt |1| hospitali sancti Iacobi de Heyno,[c] scilicet unam virgatam terre in villa de *Byfeld'*,[d] quam Radulfus filius Reineri[e] tenuit, reddendo inde annuatim quatuor sol(idos) predicto |2| hospitali, sicut carte Baldewini[f] patris mei et *Aliz* matris mee et Willelmi fratris mei testantur. Et ut hec concessio et confirmatio mea[g] rata et inconcussa perma-|3|-neat, eam sigillo meo corroboravi. Hiis[h] testibus:[i] Thurberto persona de Eyno, Ada capellano de Edb(ur)b(er)ia, Ric(ardo) de *Hinton'*, Roberto de Thurevilla, |4| Osberto filio Ric(ardi) de *Hynton'*, Waltero camerario, Roberto de Bello Monte, Rog(er)o de *Costetin'*, Warino de Vireni, Radulfo clerico de Eyno, Willelmo de *Byfeld'*, |5| Iordano qui hanc cartam scripsit, et multis aliis.

(a) Wydo *B.* — (b) Baldowinus *B.* — (c) Hayno *B.* — (d) Bifeld' *B.* — (e) Reyn(eri)*B.* — (f) Baldow<i>ni *B.* — (g) mea concessio et confirmatio *B.* — (h) His *B.* — (i) *B ends here.*

### The other son's confirmation

May those present and future know that I, Guy de la Haye, son of Baldwin de Boulogne, concede and confirm the donation that Baldwin, my father, and Alice, my mother, gave to the hospital of St James of Aynho, namely one virgate of land in the vill of Byfield, which Ralph, son of Reginer, held, thence returning 4s each year to the said hospital, as the charters of Baldwin, my father, Alice, my mother, and William, my brother, testify. And so that this my concession and confirmation remain valid and intact, I have corroborated it with my seal. With these witnesses: Turbert, parson of Aynho; Adam, chaplain of Adderbury; Richard of Hinton [in the Hedges]; Robert de Turville; Osbert, son of Richard of Hinton [in the Hedges]; Walter Chamberlain; Robert de Beaumont; Roger of the Cotentin; Warin de *Verineto*; Ralph, clerk of Aynho; William of Byfield; Jordan, who wrote this charter; and many others.

*Original.* MCA, Aynho 40. Endorsed: Eynow. Pro villa de Byfeld' (s.xv). Dimensions: 227 × 62 + 11 mm. Sealed *sur double queue*, parchment tag through three slits. Seal, round, white wax painted brown: 30 mm. A fleur-de-lis. Legend: ✠ SIGILL(*vm*) WIDONIS DE HAIA.

*Note.* Dated *c.*1215 by Macray, but likely closer in date to nos. **36–8**. The act is witnessed by Turbert, parson of Aynho, who appears as witness to the hospital's 'foundation charter' (no. **4**) and was first installed at the presentation of Ralph de Diceto in the 1160s. Unless we therefore wish to make Turbert especially long lived, this charter was likely issued around the same time as nos. **36–8**. The charter's scribe, Jordan, is perhaps the chaplain by that name who witnesses alongside Turbert in nos. **36–8**, and thus also perhaps the future master of Aynho Hospital by that name.

## 40

[May 1177 × Sep 1181]

### Carta domini Cantuariensis

Ric(ardus), Dei gratia, Cant(uariensis) archiepiscopus, tocius Anglie primas et apostolice sedis legatus, universis Christi fidelibus ad quos littere iste perve-|1|-nerint, eternam in Domino salutem. Ad omnium noticiam volumus pervenire, controversiam inter dilectos filios nostros Laur(encium) presbiterum de *Creulton'*[a] |2| et R. clericum de *Wavre*,[b] super capella sancti Michaelis de *Creult'* et pertinenciis eius motam et aliquandiu agitatam, tandem sub hac[c] transactionis |3| forma conquievisse. Predictus R. percipiet omnes decimas tocius dominii Galfridi de *Wavre*[d] et Osberti[e] filii Ric(ardi), quod est de feodo |4| comitis Willelmi de *Mandevill'*,[f] in villa de *Creult'*, a quocunque culti,[g] et omnes decimas de garbis molendinarii et firma[h] molen-|5|-dini, minute autem decime molendinarii et oblationes, apud matricem ecclesiam de *Creult'*, residebunt, ubi idem molendinarius et sui |6| spiritualia percipient. Preter hec autem percipiet ecclesia de *Creult'*, in autumpno, omnes fructus unius acre, et unum agnum, et unum por-|7|-cellum, et unum vellus, et unum caseum, annuatim, si forte de dominio predicti G. talia provenerint.[i] Omnia vero alia inde provenien-|8|-cia ad predictam capellam pertinebunt. Preterea habebit matrix ecclesia, decimas provenientes[j] de quarta parte virgate terre, ad preli-|9|-batam capellam pertinente. Prescriptus quoque R. absque[k] licencia persone ecclesie de *Creult'*, libere et sine contradictione, in pretaxata capella |10| divina faciet celebrari officia. Unde ut[l] eadem transactio que de voluntate et beneplacito predictorum G. et O. et Ric(ardi) Nigrenoctis |11| et H. *Pirun*, advocatorum ecclesie[m] de *Creult'*,[n] sicut prefati L. presbiter et R. clericus constanter nobis proposuerunt, facta est, permaneat |12| in posterum inconvulsa,[o] eam presenti scripto confirmamus et sigilli nostri apposicione[p] roboramus. His testibus:[q] magistro Ger(ardo), Willelmo archidiacono |13| Gloec(estriensi), magistro R. de Sancto Martino, magistro R. de *Roulvest'*, Nicholao Walensi, magistro R. Norwic(ensi), magistro R. |[14]| Walensi, Henrico Baioc(ensi), Ric(ardo) et Galfr(ido), clericis, Willelmo de *Sotindon*'.

(a) Croulton' *in all subsequent occurences but one, B.* — (b) Waver(e) *B.* — (c) hac *om. B.* — (d) Wavere *B.* — (e) Oseberti *B.* — (f) Mandevile *B.* — (g) cultu *B.* — (h) firmo *B.* — (i) pervenerint *B.* — (j) pertinentes *B.* — (k) asque *B.* — (l) ad *B.* — (m) eccilesie *with expunging dot under* -i-, *B.* — (n) Crolton' *B.* — (o) inconwlsa *B.* — (p) aposicione *B.* — (q) *B ends here.*

## The lord [archbishop] of Canterbury's charter

Richard, by God's grace archbishop of Canterbury, primate of all England and legate of the Apostolic See, [sends his] eternal greeting in the Lord to all the faithful in Christ whom this document may reach. We wish for notice to reach everyone that the dispute raised and pursued for some time between our beloved sons, Lawrence, priest of Croughton, and R., clerk of Wavre, concerning the chapel of St Michael of Croughton and its appurtenances, has at last been settled by way of this agreement: the aforementioned R. will receive all the tithes of all the demesne of Geoffrey de Wavre and Osbert, son of Richard, which is of the fief of Earl William de Mandeville, in the vill of Croughton, from whatever crop, and all the tithes of the miller's sheafs and the mill-house farm, but the miller's small tithes and offerings shall remain at the mother church of Croughton, where that miller and his men receive spiritual [ministrations]. Besides this, moreover, the church of Croughton shall receive in autumn each year all the fruits of an acre, and one lamb, and one piglet, and one fleece, and one cheese, if such things should be produced by the demesne of the said G[eoffrey]. Everything else accruing thereafter shall belong to the said chapel. Furthermore, the mother church will have the tithes arising from the fourth part of a virgate of land pertaining to the aforesaid chapel. The aforesaid R. may also celebrate the divine offices in the aforesaid chapel, freely and without contradiction, without license of the parson of the church of Croughton. So, on that basis, this agreement was made with the goodwill and pleasure of the aforesaid G[eoffrey] and O[sbert], and of Richard Neirenuit and H. Pirun, advocates of the church of Croughton, in the same way that the aforesaid L[awrence], the priest, and R., the clerk, have consistently declared to us, [and so that it] remains henceforth undisputed, we confirm the present document and strengthen it by the affixing of our seal. With these witnesses: Master Gerard; William, archdeacon of Gloucester; Master R. de St Martin; Master R. of Rolleston; Nicholas Walensis; Master R. of Norwich; Master R. Walensis; Henry de Bayeux; Richard and Geoffrey the clerks; William of Shottenden.

*Original.* MCA, Brackley 76A. Endorsed: Cyrencestr' (s.xiii, preceded and followed by notary's signs?); Carta de dec(imis) capelle de Crolton' (s.xiii/s.xiv). Dimensions: 188 × 110 + 20 mm. Sealed *sur double queue*, parchment tag through three slits, with seal sewn in patterned woollen bag. Pd from *A* in *EEA*, vol. 2, no. 117, pp. 95–6.

*Note.* The dates are those of William [of Northolt] as archdeacon of Gloucester.

*Cartulary marginalia.* Archiepiscopus super capellam.

## 41

[bef. 25 Oct 1202]

### Carta donatoris capelle[(a)] de *Croulton'*

**[Membrane 7]**

Sciant tam presentes quam futuri quod ego Ba[ld]uinus de Buluinia[(b)] dedi et concessi consilio |[1]| et assensu *Aliz* uxoris mee et Willelmi filii mei heredis mei capellam meam in villa de Crowltona[(c)] |[2]| cum omnibus pertinentiis hospitali sancti Iacobi de Heinoia,[(d)] in puram et perpetuam elemosinam, |[3]| pro salute anime mee et *Aliz* uxoris mee et Willelmi filii mei et Walteri filii mei et Galfridi de |[4]| *Waffre*[(e)] et Beatricis et omnium antecessorum meorum, post decessum Thome clerici, filii Laurentii |[5]| sacerdotis. Hiis[(f)] testibus:[(g)] Ricardo de Hintona, Roberto de *T(ur)vill'*, Hosberto filio Ric(ardi) de *Hint'*, Waltero ca-|[6]|-merario, Roberto de *Beaumund'*, Rog(er)o de *Costetin'*, Warino de Virineto, Philippo filio Hugonis |[7]| de *Biffeud'*, Rad(u)l(fo) clerico de Heino, Turberto persona, Iordano capellano, Laurentio persona de |[8]| Crowltona, et multis aliis.

(a) cappelli *B.* — (b) Baldwinus de Buluina *B.* — (c) Croulton' *B.* — (d) Hayno *B.* — (e) Wavere *B.* — (f) His *B.* — (g) *B ends here.*

### Charter of the donor of the chapel of Croughton

May those present and future know that I, Baldwin de Boulogne, after the death of Thomas the clerk, son of Lawrence the priest, have given and conceded, with the counsel and consent of Alice, my wife, and my son William, my heir, my chapel in the vill of Croughton, with all its appurtenances, to the hospital of St James of Aynho, in pure and perpetual alms, for the salvation of my soul and [those] of my wife Alice, my sons William and Walter, Geoffrey de Wavre and [his wife] Beatrice, and all my ancestors.

With these witnesses: Richard of Hinton [in the Hedges]; Robert de Turville; Osbert, son of Richard of Hinton [in the Hedges]; Walter Chamberlain; Robert de Beaumont; Roger of the Cotentin; Warin de *Verineto*; Philip, son of Hugh of Byfield; Ralph, clerk of Aynho; Turbert, the parson; Jordan, the chaplain; Lawrence, parson of Croughton; and many others.

*Original.* MCA, Aynho 85. Endorsed: Baldewinus. Capella de Crowlto' [...] (s.xv, badly faded); R. de Clipston' (? s.xvi, followed by notary's mark?). Dimensions: 166 × 70 + 22 mm. Sealed *sur double queue*, parchment tag through three slits, seal impression missing.

*Note.* Macray dates this act *c.*1210, but this donation must have been made before 25 October 1202, when Innocent III confirmed the hospital's possessions, including the chapel of St Michael's, Croughton (no. **1**). Many of the witnesses to this act also appear in nos. **36–9**.

## 42

[bef. 25 Oct 1202]

### Item donatio eiusdem

Sciant presentes et futuri quod ego Alicia de *Wavre,* uxor Baldowini de Balonia, dedi et concessi, consilio et assensu Willelmi filii mei, heredis mei, capellam meam in villa de *Croulton',* cum omnibus pertinentiis, hosp(itali) sancti Iacobi de Hayno, in puram et perpetuam elem(osinam), salvo servitio forinseco, pro salute anime mee et Baldowini sponsi mei, et Willelmi filii mei, et Walteri filii mei, et Galfridi de *Wavre* patris mei et Beatricis matris mee et omnium antecessorum meorum, post decessum Thome clerici, filii Laurentii sacerdotis. His testibus.

### Also [concerning] the donation of the same

May those present and future know that I, Alice de Wavre, wife of Baldwin de Boulogne, after the death of Thomas the clerk, son of Lawrence the priest, have given and conceded, with the counsel and consent of my son William, my heir, my chapel in the vill of Croughton, with all its appurtenances, to the hospital of St James of Aynho, in pure and perpetual alms, saving foreign service, for the salvation of my soul and [those] of Baldwin, my spouse, William, my son, Walter, my son, and Geoffrey de Wavre, my father, and Beatrice, my mother, and all my ancestors. With these witnesses.

*Note.* Since Baldwin de Boulogne, Alice, his wife, and William, their heir, all issued their acts concerning the land at Byfield at the same time (nos. **36–8**), using the same scribe each time, it seems reasonable to assume that they did so similarly in relation to the chapel of Croughton. This act is therefore dated the same as no. **41**.

## 43

[bef. 25 Oct 1202]

### Confi[r]matio dicte capelle

Nov<er>rint tam presentes quam futuri quod ego Willelmus de Haya concedo et confirmo et ratam habeo donat(ionem)[a] quam pater meus et mater mea fecerunt hosp(itali) sancti Iacobi de Hayno de capella in villa de *Croulton'*, cum omnibus pertinentiis, in puram et perpetuam elem(osinam), salvo forinseco servitio sicut carta patris mei Baldowini de Bolo(n)ia et carta matris mee Alic(ie) de *Wavre*[b] testantur. His testibus.

(a) meam *struck through, B.* — (b) -r- *of* Wavre *inserted in interline, B.*

### Confirmation of the said chapel

May those present and future know that I, William de la Haye, concede, confirm, and consider valid the donation my father and mother made to the hospital of St James of Aynho of a chapel in the vill of Croughton, with all its appurtenances, in pure and perpetual alms, saving foreign service, as the charter of my father, Baldwin de Boulogne, and the charter of my mother, Alice de Wavre, testify. With these witnesses.

*Note*. Dated for the same reason as nos. **41–2**.

## 44

[*c*.1215]

### Item confirmatio eiusdem

Omnibus Christi fidelibus ad quos presens scriptum pervenerit Wido de Haya eternam in Domino salutem. Discrecioni vestre notum facio me, divine pietatis intuitu, et pro salute mea et meorum et pro salute animarum antecessorum meorum concessionem et don(ationem) patris mei Baldowini et matris mee Alic(ie) de *Wavre* super capella sancti Michaelis in *Croult'* factam hosp(itali) sancti Iacobi in Ayno et fratribus ibidem commorantibus, salvo extrinseco servitio V acrarum, sigilli mei robore confirmasse, sicut carte eorum testantur. His testibus.

**Also [concerning] the confirmation of the same**

Guy de la Haye [sends his] eternal greeting in the Lord to all the faithful in Christ whom this present document may reach. I make it known to your discernment that I have confirmed with the strength of my seal, for the sake of holy piety and the salvation of my soul and the souls of my ancestors, the concession and donation of my father, Baldwin, and my mother, Alice de Wavre, concerning the chapel of St Michael in Croughton to the hospital of St James of Aynho and the brothers dwelling there, saving outside service of five acres, as their charters testify. With these witnesses.

*Note.* This act is difficult to date precisely without a witness list, but it was perhaps issued around the same time as no. **47**, in which Guy is said to have given his consent as the chapel's patron.

**45**

[bef. 25 Oct 1202 or *c.*1215]

**Item donatio dicte capelle**

Sciant presentes et futuri quod ego Robertus de Bellomonte et *Mileseynt* uxor mea dedimus et concessimus et quantum ad nos pertinet cartis nostris confrimavimus capellam sancti Michaelis de *Croult'*, cum omnibus pertinentiis suis, hosp(itali) sancti Iacobi de Hayno in puram et perpetuam elem(osinam), pro salute animarum nostrarum et omnium antecessorum nostrorum. Et ut hec don(atio) rata et inconcussa permaneat, sigillorum nostrorum apositione roboravimus. His testibus.

**Also [concerning] the donation of the said chapel**

May those present and future know that I, Robert de Beaumont, and Melisende, my wife, have given, conceded, and inasmuch as pertains to us, confirmed with our charters, for the salvation of our souls and [those] of all our ancestors, the chapel of St Michael in Croughton, with all its appurtenances, to the hospital of St James of Aynho, in pure and perpetual alms. And so that this donation remains valid and intact, we have corroborated it with the affixing of our seals. With these witnesses.

*Note.* As the husband of the other daughter of Geoffrey de Wavre, Robert may have issued this act with his wife at the same time as that of his brother-in-law, Baldwin de Boulogne (no. **41**). Alternatively, it may have been issued at the same time as Guy de la Haye's confirmation above (no. **44**).

## 46

[bef. 25 Oct 1202]

### Item donatio eiusdem

Sciant presentes et futuri quod ego Walterus camerarius et uxor mea *Roeis*[(a)] dedimus et concessimus et quantum ad nos pertinet cartis |[1]| nostris confrimavimus capellam[(b)] sancti Michaelis de Crueltona,[(c)] cum omnibus pertinentiis suis, hospitali sancti Iacobi de Heyno,[(d)] karitatis |[2]| intuitu, in puram et perpetuam elemosinam, et[(e)] pro salute animarum nostrarum et omnium antecessorum et successorum[(f)] nostrorum.[(g)] Et ut |[3]| hec donatio nostra[(h)] rata et inconcussa permaneat, sigillorum[(i)] nostrorum corroboratione corroboravimus. Hiis[(j)] testibus:[(k)] Rog(er)o decano de *Pa*-|[4]|-*teshulle*, Thurberto persona de Ehino, Willelmo persona de *Sulthorn'*, Roberto capellano de *Dadint'*, Rad(ulfo) *Neirnut*, Ric(ardo) clerico, |[5]| de C(r)uwltona, Rad(ulfo) clerico de Ehino.

(a) Yoeis *B.* — (b) ca- *written above erasure, B.* — (c) Croulton' *B.* — (d) Hayno *B.* — (e) et *om. B.* — (f) succesusorum *A.* — (g) nostrorum et successorum *B.* — (h) mea donatio *B.* — (i) *Second* -i- *of* sigillorum *inserted in interline, B.* — (j) His *B.* — (k) *B ends here.*

### Also [concerning] the donation of the same

May those present and future know that I, Walter Chamberlain, and my wife, Roeis, have given, conceded, and inasmuch as pertains to us, confirmed with our charters, for charity's sake and for the salvation of our souls and [those] of all our ancestors and successors, the chapel of St Michael in Croughton, with all its appurtenances, to the hospital of St James of Aynho, in pure and perpetual alms. And so that this donation remains valid and intact, we have corroborated it with the strengthening of our seals. With these witnesses: Roger, dean of Pattishall; Turbert, parson of Aynho; William, parson of Souldern; Robert, chaplain of Deddington; Ralph Neirenuit; Richard, clerk of Croughton; Ralph, clerk of Aynho.

*Original.* MCA, Aynho 30. Endorsed: Capella de Crolton' (s. xv). Dimensions: 204 × 55 + 15 mm. Sealed *sur double queue*, two parchment tags through three slits, one seal remaining. Three slits also in centre of fold, no tag. Seal: round, white wax painted brown: 39 mm. Stylised vines. Legend: ✠ S[IG]ILL(*vm*) W[ALTERI L]E CHA(*m*)BERLENE.

*Note.* Macray dates this act *c*.1210 × 1215, but it was likely issued around the same time as no. **41**. Some of the witnesses of this act also appear in nos. **36–9**, **41**, including Turbert, parson of Aynho, who was first installed in the 1160s.

## 47

7 February 1215 — Banbury.

### Confirmatio capelle per dominum Lincoln'

Omnibus Christi fidelibus ad quos presens scriptum pervenerit Hugo, Dei gratia, Linc(olniensi) episcopus, eternam in domino salutem. |1| Cum ea que locis religiosis rationabiliter collata sunt pium sit perpetuo roborare, nos intuitu Dei capellam de *Cro-*|2|*-ultun'*,(a) de consensu Guidonis de *la Haye*(b) patroni eiusdem cappelle, hospitali de Einho(c) in usus proprios habendam con-|3|-cedimus et episcopali auctoritate confirmamus, salvis in omnibus episcopalibus consuetudinibus et Linc(olniensis) ecclesie dignitate. Quod ut |4| perpetuam optineat firmitatem, presenti scripto sigillum nostrum apposuimus. Hiis(d) testibus:(e) Willelmo de *Tornac'* archi-|5|-diacono de Stowa, magistro Reginaldo de Cestr(iensi), Rogero cappellano, Petro de Bathon(iensi), canonicis Linc(olniensibus), magistro Roberto |6| de *G(r)avel'*, magistro Ric(ardo) de *Tinghurst'*, Rog(er)o de *Bohu(n)*, Stephano de Cicestr(iensi) et aliis. Dat(um) per manum Roberti |7| archidiaconi *Huntend'*, apud *Bannebyr'* septimo idus Februarii pontificatus nostri anno sexto.

(a) Croult' *B*. — (b) concensu Widon(is) de la Haya *B*. — (c) Hayno *B*. — (d) His *B*. — (e) *B ends here.*

### Confirmation of the chapel by the lord [bishop] of Lincoln

Hugh, by God's grace bishop of Lincoln, [sends his] eternal greeting in God to all the faithful in Christ whom this document may reach. Because it is pious to confirm in perpetuity those [things] granted in accordance with reason to holy places, we have conceded and confirmed with our episcopal authority, for the sake of God, the chapel of Croughton, with the consent of Guy de la Haye, patron of the same chapel, to the hospital of Aynho, to have for their own usage, saving all episcopal customs and the authority of the church of Lincoln. In order that this obtains perpetual strength, we have affixed our seal to the present document. With these witnesses: William de Tournai, archdeacon of Stow; Master Reginald of Chester; Roger the chaplain; Peter of Bath, canons of Lincoln; Master Robert of Graveley; Master Richard of Fingest; Roger de Bohon; Stephen of Chichester; and others. Given at Banbury by the hand of Robert, archdeacon of Huntingdon, on the seventh ides of February in the sixth year of our episcopate.

*Original.* MCA, Aynho 82. Endorsed: Confirmatio capelle de Crolton' (s.xv/s.xvi); R. de Clipston' (? s.xvi, followed by notary's mark?). Dimensions: 165 × 70 + 5 mm. Sealed *sur double queue*, parchment tag through one slit. Seal: pointed oval, fragmentary, white wax painted brown: 49 mm. A bishop standing, robed (head and feet destroyed), the Roman numeral 'ii' to his left. Legend: [...] [...]RA [...]. Counterseal: pointed oval, fragmentary: 35 mm. A bishop praying beneath the Virgin and Child. Legend: [VITA S]IT HVGONIS HIIS INFORMATA PA[TRONIS]. Pd from *A* in D. Smith (ed.) *The Acta of Hugh of Wells, Bishop of Lincoln, 1209–1235* (Woodbridge, 2000), no. 16, p. 13; copy (s.xiii) in Lincoln, Lincolnshire Archives, Add. Reg. 6 (Liber antiquus), fol. 23r, whence pd in A. Gibbons (ed.), *Liber antiquus de ordinationibus vicariarum tempore Hugonis Wells, Lincolniensis Episcopi, 1209–1235* (Lincoln, 1888), pp. 73–4.

*Cartulary marginalia.* II[a] episcopus.

## 48

[*c.*1215]

### Confirmatio eiusdem per capitulum Lincoln'

Omnibus sancte matris ecclesie filiis ad quos presens scriptum pervenerit R. decanus et ca-|[1]|-pitulum ecclesie Linc(olniensis), eternam in Domino salutem. Inspeximus cartam venerabilis patris nostri Hugonis |[2]| secundi Dei gratia Linc(olniensi) episcopi continentem quod ipse intuitu Dei capellam de *Crewelton'*[(a)] per consensum |[3]| Guidonis *de la Haie*[(b)] patroni eiusdem capelle hospitali de Einho[(c)] in usus proprios habendam |[4]| concessit et episcopali autoritate confirmavit, salvis in omnibus episcopalibus[(d)] consuetudinibus |[5]| et Linc(olniensis) ecclesie dignitate.[(e)] Nos igitur eandem concessionem gratam et ratam habemus et pre-|[6]|-senti scripto,[(f)] sigillum nostrum in huius rei testimonium apposuimus.

(a) Croulton' *B.* — (b) concensum Gwidonis de Haya *B.* — (c) Hayno *B.* — (d) episcopalibus in omnibus *B.* — (e) dignitate ecclesie *B.* — (f) scripto *inserted in interline, B.*

**Confirmation of the same by the chapter of Lincoln**

The dean, R[oger], and chapter of the church of Lincoln [send their] eternal greeting in the Lord to all children of the holy mother Church whom this present document may reach. We have examined the charter of our venerable father Hugh the second, by God's grace bishop of Lincoln, containing that he, for God's sake, has conceded and confirmed with his episcopal authority the chapel of Croughton, with the consent of Guy de la Haye, patron of the same chapel, to the hospital of Aynho, to have for their own usage, saving all episcopal customs and the authority of the church of Lincoln. We therefore consider this concession agreeable and valid [and] affix our seal to the present document in evidence of this matter.

*Original.* MCA, Aynho 81. Endorsed: Confirmacio capelle sancti Michaelis de Crolton' (s.xv/s.xvi); R. de Clipst' (? s.xvi, followed by notary's mark?). Dimensions: 154 × 59 + 10 mm. Sealed *sur double queue*, parchment tag through two slits. Seal: pointed oval, fragmentary, green wax: 65 mm. The Virgin and Child seated on a throne. Legend: destroyed. Counterseal: pointed oval, fragmentary: 50 mm. The Annunciation. Legend: ✠ AVE : MARIA : GR[ATIA : PL]ENA : DOMINUS : TECVM.

*Cartulary marginalia.* Capit(ulum) Linc(olnienses) II[a].

**49**

[*c.*1250 × *c.*1260/70]

Sciant presentes et futuri quod ego Ricardus de *Beaumund* dedi, concessi et presenti carta confirmavi Roberto de *Seringes*, pro homagio et servicio suo, quinque acras terre de dominico meo in campo de *Crowlton'*, videlicet in campo de *Sehu* tres acras in loco qui vocatur *Fhurteneakeres* inter terram Nicholai de *Grimescot'* et terram Galfridi *Beaumund*, in campo *del Norht* duas acras scilicet in *Eastbernel'* inter terram dicti Nicholai et dicti Galfridi, habendas et tenendas de me et heredibus meis sibi et heredibus suis vel cuicumque vel quomodocumque dare vel assignare voluerit, libere et quiete, bene et in pace, reddendo inde annuatim mihi et heredibus meis ipse et heredes sui unum den(arium) in die natalis Domini ad oblat(ionem) pro omnimodis serviciis. Pro hac autem donacione, concessione et presentis carte confirmatione dedit mihi prefatus Robertus duas marcas sterlingorum. Et ego Ricardus et heredes mei warantizabimus dicto Roberto et heredibus vel assignatis suis dictam terram cum pertin(enciis) contra omnes gentes per predictum servicium. Et ut hec donatio, concessio et presentis carte confirmatione perpetuum robur optineat, hanc cartam sigillo meo roboravi. Hiis testibus.

May those present and future know that I, Richard de Beaumont, have given, conceded, and confirmed with this my present charter to Robert of Sheering, for his homage and service, five acres of land from my demesne in the field of Croughton, namely three acres in the southern field in the place called *Fhurteneakeres*, between the land of Nicholas of Grimscote and the land of Geoffrey Beaumont, [and] two acres in the northern field, namely in *Eastbernel'*, between the lands of the said Nicholas and the said Geoffrey, to have and to hold from me and my heirs by him and his heirs, and to give or assign to whomever and in whatever way he wants, free and quit, well and in peace, he and his heirs thence rendering to me and my heirs 1d each year on Christmas Day, as an offering for services of every sort. For this donation, concession, and present charter's confirmation, the aforementioned Robert gave me two marks in silver. And I, Richard, and my heirs will warrant the said land, with all its appurtenances, to the said Robert and his heirs or assignees against all people on account of the aforementioned service. And so that this donation, concession, and present charter's confirmation obtains perpetual strength, I have strengthened this charter with my seal. With these witnesses.

*Note*. This and the following act are written by a continuator (Scribe B), who is also the scribe responsible for the original of no. **32**. It is difficult to date precisely without a witness list. The *terminus a quo* is given by the earliest mention of Richard de Beaumont and the *terminus ad quem* by the date at which Scribe B was working. It must also have been issued around the same time as no. **50**, which concerns the same property.

## 50

[*c*.1250 × *c*.1260/70]

Sciant presentes et futuri quod ego Robertus de *Seringes* dedi, concessi et presenti carta confirmavi Deo et beate Marie et hospitali sanctorum Iacobi et Iohannis de Eynh(o) et fratribus ibidem Deo servientibus quinque acras terre in campo de *Crowlt'* quas emi de Ric(ardo) de *Beaumund*, prout carta ipsius testatur, quam predicti fratres penes se habent, videlicet in campo australi tres acras in loco qui vocatur *Fhurteneakeres* inter terram Nicholai de *Grimescote* et terram Galfridi de *Beaumund* et in campo aquilonari duas acras in *Eastbernel'* inter terram dicti Nicholai et dicti Galfr(idi), habendas et tenendas de me et heredibus meis predicto hospitali et dictis fratribus et eorum successoribus inperpetuum, libere, quiete, bene et in pace, reddendo inde annuatim mihi et heredibus meis predicti fratres et eorum successores unum den(arium) in die natalis Domini, pro omnibus serviciis, sectis curiarum, exactionibus et demandis. Et ego Robertus de *Seringes* et heredes mei warantizabimus dicto hospitali et dictis fratribus et eorum successoribus dictam terram cum pertinentiis contra omnes gentes et de omni terreno servicio per predictum servicium defendemus et adquietabimus. Pro hac autem donatione, concessione, presentis carte confirmatione et warantizatione dederunt mihi predicti fratres duas marc(as) sterlingorum. Et ut hec donatio, concessio, presentis carte confirmatio et warant(izatio) perpetuum robur optineat, hanc cartam sigilli me inpressione corroboravi. Hiis testibus.

May those present and future know that I, Robert of Sheering, have given, conceded, and confirmed with this my present charter to God and blessed Mary, and to the hospital of saints James and John of Aynho, and the brothers who serve God there, five acres of land in the field of Croughton that I bought from Richard de Beaumont, as his charter testifies, which the aforementioned brothers have in their possession, namely three acres in the southern field in the place called *Fhurteneakeres*, between the land of Nicholas of Grimscote and the land of Geoffrey de Beaumont, and two acres in the northern field in *Eastbernel'*, between the lands of the said Nicholas and the said Geoffrey, to have and to hold by the said hospital, and its brothers and their successors, from me and my heirs in perpetuity, free, quit, well and in peace, with the said brothers and their successors thence rendering 1d to me and my heirs each year on Christmas Day, for all services, court obligations, exactions, and demands. And I, Robert of Sheering, and my heirs will warrant the said land, with its appurtenances, to the said hospital, its brothers and their successors, release it from all earthly services on account of the aforementioned service, and defend it against all people. For this donation, concession, [and] present charter's confirmation and warranty, the aforementioned brothers gave me two marks in silver. And so that this donation, concession, and present charter's confirmation and warranty obtains perpetual strength, I have strengthened this charter with the impression of my seal. With these witnesses.

*Note*. This act is difficulty to date precisely without a witness list. The *terminus a quo* is given by the earliest mention of Robert of Sheering and the *terminus ad quem* by the date at which Scribe B, who copied this act in the cartulary, was likely working (see Chapter 4).

**51**

[*c*.1250 × 1260]

Sciant presentes et futuri quod ego Paulinus de *Merlawe* dedi, concessi[(a)] et hac carta[(b)] confirmavi hospitali sanctorum Iacobi et Iohannis de Eyno tres acras terre mee in villa de *Crowlton'*, scilicet unam acram que se extendit |[1]| usque in *Horsemor* ex parte occidentis iuxta *la Hydeacre*[(c)] et aliam acram in eodem campo, scilicet in campo australi que se extendit ultra *le Smaleweye* et abutat super foreram Thome *Botyld* iuxta terram |[2]| dicti hospitalis de Eyno, et unam acram que iacet super culturam que vocatur *Sefneacres*[(d)] inter terram que fuit Thome molendinarii quam Nicholaus *Bastard* tenet et terram Ricardi *le Machun*, ha-|[3]|-bendas et tenendas de me et heredibus meis dicto hospitali inperpetuum, libere, quiete, bene et[(e)] in pace, reddendo inde annuatim mihi et heredibus meis tres denarios ad festum beate Marie in Marcio, pro omni |[4]| servicio seculari, secta curie, et omnibus aliis demandis, salvo forinseco servicio quantum pertinet ad tantam terram eiusdem feodi. Et ego predictus Paulinus et heredes mei predicto hospitali predictas tres |[5]| acras terre per predictum servicium contra omnes imperpetuum warantizabimus[(f)] et defendemus et ab omni secta cuiuscumque curie aquietabimus. Et ut hec mea donacio, concessio[(g)] et presentis carte mee confirmacio |[6]| robur obtineant,[(h)] hanc cartam sigilli mei inpressione[(i)] roboravi. Hiis[(j)] testibus:[(k)] Willelmo de *la Haye*, Nicholao de *Grymescote*, Ricardo *Beaumund*, Roberto *Beaumund*, Roberto de *Seringes*, |[7]| Huberto de Eyno, Galfrido *Marcward*, Iohanne de *Sutt'* clerico, et aliis.

(a) consessi *B*. — (b) mea *add. B*. — (c) Lahydeacre *B*. — (d) Sef(e)neacres *B*. — (e) et *om. B*. — (f) in perpetuum warentizabimus *B*. — (g) consessio *B*. — (h) brobur *corrected to* robur *by partial erasure of* b-, *and* optineant *B*. — (i) inprecione *B*. — (j) His *B*. — (k) *B ends here*.

May those present and future know that I, Paulinus of Marlow, have given, conceded, and confirmed with this charter to the hospital of saints James and John of Aynho three acres of my land in the vill of Croughton, namely one acre that extends as far as *Horsemor* on the eastern side next to *la Hydeacre*, and another acre in the same field, that is, in the southern field, which extends beyond *le Smaleweye* and abuts on the headland of Thomas Botild next to the land of the said hospital of Aynho, and one acre situated above the ploughland known as *Sefneacres*, between the land that was Thomas the miller's, which Nicholas Bastard holds, and the land of Richard le Machun, to have and to hold in perpetuity by the said hospital from me and my heirs, free, quit, well and in peace, thence rendering unto me and my heirs 3d each year at the feast of blessed Mary, for all secular services, court obligations, and all other demands, saving foreign service inasmuch as it pertains to the land of that fief. And I, the aforementioned Paulinus, and my heirs will warrant the said three acres of land to the aforementioned hospital on account of the said service, and defend and release them from whatever court obligations, in perpetuity. And so that this my donation, concession, and present charter's confirmation obtains strength, I have strengthened this charter with the impression of my seal. With these witnesses: William de la Haye; Nicholas of Grimscote; Richard Beaumont; Robert Beaumont; Robert of Sheering; Hubert of Aynho; Geoffrey Markward; John of [King's] Sutton, clerk; and others.

*Original.* MCA, Aynho 58. Endorsed: Paulinus Merlaw'. Crowlton' (s. xv). Dimensions: 282 × 74 + 12 mm. Sealed *sur double queue*, parchment tag through one slit. Parchment used for tag taken from existing charter, written in the same hand as this act, with the following text visible: 'Sciant presentes et futuri quod ego Paulinus [...] [vill]a de Crowlton', scilicet unam acram que se exten[dit]'. Seal: oval, white wax painted brown: 29 × 19 mm. A fleur-de-lis. Legend: indistinct. The scribe of this act also wrote no. **A9**.

*Cartulary marginalia.* V acre.

## 52

[1270 × 1280]

Universis Christi fidelibus presentes litteras[a] inspecturis, Robertus de *Scyring'*,[b] salutem[c] |1| in Domino. Noveritis me relaxasse et[d] quietum clamasse pro me et heredibus meis et |2| meis assignatis Iohanni de *Graham*, dicto magistro[e] hospitalis de Eyno,[f] et fratribus |3| ibidem Deo servientibus tres[g] denariatos annui redditus quos michi[h] debuerunt[i] |4| pro terris quas de me tenuerunt in territorio de *Crowethon'*.[j] Et ut hec mea dona-|5|-cio et relaxacio et concessio et presentis carte[k] mee confirmacio robur inperpetuum |6| optineat, presens scriptum sigilli mei inpressione coroboravi.[l] Hiis testibus: |7| Reginaldo de Bello Campo, Willelmo *Wakelin'*,[m] Willelmo de Haya, Ric(ardo) de |8| *Beumont*[n] et aliis.

(a) literas *B*. — (b) Scyringes *B*. — (c) saltutem *A*. — (d) omnino *add. B*. — (e) dictus magister *B*. — (f) Haynho *B*. — (g) III *B*. — (h) mihi *B*. — (i) solvere *add. B*. — (j) Croultone *B*. — (k) ca<r>te *B*. — (l) roboravi *B*. — (m) Willelmo Wakelin' *om. B*. — (n) Beumunt *B*.

Robert of Sheering [sends his] greeting in the Lord to all the faithful in Christ who may examine this present document. May you know that I have released and quit-claimed on behalf of myself, my heirs, and my assignees to John of Graham, said master of the hospital of Aynho, and the brothers who serve God there, the annual rent of 3d they owed me for the lands they held from me in the territory of Croughton. And so that this my donation, release, concession, and my present charter's confirmation obtain strength in perpetuity, I have corroborated the present document with the impression of my seal. With these witnesses: Reginald de Beauchamp; William Wakelin; William de la Haye; Richard de Beaumont; and others.

*Original.* MCA, Aynho 55. Endorsed: Quieta clamacio Roberti de Scyringes de .iii. d. annui redditus (s.xiii, hand of scribe responsible for copying this act into the cartulary). Dimensions: 155 × 85/74 mm. Sealed *sur simple queue*; tongue 148 mm, seal impression missing. Wrapping tie fragment. The scribe of this act also wrote nos. **A13–A14**, **A18**.

[[**Reverse**]]

**53**

25 Oct [1202] — Lateran.

See no. **1**

**54**

27 Nov [1215] — Latcran.

See no. **2**

**55**

[*c.*1250 × *c.*1270]

Sciant presentes et futuri quod ego Robertus de *Schiringe* dedi et concessi et presenti carta confirmavi magistro et fratribus hospitalis beatorum apostolorum Iacobi et Iohannis de Eynho duas acras terre in campis de *Croweltune*, quarum una acra iacet in campo australi apud *þickeþorne* iuxta terram Petri *le Barun* et alia acra iacet in campo boreali apud *Siche*, scilicet acra capitalis iuxta terram ecclesie, habendas et tenendas de me et heredibus meis dictis magistro et fratribus et eorum successoribus, libere et quiete, reddendo inde annuatim mihi et heredibus meis unum denarium ad Pasca, pro omnimodis serviciis et demandis et omnium curiarum sectis. Pro hac autem donatione, concessione et presentis carte confirmatione dederunt michi predicti magister et fratres viginti solidos sterlingorum. Et ego Robertus de *Schiringes* et heredes mei warantizabimus ecciam de dominica terra nostra si necesse fuerit et defendemus duas predictas acras terre, cum pertinenciis suis, dictis fratribus et eorum successoribus per predictum servitium contra omnes gentes inperpetuum. Quod ut ratum sit, presentem cartam sigilli mei inpressione confirmavi. Hiis testibus.

May those present and future know that I, Robert of Sheering, have given, conceded, and confirmed with the present charter to the master and brothers of the hospital of the blessed Apostles James and John of Aynho two acres of land in the fields of Croughton, of which one lies in the southern field at Thickthorn, next to the land of Peter Baron, and the other in the northern field at *Siche*, namely the acre of headland next to the land of the church, to have and to hold by the said master and brothers and their successors from me and my heirs, free and quit, thence rendering to me and my heirs 1d each year at Easter for every sort of service and demand and all court obligations. For this donation, concession, and present charter's confirmation, the aforementioned master and brothers gave me 20s in silver. And I, Robert of Sheering, and my heirs will also warrant the aforementioned two acres, with their appurtenances, from our demesne land, if necessary, to the said brothers and their successors on account of the said service and defend them against all people in perpetuity. In order that this is valid, I have confirmed the present charter with the impression of my seal. With these witnesses.

*Note.* This act is difficulty to date precisely without a witness list. The *terminus a quo* is given by the earliest mention of Robert of Sheering and the *terminus ad quem* by the date at which Scribe E, who copied this act in the cartulary, was likely working (see Chapter 4).

## 56

[*c*.1260]

Omnibus Christi fidelibus presentem cartam inspecturis vel audituris Tomas de *Crewelt'*(a) filius Roberti *Ni*{*w*}*eman* de *Frutewelle*, salutem. No-|1|-veritis me pro salute anime mee et pro salute anime Margarete uxoris mee {et} pro animabus antecessorum et successorum meorum dedisse et concessisse et hac |2| carta confirmasse Deo et beate Marie {et} magistro et fratribus hospital(is)(b) beatorum apostolorum Iacobi et Iohannis de Heyno(c) duas acras terre mee et unam rodam |3| arabiles {in villa de} *Crewelt'*,(d) scilicet unam acram iacentem(e) in campo australi(f) cuius dimidia acra iacet ex parte occidentali de *Hor*{*semor* inter ter}ram |4| Robeia[ce] et t[erram] Wilelmi *Cosin*, et altera dimidia acra iacet versus orientem de *Stanihulle* {iuxta terram eius}dem hospitalis et terram predicti |5| Tom[e], et unam acram iacentem in campo(g) boreali(h) cuius {dim}idia acra et una roda iacet in *Gateris* inter terras predicti Tome, et altera dimidia acra |6| iacet super *Smalebrochulle* inter terram eiusdem hospitalis et terram predicti Tome, habendas et tenendas dictis magistro et fratribus et eorum successo-|7|-ribus, libere et quiete, bene et in pace, absque omni seculari servitio, consuetudine, sectis curie, et demandis mihi vel alicui pertinentibus inperpetuum, |8| in liberam et puram et perpetuam elemosinam, sicut aliqua {e}lemosina melius et liberius dari vel conferri potest, ita tamen quod omnibus et singulis |9| annis celebretur anniversarius dies {M}argarete comitisse de *Kent*, defuncte, pro salute anime eius in dicto hospitali, die sancti Macuti episcopi et con-|10|-fessoris, quo die omnibus et singulis annis fratres dicti hospitalis habebunt de eadem terra pitanciam ad precium duo{de}cim den(ariorum). Et ego |11| Tomas et heredes mei predictas duas acras et rodam dictis magistro et fratribus et eorum {su}ccessoribus contra omnes gentes warantizabimus et |12| defendemus et de omni servicio aquietabimus. Quod ut ratum {si}t, presenti scripto sigilli mei inpressionem apposui. Hiis testibus:(i) |13| Willelmo de *la Haye*, Nicolao de *Grimescote*, Roberto de *Syringe*, Ric(ardo) *Beumund*, Roberto *Beumund*, Paulino de *Merlaue*, |14| Huberto de Heyno, Ricardo filio Iohannis, Rog(ero) Coco, Galfrido *Marcward'*, et aliis.

(a) Crowelt' *B.* — (b) hospitalis *om. B.* — (c) Eynho *B.* — (d) Crowelt' *B.* — (e) <i>acentem *B.* — (f) a<u>strali *B.* — (g) in campo *repeated in error, B.* — (h) boriali *AB.* — (i) *B ends here.*

Thomas of Croughton, son of Robert Newman of Fritwell, [sends his] greeting to all the faithful in Christ who may examine or hear the present charter. May you know that I have given, conceded, and confirmed with this charter, for the salvation of my soul and the soul of my wife, Margaret, and the souls of my ancestors and successors, to God and blessed Mary, and to the master and brothers of the hospital of the blessed Apostles James and John of Aynho, two acres of my land and one rood of arable land in the vill of Croughton: namely one acre lying in the southern field, of which one half acre lies on the western side of *Horsemor* between the land of Robeiace and the land of William Cosin, and the other half acre lies towards the east of *Stanihulle* next to the land of that hospital and the land of the aforementioned Thomas, and one acre lying in the northern field, of which one half acre and rood lie in Gateridge, between the lands of the said Thomas, and the other half acre above *Smalebrochulle*, between the land of the same hospital and the land of the said Thomas, to have and to hold by the said master and brothers and their successors, free and quit, well and in peace, free from all secular service, custom, and court obligations and demands pertaining to me or anyone else, in perpetuity, in free and perpetual alms, just as all alms should best and freely be given and conferred, on condition that the anniversary day of Margaret, countess of Kent, deceased, is celebrated for the salvation of her soul in the said hospital, each and every year, on the [feast] day of St Malo, bishop and confessor [15 November], [on] which day each and every year the brothers of the said hospital will have from that land a pittance to the value of 12d. And I, Thomas, and my heirs will warrant the aforementioned two acres and rood to the aforementioned master and brothers and their successors, release them of all service, and defend it against all people. In order that this is valid, I have affixed to the present document the impression of my seal. With these witnesses: William de la Haye; Nicholas of Grimscote; Robert of Sheering; Richard Beaumont; Robert Beaumont; Paulinus of Marlow; Hubert of Aynho; Richard, son of John; Roger Cook; Geoffrey Markward; and others.

*Original.* MCA, Aynho 36. Endorsed: Carta Thome de Crolton' filii Roberti Newman de Frytwell de duabus acris terre et una roda (s.xv/xvi). Dimensions: 220 × 131 + 17 mm. Sealed *sur double queue* through one slit, tag and seal impression missing. A loose fragment of parchment tag, as well as a blank piece of seal, is to be found among the Aynho deeds. The reverse of the tag contains the following text, written in the same hand as this act: '[...] Tomas de Criweltune filius Rob[erti] [...] animabus antecessorum et successorum [...]'. These fragments are likely all that remains of the tag and seal of this act.

*Note.* This act must have been issued after the death of Margaret (of Scotland), countess of Kent, on 25 November 1259, while Paulinus of Marlow does not appear in the record beyond *c*.1260. Taken together, these two chronological points gives us the approximate date of this act. Thomas of Croughton appears in other Aynho charters, always as Thomas Newman (nos. **A11–A12, A15, A17–A18**). That this Thomas is the same as the one above is proved by no. **A21**. The scribe responsible for the original charter is the same as the one who copied the act in the cartulary (Scribe E). He also wrote no. **A8**.

## 57

[*c*.1260]

Omnibus Christi fidelibus presentem cartam inspecturis vel audituris, Wilelmus de *T*(*u*)*rvile*, salutem. Noveritis me pro salute anime mee et pro salute anime uxoris mee et pro animabus antecessorum et successorum meorum dedisse et concessisse et hac carta confirmasse Deo et beate

Marie et magistro et fratribus hospital(is) beatorum apostolorum Iacobi et Iohannis de Eynho dimidiam virgatam terre in villa de *Crowelt'*, illam scilicet quam Walterus[(a)] de *Caudecot'* tenuit et Ricardus filius eius post ipsum, cum quodam mesuagio in eadem villa,[(b)] quod iacet inter viam regiam et terram [...],[(c)] habendam et tenendam dictam dimidiam virgatam terre cum omnibus pertinentiis suis integre, libere et quiete, bene [et in pace], in pratis et pascuis, in viis et semitis, et in omnibus libertatibus predicte terre pertinentibus, absque omni seculari ser[vitio, cons]uetudine, sectis curie, et demandis mihi vel alicui pertinentibus in perpetuum, in liberam et puram et perpetuam elemosinam, sicut aliqua elemosina melius et liberius dari vel conferri potest. Et ego Wilelmus de *T(u)rvile* et heredes mei predictam terram cum omnibus pertinenciis suis dictis magistro et fratribus et eorum successoribus contra omnes gentes warantizabimus et defendemus et de[(d)] omni servicio aquietabimus. Quod ut ratum sit, presenti scripto sigilli mei inpressionem apposui. Hiis testibus.

(a) Waliterus *with expunging dot under* -i-, *B.* — (b) willa *B.* — (c) *Text missing due to parchment damage, B.* — (d) def *with expunging dot under* -f, *B.*

William de Turville [sends his] greeting to all the faithful in Christ who may examine or hear the present charter. May you know that I have given, conceded, and confirmed with this charter, for the salvation of my soul and the soul of my wife, and [those] of my ancestors, and successors, to God and blessed Mary, and to the master and brothers of the hospital of the blessed Apostles James and John of Aynho, a half virgate of land in the vill of Croughton, namely that which Walter of Caldecote held and his son Richard after him, with a certain messuage in the same vill, which is situated between the king's highway and the land [...], to have and to hold the said half virgate of land, with all its appurtenances, in full, free and quit, well and in peace, in meadows and pastures, roads and paths, and in all freedoms pertaining to the aforementioned land, free from all secular service, custom, court obligations, and demands pertaining to me or anyone else in perpetuity, in free and perpetual alms, just as all alms should best and freely be given and conferred. And I, William de Turville, and my heirs will warrant the aforementioned land, with all its appurtenances, to the aforementioned master and brothers and their successors, release them of all service, and defend it against all people. In order that this is valid, I have affixed to the present document the impression of my seal. With these witnesses.

*Note.* This act is difficult to date precisely without a witness list, but if the half virgate of land and messuage granted here is the same as that in no. **58**, which seems to have been issued to provide reassurance to the hospital in light of the upheaval of the Second Barons' War, then the act here presumably predates the one that follows below.

**58**

[1263 × 1265]

Universis Christi fidelibus presens scriptum audituris, Wilelmus de *T(u)rvile* salutem. Noveritis me dedisse Deo et beate Marie et hospitali sanctorum Iacobi et Iohannis de Eynho et fratribus ibidem Deo servientibus et eorum successoribus dimidiam virgatam terre et unum mesuagium in villa de *Croultun'*, cum omnibus suis pertinenciis, in puram et liberam et perpetuam elemosinam, sicut carta mea inde confecta plenius testatur. Et ego Wilelmus de *T(u)rvile* et heredes mei de ingressu dicte dimidie virgate terre et mesuagii contra dominum comitem *Leycestr'* et heredes suos et contra quoslibet alios defendemus et aquietabimus, sine omni occasione et calumpnia[(a)] quam ego vel heredes mei poterimus demandare. Et si forte contigerit quod dictus comes vel heredes sui vel quicumque alii pro dicta terra averia dicti hospitali inparcaverint vel aliquam molestiam intulerint, ego et heredes mei propria averia nostra pro eorum averiis inparcabimus et in omnibus indemnes conservabimus. In cuius rei testimonium huic scripto impressionem sigilli mei apposui. Hiis testibus.

(a) -p- *of* calumpnia *inserted in interline, B.*

William de Turville [sends his] greeting to all the faithful in Christ who may hear the present document. May you know that I have given to God and blessed Mary, and to the hospital of saints James and John of Aynho, and the brothers who serve God there and their successors, a half virgate of land and a messuage in the vill of Croughton, with all its appurtenances, in pure, free, and perpetual alms, just as my charter hereby granted amply testifies. And I, William de Turville, and my heirs will defend and release the entry of the said half virgate of land and messuage against the lord earl of Leicester, his heirs, and anyone else, without any pretext or charge, whenever I or my heirs can commit to it. And if it happens that, on account of the said land, the said earl or his heirs or anyone else should impound the hospital's animals or otherwise raise trouble, my heirs and I will impound our own animals on account of theirs and keep them safe in all things. In evidence of this matter, I have affixed the impression of my seal to this document. With these witnesses.

*Note*. This act is difficult to date precisely without a witness list, but the stipulation made in relation to the earl of Leicester perhaps suggests that it was issued when Simon de Montfort, earl of Leicester (1239–65), a significant landholder in and around Aynho, including at Croughton, was in open rebellion against the king during the Second Barons' War.

# Appendix

# ORIGINAL CHARTERS NOT TRANSCRIBED IN THE AYNHO CARTULARY (*c*.1190–*c*.1285)

The editorial principles used here are the same as those for the cartulary. Dates are those assigned by William Macray in the mid-nineteenth century, although these are refined/revised wherever possible.

## A1

[*c*.1190 × 1200, perhaps 1194 × 1202]

*Act by which Turbert, son of Turbert, rector of the church of Aynho, makes it known that, as rector, he has no right in the custody and governance of the hospital of Aynho, save only at the request of lord Robert Fitz Roger and then only for as long as it should please him. Turbert also declares that his successors in the rectory may not hereafter claim for themselves any right over the hospital. Witnesses: Roger, dean of Pattishall, Ingeram, parson of Marston [St Lawrence], Lawrence, parson of Croughton, Thomas, clerk of Brackley, Roger, chaplain of Newbottle, Richard, chaplain of Aynho, Ralph, clerk of Aynho, Robert of Burnham, parson of Iver, Master Hugh de* Castref' *[? Castleford].*

*A*. MCA, Aynho 68. Endorsed: Carta Turberti de Einho de hospit' de Einho (s.xiii); Remit' iuris rectoris de Ayno super hospitalis sancti Iacobi et Iohannis (s.xv/s.xvi). Dimensions: 176 × 83 + 29 mm. Sealed *sur double queue*, parchment tag through three slits, seal impression missing.

Omnibus Christi fidelibus ad quos presens scriptum pervenerit, T(ur)-bert(us) filius T(ur)berti, rector ecclesie de Eynho, salutem. |[1]| Noverit presens universitas et subsecuta posteritas me nichil iuris habere vel unquam habuisse in custodia et gu-|[2]|-bernatione hospitalis sancti Iacobi de Eynho occasione predicte ecclesie de Eynho, nisi ad petitionem et commen-|[3]|-dationem domini Roberti filii Rog(er)i, quamdiu ei placuerit.

Et ne successores mei rectores ecclesie de Eyn-|[4]|-ho aliqui iuris possint sibi vendicare in predicto hospitali. Quia non minus delinqui qui veritatem occultat quam |[5]| qui falsum astruit, testimonium perhibemus veritati in eo qui est in celis testis fidelis. Et ut hec testi-|[6]|-monium verum et manifestum permaneat, scripti nostri attestatione et sigilli nostri munimine roboravimus. H-|[7]|-iis testibus: Rog(er)o decano de *Pateshill'*, Ingera(m)mo persona de *Merston'*, Laurencio persona de *Croulton'*, |[8]| Thome clerico de *Brackel'*, Rog(ero) capellano de *Neubotle*, Ric(ardo) capellano de Eynho, Rad(ulfo) clerico de |[9]| Eynho, Roberto de *Burneha(m)* persona de *Evre*, magistro Hugone de *Castref'*, et multis aliis.

*Note.* Macray dates this *c.*1190 × 1200, but the presence of Robert of Burnham, parson of Iver, suggests this charter was likely issued after the grant of the manor of Iver by Richard the Lionheart to Robert Fitz Roger in 1194. The *terminus ad quem* is only approximate, but, if Turbert, son of Turbert, is the T., proctor of the hospital, addressed in Innocent III's bull of 25 October 1202 (no. **1**), as seems likely, then he must have still been alive at this point. That said, since Turbert was first instituted in the church of Aynho in the 1160s, he cannot have lived much beyond this date.

## A2

[*c.*1200]

*Act by which Alice de Wavre, daughter of Geoffrey de Wavre, grants the chapel of St Michael in the vill of Croughton, which is in her inheritance, to Osmund the clerk, in perpetual alms. Witnesses: Roger, dean of Pattishall, Robert, parson of Moreton [Pinkney], Robert, parson of Farthinghoe, Simon, chaplain of Hinton [in the Hedges], Payn, chaplain of Steane, Adam, chaplain of Stuchbury.*[2]

A. MCA, Aynho 83. Endorsed: Capella de Crolton' (s.xv/s.xvi). Dimensions: 155 × 76 + 28 mm. Sealed *sur double queue*, parchment tag through three slits. Seal: pointed oval, white wax painted brown: 40 × 22 mm. A fleur-de-lis. Legend: ✠ SIGILL(*vm*) ALIZ DE WAVERE (indistinct). The scribe is perhaps the same as that responsible for no. **39** and is definitely the same as that of no. **A3**.

Omnibus ad quos presens scriptum pervenerit, *Aliz* de *Wavere*, filia Galfridi de *Wavere*, salutem in Domino. No-|[1]|-verit universitas vestra me divine pietatis intuitu capellam sancti Michaelis in villa de *Crewelt'* in hereditate

[2] This is presumably the future master of Ayhno Hospital by this name (see Table 1.1).

|[2]| mea sitam Osmundo clerico concessisse. Et quantum ad patronam et ad ius patronatus pertinet, in perpetuam |[3]| elemosinam contulisse. Et ut hec concessio et donatio mea perpetue commendetur memorie, sigilli mei mu-|[4]|-nimine confirmavi. Hiis testibus: Rogero decano de *Pateswlle*, Roberto persona de *Mort*(*u*)*n*, Roberto persona de |[5]| *Farnigho*, Simone capellano de *Hinton'*, Pagano capellano de *Stanes*, Ade capellano de *Stutes-b*(*ur*)*i*, et aliis.

**A3**

[*c*.1200]

*Act by which Guy de la Haye, son of Alice de Wavre, confirms to Osmund the clerk the grant made to him by his mother of the chapel of St Michael's, Croughton. Witnesses: Roger, dean of Pattishall, Robert, parson of Moreton [Pinkney], Robert, parson of Farthinghoe, Simon, chaplain of Hinton [in the Hedges], Payn, chaplain of Steane, Adam, chaplain of Stuchbury, W., chaplain of Weedon [Lois], W., chaplain of Woodford [Halse].*

*A*. MCA, Aynho 34. Endorsed: Capella de Crolton' (s.xv/s.xvi). Dimensions: 128 × 78 + 15 mm. Sealed *sur double queue*, parchment tag through three slits. Seal: round, white wax painted brown: 34 mm. A fleur-de-lis. Legend: ✠ SIGILL(*vm*) WIDONIS DE L[A] HAYE. The seal is seemingly Guy's first, as it differs from that affixed to no. **29**, which has an heraldic motif. The scribe is perhaps the same as that responsible for no. **39** and is definitely the same as that of no. **A2**.

Sciant presentes et futuri quod ego Wido de *la Hay* filius *Alis* de *Wavere* eandem con-|[1]|-cessionem et donationem capelle sancti Michaelis de *Creuult'* quam *Alis* mater mea, divine |[2]| pietatis intuitu, Osmundo clerico contulit, pro salute mea et pro animabus antecessorum |[3]| meorum ipsi O. clerico sigilli mei robore in perpetuam elemosinam confirmavi.[(a)] Hiis testibus: |[4]| Rogero decano de *Pateswlle*, Roberto persona de *Mortu*(*n*), Roberto persona de *Faringho*, Symone |[5]| capellano de *Hintu*(*n*), Pagano capellano de *Stanes*, Ade capellano de *Stutesb*(*ur*)*i*, W. capella-|[6]|-no de *Vedun'*, W. capellano de *Vodeford*, et multis aliis.

(a) confirmavi *written over an erasure in lighter ink and a different hand, A.*

## A4

[*c*.1200]

*Act by which William [I] de la Haye, son of Alice de Wavre, confirms to Osmund the clerk the grant made to him by his mother of the chapel of St Michael's, Croughton. Witnesses: Roger, dean of Pattishall, Robert, parson of Moreton [Pinkney], Robert, parson of Farthinghoe, Simon, chaplain of Hinton [in the Hedges], Payn, chaplain of Steane, Adam, chaplain of Stuchbury, W., chaplain of Weedon [Lois], W., chaplain of Woodford [Halse], W. of Wardington, I. of Appletree.*

A. MCA, Aynho 84. Endorsed: Capella de Crolton' (s.xv/s.xvi). Dimensions: 161 × 88 + 16 mm. Sealed *sur double queue*, parchment tag through three slits. The tag has been fashioned from an existing document, with the following text still visible: '... sive [?] ius non facias per duo die[s] ...', beneath which is a word it has not been possible to decipher. Seal: round, white wax painted brown: 40 mm. A mythical creature or perhaps a lion or a wolf. Legend: ✠ SIGILLVM WILLELMI DE HAIA.

Sciant presentes et futuri quod ego Willelmus de *la Hay* filius *Alis* de *Wavre* eandem concessionem |[1]| et donationem capelle sancti Michaelis de *Creueltun'* quam *Aliz* mater mea divine pietatis intu-|[2]|-itu Osmundo clerico contulit, pro salute mea, et pro animabus antecessorum meorum ipsi O. clerico, sigil-|[3]|-li mei robore in perpetuam elemosinam confirmavi. Hiis testibus: Rog(er)o decano de *Pates*-|[4]|-*wlle*, Roberto persona de *Mortun'*, Roberto persona de *Faringho*, Symone capellano de *Hi*(*n*)*ctun'*, |[5]| Pagano capellano de *Stanes*, Ade capellano de *Stuteb*(*ur*)*i*, W. capellano de *Wedun'*, W. capellano |[6]| de *Wdeford*, W. de *Wardint'*, I. de *Apeltre*, et multis aliis.

## A5

[*c*.1240]

*Act by which William of Turweston gives, concedes, and quit-claims to Hugh Fiddler of Hinton [in the Hedges], in consideration of the receipt of 6s 4d, a messuage with a courtyard in Brackley, which William holds from the hospital of Aynho, between the messuages held formerly by Richard Kay and Odo Cooper, paying annually 3d to the earl of Winchester and 15d to the hospital of Aynho. Witnesses: lord Arnulf le Goer, lord Andrew Bonvahtleht, Robert the vintner, Richard the clerk, Rannulf of Brackley, Adam, son of William, son of Ralph.*

*A*. MCA, Aynho 13. Endorsed: no endorsements. Dimensions: 166 × 78 + 11 mm. Sealed *sur double queue*, parchment tag through one slit. Seal: pointed oval, white wax painted brown: 27 × 15 mm. A fleur-de-lis. Legend: ✠ SIGILL(*vm*) WILLELMI DE TORVESTV(*n*).

Sciant presentes et futuri quod ego Willelmus de *Turveston'* dedi et concessi et hac presenti carta mea confirmavi et quiete clamavi plenarie |1| Hugoni Viellatori de *Hynton'* pro sex solid(orum) argenti et quatuor denar(iorum) quos michi premanibus dedit, illud mesuagium cum curia |2| in *Brakkel'*, quod ego aliquando tenui de hospitalario de Aynho, quod scilicet est inter mesuagium quod Ric(ardus) *Kay* quandoque tenuit et |3| mesuagium quod Odo *le Cupper* quandoque tenuit, videlicet quod ego Willelmus de *Turveston'* quiete clamavi dicto Hugoni de *Hyn*-|4|-*ton'* totum illud ius predicte domus cum libertatibus quod habui vel habere potui, tenendum et habendum in feodo et hereditate |5| de hospitalario de Aynho sibi et heredibus suis vel cuicumque dare vel legare vel assignare voluerit, libere et quiete bene et |6| in pace, sine aliqua contradictione de me vel heredibus meis in posterum, reddendo inde annuatim ipse et heredes sui vel assignati |7| sui, sicut ego quandoque reddidi comiti scilicet *Winton'*, tres denar(ios) et hospit(ali) de Aynho quindecim denar(ios) ad tres t(erm)i(n)os annui, scilicet |8| ad purificationem beate Marie comiti *Wint'* unum denar(ium) et hospit(ali) de Aynho quinque den(arios), ad Pentecostn' com(iti) *Wint'* unum |9| den(arium) et hospit(ali) de Aynho quinque den(arios), ad festum beati Michaelis, com(iti) *Wint'* unum den(arium) et hospit(ali) de Aynho quinque den(arios). In cuius rei |10| testimonium presentem cartam in modum quiete clamationis confectam, sigillo meo roboravi. Hiis testibus: domino Arnulfo *le Goer*, |11| domino Andreo *Bonvahtleht*, Roberto vinitario, Ric(ardo) clerico, Ranulfo de *Brakkel'*, Ada(m) *Wigod*, Ada(m) filio Willelmi filii Rad(ulfi), et aliis.

## A6

[*c*.1250]

*Act by which Paulinus of Marlow gives, concedes, and confirms to Simon, son of Geoffrey Bonknit of Croughton, in consideration of the receipt of two marks and at an annual rent of 3d, three acres of land in the fields of Croughton, of which one acre extends to* Horsemor *from the western part up to* la Hydeacre, *and another extends beyond* le Smaleweye, *abutting upon the headland of Thomas Botild next to the land of Aynho Hospital, and another lies above the ploughland called* Sefneacres *between the land that was Thomas the miller's, which Nicholas Bastard holds, and the land of Richard le Machun. Witnesses: William de la Haye, Nicholas of Grimscote, Richard de Beaumont, Robert of Sheering, Henry Botild, Hubert of Aynho, Randulf Crasso of Astwick.*[3]

*A.* MCA, Aynho 59. Endorsed: Carta Paulini de Merlawe de tribus acris terre (s.xv). Dimensions: 192 × 140 + 14 mm. Sealed *sur double queue*, parchment tag through one slit, seal impression missing. This charter is in the hand of the clerk Ralph Albrith (see Chapter 3).

Sciant presentes et futuri quod ego Paulinus de *Merlawe* dedi, concessi et hac presenti carta mea con-|[1]|-firmavi Symoni filio Galfridi *Bonknit* de *Crowelton'* tres acras terre mee in campis de *Crowelton'*, scilicet |[2]| unam acram que se extendit usque in *Horsemor* ex parte occidentali iuxta *la Hydeacre*, et aliam acram in eodem campo |[3]| scilicet in campo australi que se extendit ultra *le Smaleweye* et abuttat super foreram Thome *Botild'* iuxta |[4]| terram hospitalis de Ayno et unam acram que iacet super culturam que vocatur *Sefneacres* inter terram que |[5]| fuit Thome molendinarii quam Nicholas *Bastard* tenet et terram Ric(ardi) *le Machun*, habendas et tenendas |[6]| de me et heredibus meis predicto Symoni et heredibus suis vel cuicunque predictas tres acras terre dare, legare, vendere, |[7]| vel assignare voluerit, libere, quiete, bene et in pace, reddendo inde annuatim ipse et heredes sui vel |[8]| sui assignati mihi et heredibus meis tres denarios, scilicet ad festum beate Marie in marcio pro omni servicio seculari, |[9]| secta curie et omnibus aliis demandis, salvo forinseco servicio quantum pertinet ad tantam terram eiusdem feodi. |[10]| Et ego predictus Pawlinus et heredes mei predictas tres acras terre antedicto Symoni et heredibus suis vel quibus-|[11]|-cumque suis assignatis per predictum servicium contra omnes homines et feminas inperpetuum warantizabimus et defende-|[12]|-mus et ab omni secta cuiuscumque curie aquietabimus. Pro hac autem donatione, concessione et presentis carte |[13]| mee confirmacione dedit michi predictus Symon duas marcas argenti premanibus in gersumam. Et ut hec |[14]| mea donatio, concessio et presentis carte mee confirmacio rate et stabiles inperpetuum permaneant, hanc car-|[15]|-tam sigilli mei inpressione roboravi. Hiis testibus: Willelmo de *la Haye*, Nicholao de *Grymescote*, Ric(ardo) |[16]| de *Bewmu(n)d*, Roberto de *Seringes*, Henrico *Botild'*, Huberto de Ayno, Rand(ulf)o Crasso de *Astwik*, et aliis.

3 The medieval village of Astwick lay some 2 km to the east of Croughton approximately where the modern 'Astwick Farm' is located.

**A7**

[*c.*1250 × 1260]

*Act by which William [II] de la Haye of Croughton gives, concedes, and confirms to the master and brothers of Aynho Hospital one half acre out of three half acres of his outlying meadows situate in the meadow of Croughton near the Cherwell, with William and his heirs choosing annually at mowing time the best half acre of the three, and the hospital taking the second best, for the maintenance of a lamp before its altar of the blessed Mary. Witnesses: Henry Pirun of Croughton, Nicholas of Grimscote, Robert of Sheering, Hubert of Aynho, Nicholas of Aynho, clerk, John of Aynho, clerk, Geoffrey Beaumont.*

*A*. MCA, Aynho 66. Endorsed: no endorsements. Dimensions: 178 × 120 + 18 mm. Sealed *sur double queue*, parchment tag through one slit, seal impression missing.

Omnibus sancte matris ecclesie filiis ad quos presens scriptum pervenerit, Willelmus de *la Haye* de *Croulton*', salutem eternam in |[1]| Domino. Noverit universitas vestra me pro salute anime mee et pro animabus antecessorum meorum dedisse, concessisse et presenti car-|[2]|-ta mea confirmasse Deo et beate Marie et magistro et fratribus hospitalis de Eyneho, unam dimidiam acram prati |[3]| scilicet de tribus dimidiis acris prati de prato meo forinseco que iacent in prato de *Creulton*' iuxta *Charewell*', habendam et tenen-|[4]|-dam dictam dimidiam acram prati sine aliquo retenemento dictis magistro et fratribus et eorum successoribus de me et here-|[5]|-dibus meis vel assignatis libere et quiete, bene et in pace, in perpetuum in liberam et puram et perpetuam elemosinam |[6]| sicut aliqua elemosina purius et liberius dari potest, sine sectis curie cuiuslibet consuetudine et demanda quibuslibet, |[7]| ita tamen quod ego Willelmus et heredes mei singulis annis tempore falcationis de illis dictis tribus dimidiis acris prati habebi-|[8]|-mus primam meliorem dimidiam acram quamcumque eligere voluerimus et dicti magister et fratres et eorum successores singu-|[9]|-lis annis inperpetuum habebunt secundam meliorem dimidiam acram de dictis tribus dimidiis acris quamcumque eligere, vo-|[10]|-luerint, sine aliquo impedimento, ad sustentacionem unius lamp(adis) in ecclesia dicti hospitalis coram altaris beate Ma-|[11]|-rie in perpetuum. Ego et heredes mei vel assignati dictam dimidiam acram prati ut pre[n]ominatum est dictis magistro et fra-|[12]|-tribus et eorum successoribus contra omnes gentes inperpetuum warantizabimus, acquietabimus et defendemus. In cuius rei |[13]| testimonium presentem cartam sigilli mei inpressione duxi roborandam. Hiis testibus: H(e)nr(ico) *Pyrun* de *Croultun*', Nicholao |[14]| de *Grimescote*, Roberto de *Shering*', Huberto de Eyneho,

Nicholao de Eyneho, clerico, Iohanne de Eyneho, clerico, Galfrido |15| *Beumund*, et aliis.

## A8

[*c*.1260]

*Act by which Peter [of Windsor], master of Aynho Hospital, and the brothers of that place give, concede, and confirm to Roger of Leyton, cook, in consideration of the receipt of 20s and an annual rent of 2s, a messuage with its curtilage and appurtenances, held formerly by Richard Sewat, which lies between the hospital's land near the house held of it by John Payn and the king's way, and abutting the king's way to the land of Alvred son of Philip. The aforementioned 2s are to be paid at four terms, namely: 6d at the feast of St Thomas the Apostle, 6d at the feast of the Virgin Mary in March, 6d at the Nativity of John the Baptist, and 6d at the feast of St Michael. Witnesses: William de la Haye, Nicholas of Grimscote, Hubert of Aynho, Richard son of John, Walter West of Walton [Grounds], Geoffrey Markward of [King's] Sutton, Henry Morel.*

*A*. MCA, Aynho 38. Endorsed: no endorsements. Dimensions: 209 × 118 + 18 mm. Sealed *sur double queue*, parchment tag through three slits, seal impression missing. Bundle of tow around tag. This act is in the hand of one of the cartulary continuators (Scribe E).

Omnibus Christi fidelibus ad quos presens scriptum pervenerit, Petrus dictus magister hospitalis beatorum apostolorum Iacobi et Iohannis de Heynho, |1| et fratres eiusdem loci, salutem. Noveritis nos dedisse et concessisse et presenti carta confirmasse unum mesuagium cum curtilagio et pertinentiis in vil-|2|-la de Heyno Rog(er)o de *Leyhtun'* coco et heredibus suis illud scilicet mesuagium quod Ricardus *Sewat* aliquando tenuit, quod iacet inter terram predicti hospita-|3|-lis iuxta domum Iohannis *Payn,* quam tenuit de predicto hospitali, et viam regiam, et abutat se a via regia usque ad terram Alvredi filii Philippi, |4| habendum et tenendum sibi et heredibus suis, libere et quiete, pro omni servicio, reddendo inde annuatim dicto hospitali duos solidos per an-|5|-num ad quatuor terminos anni, scilicet sex den(arios) ad festum beati Thome apostoli et sex den(arios) ad festum Marie beate virginis in marcio et sex den(arios) ad nati-|6|-vitate beati Iohannis Baptiste et sex den(arios) ad festum beati Michaelis, pro omni servicio seculari, exactione, demanda et secta curie. Pro hac autem |7| donatione et concessione et carte nostre confirmatione dedit nobis predictus Rog(er)us viginti solidos in gersumam. Nos autem predicti magister et[(a)] |8| confratres predictum mesuagium cum pertinentiis dicto Rog(er)o et heredibus suis warantizabimus et defendemus et per predictum servicium aquietabimus contra |[9]| omnes gentes inperpetuum. Et ut hec nostra donatio et concessio et carte nostre confirmacio stabile robur optineant, presens scriptum inpressi-|[10]|-one comunis sigilli predicti hostpitalis corroboravimus. Hiis testibus: Wilellmo de *la Haye*, Nicolao de *Grimmescot'*, Huberto de Heynho, |[11]| Ricardo filio Iohannis, Waltero *West* de *Walt'*, Galfrido *Markward* de *Suttune*, Henrico *Morel*, et aliis.

(a) et *repeated in error, A.*

**A9**

[1265]

*Act by which William Wakelin and Joan, his wife, daughter and heir of Henry Pirun, quit-claim to the master and brothers of Aynho Hospital, in consideration of the receipt of one mark, all the land they have in Croughton of the fief of Henry Pirun, from the forty-ninth year of the coronation of King Henry III to the feast of the blessed Mary in March next ensuing. Witnesses: William de la Haye, Nicholas of Grimscote, Robert Beaumont, Richard Beaumont, Hubert of Aynho, Richard of Aynho, clerk, Geoffrey Markward of [King's] Sutton, Walter West of Walton [Grounds], John the clerk, who wrote the charter.*

*A.* MCA, Aynho 37. Endorsed: no endorsements. Dimensions: 204 × 85 + 14 mm. Sealed *sur double queue*, two parchment tags through one slit, seal impressions missing. The scribe of this act also wrote no. **51**.

Omnibus Christi fidelibus ad quos presentes littere pervenerint, Willelmus *Waukelin* et Iohanna, uxor eius, filia et heres Henrici *Pirun*, in Domino salutem. |[1]| Noveritis nos quietos clamasse magistrum et fratres hospitalis de Eyno pro nobis et heredibus nostris de tota terra quam habent in villa de *Crowet'* |[2]| de feudo Henrici *Pirun* ab anno coronationis domini regis Henrici tercii quadragesimo nono usque ad proximum festum beate Marie in |[3]| martio sequens. Pro hac autem quieta clamatione dederunt magister et dicti fratres nobis unam marcam argenti. Nos vero dictam quietam |[4]| clamationem warantizabimus pro nobis et heredibus nostris et defendemus contra omnes imperpetuum, libere et quiete, absque omni seculari exactione |[5]| et omnibus sectis curie nobis vel heredibus nostris pertinentibus. Ut autem hec quieta clamatio de terra predicti feudi inconcussa et stabilis perma-|[6]|-neat, presenti scripto signorum nostrorum inpressionem apposuimus. Hiis testibus: Willelmo de Haya, Nicholao de *Grimescote*, Roberto |[7]| *Beaumu(n)d*, Ricardo *Beaumund*, Huberto de Eyno, Ricardo de Eyno, clerico, Galfrido *Markeward* de *Sutt'*, Waltero |[8]| *West* de *Walt'*, Iohanne clerico qui hanc litteram scripsit, et aliis.

### A10

[*c*.1268 × *c*.1270]

*Act by which Robert [II] Fitz Roger grants to Aynho Hospital and the brothers who serve God there 40s of annual rent from his mill in Aynho called* Godboldesmilne, *to be paid at four terms, namely: 10s at the feast of St Michael, 10s at Christmas, 10s at the feast of the Annunciation, and 10s at the feast of John the Baptist. In return, the brothers and their successors are held in perpetuity to support a suitable chaplain, who will be elected and presented by Robert and his successors, and who will celebrate the divine office for the soul of his grandmother, Euphemia, former countess of Dunbar, and for the souls of his ancestors and successors. Should it transpire that the aforesaid rent is lacking from that mill, whether through misfortune or some other reason, then Robert and his successors hold themselves to compensate the brothers fully from elsewhere. Witnesses: lords Walter of Bibbesworth, Hugh Gubiun, John de Mohaut, knights, Hubert of Aynho, William de la Haye, John Bayard, William of Overton, William Abbot.*

*A*. MCA, Aynho 51. Endorsed: Aynho pro molendino (s.xvii). Dimensions: 230 × 106 + 17 mm. Sealed *sur double queue*, parchment tag through one slit, sealing impression missing.

Omnibus Christi fidelibus presens scriptum visuris vel audituris Robertus filius Rogeri, salutem in Domino. Noveritis me concessisse, dedisse et hac |[1]| presenti carta mea confirmasse Deo et hospitali beati Iacobi de Aynho et fratribus ibidem Deo servientibus et servituris quadraginta sol(idos) |[2]| annui redditus annuatim percipiendas de molendino meo quod vocatur *Godboldesmilne* [in] eadem villa, ad quatuor anni terminos, vide-|[3]|-licet ad festum sancti Michaelis decem sol(idos), ad Natale Domini decem sol(idos), ad festum Annunciacionis beate Marie decem sol(idos), et ad festum sancti Iohannis Baptiste |[4]| decem sol(idos), per manum servientis de Aynho qui pro tempore fuerit, habendas et tenendas eisdem fratribus et successoribus suis in puram et perpetuam |[5]| elemosinam inperpetuum. Pro hac autem concessione et donatione dicti fratres tenentur [in perp]etuum sustinere unum capellanum idoneum per me vel he-|[6]|-redes meos electum et presentatum ad celebrandum divina pro anima Eu[phemiae] quondam comitisse de *Dumbar*, avie mee, et ante-|[7]|-cessorum et successorum meorum. Et si contingi[t quod pre]dictus redditus quadrag[inta solidos in] dicto molendino per infortunum vel aliquo casu defici-|[8]|-at, concedo pro me et heredibus meis quod teneamur dictum redditum dictis fratrib[us … …]m[(a)] villa in alio competenti loco plenarie restituere |[9]| et annuatim persolvere. Et ego dictus Robertus et heredes mei vel mei assignati w[ara]-ntizabimus, defendemus et adquietabimus dictis |[10]| fratribus predictum redditum contra omnes homines inperpetuum. In cuius rei testimonium presenti scripto sigillum meum apposui. Hiis testibus: dominis |[11]| Waltero de *Bybeswrd'*, Hugone *Gubiun*, Iohanne de *Muhault*, militibus, Huberto de A[y]nho, Willelmo de la Haye, Iohanne *Bayard*, |[12]| Willelmo de *Overto(n)*,[(b)] Willelmo *Abot*, et aliis.

(a) *Text missing due to parchment damage, A.* — (b) Willelmo de Overton' *repeated in error, A.*

*Note.* Macray dates this act *c.*1270 × 1280, but the presence among the witnesses of Walter of Bibbesworth, the celebrated Anglo-Norman knight and poet, suggests it was issued closer to 1270, the date at – or shortly after – which Walter is thought to have died (T. Hunt, 'Bibbesworth, Walter of', in *ODNB*, vol. 5, p. 639). Robert Fitz Roger came of age in 1268/9, which provides the *terminus a quo*. Robert likely knew Walter of Bibbesworth through his former guardian, William de Valence (see Chapter 1).

## A11

[*c.*1270]

*Act by which John de la Haye of Croughton concedes, gives, and confirms to Aynho Hospital one acre of arable land in Croughton, half of which lies in the north field between the land of the hospital and that of Thomas, son of the parson of Croughton, in the place called* Hollemor, *and the other half lying in the south field in the place called* le Breche, *near the land of Philip le Beaumont, one end abutting above the pit of William Cosin. Witnesses: William Wakelin, John Sheering, Phillip le Beaumont, Hubert of Aynho, Thomas Newman of Croughton.*

*A*. MCA, Aynho 8. Endorsed: Carta Iohannis de la Hay de una acra terre in puram et perptuam elemosinam (s.xv). Dimensions: 195/210 × 134 + 11 mm. Sealed *sur double queue*, parchment tag through one slit. Seal: round, white wax painted brown: 40 mm. Shield-shaped impression with indistinct patterning and no legend. (This seal is most unusual and is perhaps nothing more than the result of a finger ring having been impressed into the wax.) The scribe of this act also wrote no. **A17**.

Sciant presentes et futuri quod ego Iohannes de Haya de *Crouletone* consessi, dedi et hac presenti carta mea |[1]| confirmavi, pro salute anime mee et animarum antecessorum meorum, Deo et beate Marie et hospitali sanctorum Iacobi |[2]| et Iohannis de Eynho, et magistro et fratribus ibidem Deo devote servientibus, in liberam et perpetuam elemosinam, unam |[3]| acram terre arabilis iacentem in villa de *Crouletone*, cuius una dimidia acra iacet in campo aquilonari, scilicet |[4]| inter terram predicti hospitalis versus austrum et terram Thome filii p(er)sone de *Crouletone*, versus aquilonem, in loco qui vocatur |[5]| *Hollemor*, et alia dimidia acra iacet in campo australi, scilicet in loco qui vocatur *le Breche*, iuxta terram |[6]| Filippi *le Beumund* versus aquilonem, cuius unum caput abuttat super foveam Willelmi *Cosyn* versus orientem |[7]| et aliut caput super campum de Eynho versus occidentem, habendam et tenendam predictam acram terre, cum omnibus |[8]| suis pertinenciis, de me et heredibus meis vel meis assingnatis predicto hospitali et dictis magistro et fratribus |[9]| ibidem Deo servientibus et eorum successoribus, libere, quiete, bene et in pace, in liberam et perpetuam elemosinam, |[10]| reddendo inde ad scutagium domini regis quando evenerit unum obol(atum) tantum pro omnibus serviciis, consuetu-|[11]|-dinibus, exactionibus et secularibus demandis et sectis cuiuslibet curie. Et ego predictus Iohannes et heredes |[12]| mei aut mei assingnati warantizabimus, acquietabimus et defendemus predictam acram terre, cum pertinenciis |[13]| predicto hospitali et dictis magistro et fratribus ibidem Deo servientibus et successoribus eorum contra omnes gentes |[14]| inperpetuum. Et ut hec mea donacio elemosinata rata maneat et stabilis inperpetuum, presenti scripto |[15]| sigillum meum apposui. His testibus: Willelmo *Wakelin*, Iohanne *Schiring*, Filippo *le Beumund*, Huberto |[16]| de Eynho, Thoma *le Neuman* de *Crouletone*, et aliis.

## A12

[*c*.1270]

*Act by which Thomas Newman of Croughton gives, concedes, and confirms to lord John of Gra(nt)ham, master of Aynho Hospital, and to the brothers of that place, in consideration of the receipt of one iron needle and 18s, one acre of his arable land in the northern field of Croughton, of which one half acre lies above* le Mores *between the land of* la Hyde *and that of Geoffrey Skilleman, and of which the other half lies above* le Blyndewell' *between the land of Robert Sergeant and that of Walter Wit. Witnesses: William de la Haye, Robert Sheering, Richard de Beaumont of Croughton, Hubert of Aynho, John Bayard, Richard son of John, clerk of Aynho.*

*A*. MCA, Aynho 45. Endorsed: T. Newman. Crowlto' (s.xv). Dimensions: 206 × 105 + 18 mm. Sealed *sur double queue*, parchment tag through one slit. Seal: pointed oval, white wax painted brown: 35 × 22 mm. A fleur-de-lis. Legend: ✠ S' TOME LE NOVMAN.

Sciant presentes et futuri quod ego Thomas *le Neweman* de *Crowelton'* dedi, concessi et hac presenti carta mea confirmavi domino |[1]| Iohanni de *Graham* dicto magistro hospitalis apostolorum Iacobi et Iohannis de Eynho et fratribus eiusdem loci unam acram terre mee arabilis in |[2]| campo boriali de *Crowelton'*, una dimidia acra iacet supra *le Mores* inter terram de *la Hyde* et terram Galfridi *Skileman* |[3]| et dimidia acra iacet supra *le Blyndewell'* inter terram Roberti *le Serjant* et terram Walteri *Wit*, tenendam et habendam de me |[4]| et her(edibus) meis vel meis assignatis dictis magistro et fratribus et eorum successoribus et cuicumque vel quibuscumque et quandocumque dictam acram cum omnibus |[5]| suis pertin(entiis) dare, vendere vel assignare sive aliquo alio modo de se alienare voluerint libere, quiete, integre et pacifice, cum libero |[6]| introitu et libero exitu, et cum omnibus libertatibus et aysiamentis ad predictam acram spectantiibus, reddendo inde annuatim mihi et her(edibus) |[7]| meis vel meis assignatis ipsi et eorum successores ad Nativitatem Domini, unam acum ferream, pro omni seculari servicio, secta cuiuscumque |[8]| curie, exactione et demanda. Et ego predictus Thomas et her(edes) mei vel mei assignati predictam acram in campo de *Crowelton'* cum omnibus |[9]| suis pertin(entiis) et libertatibus eisdem magistro et fratribus et eorum successoribus contra omnes homines mares et feminas warantizabimus, aquie-|[10]|-tabimus et defendemus in perpetuum. Pro hac autem donacione, concessione et carte mee confirmacione necnon warantizacione dederunt mihi |[11]| dicti magister et fratres octodecim solidos premanibus. Et ut omnia supradicta firmitatis robur optineant presentem cartam sigilli mei |[12]| munimine corroboravi. Hiis testibus: Willelmo de *la Haye*, Roberto *Scheringe*, Ricardo de Bello Monte de *Croweltone*, |[13]| Huberto de Eynho, Iohanne *Bayard*, Ricardo filio Iohannis clerici de Eynho, et multis aliis.

## A13

[*c*.1270 × 1280]

*Act by which Richard de Beaumont of Croughton concedes, gives, and confirms to John of Gra(nt)ham, master of Aynho Hospital, in consideration of the receipt of 20s and one half quarter of corn, one acre of his land situate in the territory of Croughton, of which one rood lies at* Astermere *between the land of Robert le Modye and that of the master of Aynho, one rood in*

Helkesden *between the land of William de la Haye and the* Skillisman' *land, and one half acre lying in* le Estemede *between the land of William de la Haye and the* Pongyant *land. Witnesses: Reginald de Beauchamp, William Wakelin, William de la Haye, Ralph of Weedon [Lois], Robert Sheering, Hubert of Aynho.*

*A*. MCA, Aynho 18. Endorsed: no endorsements. Dimensions: 173 × 138 + 20 mm. Sealed *sur double queue*, parchment tag through one slit. Seal: round, fragmentary, white wax painted brown: 30 mm. Image destroyed. Legend: ✠ SI[GILLVM] [...] BEAVM(*vnt*). The scribe of this act also wrote nos. **52, A14, A18.**

Sciant presentes et futuri quod ego Ric(ardus) de Bello Monte de *Crowelthon'* concess-|1|-i et dedi et hac presenti carta mea confirmavi Iohanni de *Graham*, dicto magistro de |2| hospitali de Eyno, unam acram terre mee, in territorium de *Crowelton'* iacentem, de qua |3| una roda iacet ad *Astermere*, inter terram Roberti *le Modye* <et> terram magistri de Eyno |4| et .I. roda iacet in *Helkesden* inter terram Willelmi de *Haye* et terram *Skillisman'* et di(midia) acra |5| iacet in *le Estemede* inter terram Willelmi de *la Haye* et terram *Pongyant*, habendam |6| et tenendam dictis magistro et fratribus et eorum successoribus de predicto Ric(ardo) et hered(ibus) suis inperpetuum |7| bene, libere, quiete et in pace, in feodo et hereditate, cum omnibus suis pertinentiis, libertatibus et |8| asiamentis. Pro hac vero donatione, concessione et presentis carte confirmatione dederunt |9| michi predicti magister et fratres viginti solidos et di(midium) quarterium fr(umenti) in gersumma. Et ego |10| predictus Ric(ardus) de Bello Monte et heredes mei predictam acram terre cum omnibus pertinentiis |11| sicut predictum est predictis magistro et fratribus et eorum successoribus warantizabimus contra |12| omnes homines et in perpetuum defendemus et ab omnibus servitiis secularibus adquietabimus |13| in perpetuum, excepto forinseco servicio. In huius rei testimonium presenti scripto sigillum |14| meum apposui. Hiis testibus: Reginaldo de Bello Campo, Willelmo *Walkelin*, Willelmo |15| de Haya, Rad(uflo) de *Wedon'*, Roberto *Schering'*, Huberto de Eyno, et aliis.

## A14

[*c*.1270 × 1280]

*Act by which Robert of Sheering gives, concedes, and confirms to the master and brethren of Aynho Hospital, in consideration of the receipt of 40s, an acre of land in the territory of Croughton adjacent to the northern field above*

Chereslawe, *between the land of the church and that of Peter Baron, with all its appurtenances, which Robert had bought from Paulinus of Croughton. Witnesses: Reginald de Beauchamp, William Wakelin, William de la Haye, Ralph of Weedon [Lois], Robert of Beaumont, Hubert of Aynho, John Bayard, Richard, clerk of Aynho.*

*A*. MCA, Aynho 39. Endorsed: [C]arta Roberti de Scyringes de una acra terre (s.xiii). Dimensions: 196 × 95/104 + 24 mm. Sealed *sur double queue* through one slit, tag and seal impression missing. The scribe responsible for the endorsement is one of the cartulary continuators (Scribe D). The scribe of this act also wrote nos. **52, A13, A18.**

Sciant presentes et futuri quod ego [R]obertus de *Schering'* dedi, concessi et hac presenti carta mea confirmavi |[1]| Deo et beate Marie <et> magistro et fratrib[us] hospitalis sanctorum Iacobi et Iohannis apostolorum de Eyno unam acram terre in territorio |[2]| de *Crowelthon'* iacentem in campo boreali super *Chereslawe* inter terram ecclesie et terram Petri *Baron*, cum omnibus |[3]| pertinentiis suis, quam quidem acram emi de Paulino de *Crow-elthon'*, habendam et tenendam predictis magistro et fratribus |[4]| et eorum successoribus inperpetuum [d]e me et heredibus meis, bene et in pace, cum omnibus pertinentiis suis, libertatibus et asiamentis |[5]| infra villam et extra de *C*[*ro*]*welthon'*, videlicet in pratis, pasturis, pascuis, pasturis [*sic*] ad tantum terre pertinentibus, reddendo |[6]| inde annuatim mihi [et] he[r]-edibus me[is] unum [obulum] ad Pascha pro omnibus serviciis et exaction-ibus secularibus et sectis curie |[7]| ad dictam terram pertinentibus. Pro hac vero concessione, donatione et presentis carte mee confirmacione dederunt mihi predicti |[8]| magister et fratres quadragin[ta so]lidos in gersumma. Et ego predictus Robertus de *Schering'* et heredes mei predictam |[9]| acram terre cum omnibus pertinent[iis sicut] predictum est, predictis magistro et fratribus et eorum successoribus inperpetuum warantizab-|[10]|-imus contra omnes homines defe[nde]mus et ab omnibus serviciis et secular-ibus exactionibus adquietabimus. In huius rei |[11]| testimonium presenti scripto sigill[um m]eum apposui. Hiis testibus: Reginaldo de Bello Campo, Willelmo *Walkelin*, |[12]| Willelmo de Haya, Rad(ulfo) de *Wedon'*, [Rober]tus de Bello Monte, Huberto de Eyno, Iohanne *Bayard*, Ric(ardo) clerico de Eyno et |[13]| multis aliis.

**A15**

[*c*.1270 × 1280]

*Act by which Thomas Newman of Croughton gives, concedes, and confirms to the master and brethren of Aynho Hospital two acres of his land in the territory of Croughton, of which half an acre lies in Croughton's northern field above* Coliersforlong, *between the land of Walter son of Margaret and that of William son of Philip, and of which the other half lies above* le Syche *between the land of Ralph of Weedon [Lois] and that of Robert Bend; in the southern field, half an acre that lies beyond* le Smaleweye *next to the land of Reginald de Beauchamp, and half an acre at* Westbithebroc *between the land of Ralph of Weedon [Lois] and that of Geoffrey at Cross, with the meadow adjacent, and all its appurtenances. Witnesses: William Wakelin of Croughton, William de la Haye of Croughton, Robert Sheering of Croughton, Hubert of Aynho, Geoffrey Markward of [King's] Sutton, Richard of Bedford of [King's] Sutton, Richard of Aynho, clerk, son of John the clerk.*

*A*. MCA, Aynho 46. Endorsed: T. Newman. Crowlton'. II acras terre cum prato (s.xv). Dimensions: 190 × 144 + 22 mm. Sealed *sur double queue*, parchment tag through one slit, seal impression missing. The scribe of this act is the same as that of nos. **A16**, **A19**.

Sciant presentes et futuri quod ego Thomas *le Neweman* de *Crewelton'* dedi, concessi et hac presenti |[1]| carta mea confirmavi magistro et fratribus hospitalis sanctorum apostolorum Iacobi et Iohannis de Eynho in liberam, |[2]| puram et perpetuam elemosinam duas acras terre mee in territorio de *Crowelton'* de quibus dimidia acra |[3]| iacet in campo boriali de *Crowelton'* super *Coliersforlong* inter terram Walteri filii Margarete et terram Willelmi filii |[4]| Philippi, et dimidia acra iacet ultra *le Syche* inter terram Rad(ulfi) de *Wedon'* et terram Roberti *le Bende*, in campo |[5]| vero australi dimidia acra iacet ultra *le Smaleweye* iuxta terram Reginaldi de Bello Campo, et dimidia |[6]| acra *Westbithebroc* iacet inter terram Rad(ulfi) de *Wedon'* et terram Galfridi ad crucem, cum prato eidem dimidiae |[7]| acre adiacente, et cum omnibus pertinenciis, habendas et tenendas imperpetuum dictas duas acras terre cum prato |[8]| et cum omnibus pertinentiis dicto magistro et fratribus eiusdem hospitalis bene, libere, quiete ab omni servicio secularis |[9]| exactione et demanda, in liberam, puram et perpetuam elemosinam sicut aliqua elemosina liberius et melius |[10]| dari poterit. Et ego predictus Thomas et heredes mei dictas duas acras terre cum prato et omnibus pertinentiis predicto |[11]| magistro et fratribus et eorum successoribus contra omnes homines imperpetuum warentizabimus et defendemus, et |[12]| ab omnibus serviciis secularibus et demandis aquietabimus. In huius rei testimonium presenti scripto |[13]| sigillum meum apposui. Hiis testibus: Willelmo *Walkelin* de *Crewelton'*, Willelmo de *la Haye* de eadem |[14]| villa, Roberto *Shering'* de eadem villa, Huberto de Eynho, Galfrido *Markward* de *Sutton'*, Ricardo |[15]| de *Bedeford'* de eadem villa, Ricardo de Eynho clerico filio Iohannis clerici, et multis aliis.

## A16

[*c.*1270 × 1280]

*Act by which Richard de Beaumont of Croughton gives, concedes, and confirms to Aynho Hospital and the brothers who serve God there, in consideration of the receipt of 6s 4d and at a quit-rent of a halfpenny, four acres of his arable land in the territory of Croughton, situate in the following places: in the northern field, one half acre lying in* Foxholeforlong *between the land of William de la Haye and that of Walter Osmund, and another half acre lying above* Roulowe *between the rector of Croughton's land and that of William de la Haye, and another half acre lying above* Swynestiforlong *between the lands of the aforesaid rector and William, and one rood below* la Blakemore *between the land of the aforesaid William and that of Geoffrey the provost, and one rood next to the road to Hinton [in the Hedges] adjacent to the land of William de la Haye; in the southern field, one half acre below* Alnettesaker *between the land of the aforesaid William and the rector of Croughton, and one half acre above* Alnettesaker *next to the land of William de la Haye on the other side, and one half acre of land below* Schortehanginde *between the land of the aforesaid William and the land of Aynho Hospital, and one half acre below* Dunam *between the land of the aforesaid William and that of Ralph of Astwell, and two headlands that pertain to half a virgate of Richard's land that lies above* Smethenhulle *and* Radewellehoke. *Witnesses: Reginald de Beauchamp, William Wakelin of Croughton, William de la Haye of Croughton, Ralph of Astwell of Croughton, Robert Sheering of Croughton, Hubert of Aynho, John Baard of Aynho.*

*A*. MCA, Aynho 24. Endorsed: no endorsements. Dimensions: 215 × 145 + 11 mm. Sealed *sur double queue*, parchment tag through one slit, seal impression missing. The scribe of this act is the same as that of nos. **A15**, **A19**.

Sciant presentes et futuri quod ego Ricardus de Bello[(a)] Monte de *Crowelton'* dedi, concessi et hac presenti carta mea confirmavi |[1]| magistro hospitalis sanctorum Iacobi et Iohannis apostolorum de Eynho et fratribus eiusdem hospitalis ibidem Deo servientibus quatuor acras terre mee |[2]| arabilis in territorio de *Crowelton'*, iacentes in talibus locis subscriptis: de quibus in campo boriali dimidia acra iacet in |[3]| *Foxholeforlong*, inter terram Willelmi de *la Haye* et terram Walteri *Osemu(n)d*, et alia dimidia acra iacet super *Roulowe* inter |[4]| terram rectoris ecclesie de *Crowelton'* et terram Willelmi de *la Haye*, et alia di<mi>dia acra iacet super *Swynestiforlong* inter terras |[5]| dicti recotoris et dicti Willelmi, et una roda iacet subtus *la Blakemore* inter terram dicti Willelmi et terram Galfridi prepositi, |[6]| et una roda iacet iuxta viam de *Hinton'* iuxta terram dicti Willelmi de *la Haye*; in campo vero australi dimidia acra |[7]| iacet subtus *Alnettesak*[*er*] inter terram dicti Willelmi et dicti rectoris de *Crowelton'*, et dimidia acra iacet super *Alnettesaker* |[8]| iuxta [t]erram dicti Willelmi de *la Haye* ex utraque parte, et di<mi>dia acra iacet subtus *Schortehanginde* inter terram dicti Willelmi et terram |[9]| hospitalis de Eynho, et di<mi>dia acra iacet subtus Duna(m) inter terram dicti Willelmi et terram Rad(ulfi) de [*E*]*stwelle*, et duo capita prati |[10]| que pertinent ad di<mi>diam virgatam terre mee que iacent super *Smethenhulle* et *Radewellehoke*, habendas et tenendas dictis magistro et |[11]| fratribus et eorum successoribus imperpetuum de me et heredibus meis libere, quiete, bene et in pace in feodo et hereditate cum omnibus |[12]| pertinentiis suis et aysiamentis infra villam de *Crowelton'* et extra, redendo michi annuatim et heredibus meis unum ob(ulum) ad |[13]| festum sancti Michaelis pro omnibus serviciis, consuetudinibus et demandis secularibus et sectis curie, salvo forinseco servicio. Pro hac vero con-|[14]|-cessione, donatione et presentis carte mee confirmatione dederunt mihi predicti magister et fratres quadraginta sex solid(os) et octo denar(ios) sterlingorum |[15]| in gersuma. Et ego predictus Ric(ardus) et heredes mei predictas quatuor acras terre cum prato prenominato et pastura adiacente et cum omnibus pertin(entiis) |[16]| predictis magistro et fratribus et eorum successoribus contra omnes homines et feminas imperpetuum warentizabimus et defendemus. In huius rei testimonium |[17]| presenti scripto sigillum meum apposui. Hiis testibus: Reginaldo de Bello Campo, Willelmo *Walkelin* de *Crowelton'*, Willelmo de *la* |[18]| *Haye* de eadem, Rad(ulfo) de *Estwelle* de eadem villa, Roberto *Shering'* de eadem, Huberto de Eynho, Iohanne *Baard* de eadem, et multis aliis.

(a) Bollo *A*.

*Note*. Macray dates this act *c*.1260, but since its scribe is the same as that responsible for nos. **A15** and **A19**, both of which date to the final quarter of the thirteenth century, it seems more likely to be contemporaneous to them, especially since many of its witnesses also appear in Aynho acts at this time.

## A17

[*c*.1270 × 1280]

*Act by which Thomas Newman concedes, gives, and confirms to John of Gra(nt)ham, master of Aynho Hospital, and to its brothers, two acres of his arable land, of which one lies in Croughton's southern field, between the land of Geoffrey Skilleman towards the north and that of Osbern Giffard towards the south, one end abutting on the land of the lord William de Turville towards the east, namely between the road that leads from Croughton to Brackley, towards the south, and the land of Geoffrey de Cross*[4] *towards the north, one end abutting the land of William Wakelin which is called* Otindene *towards the east. Witnesses: lord William de Turville, lord Reginald de Beauchamp, knights, William de la Haye, Hubert of Aynho, Robert of Sheering, Richard de Beaumont, Theobald of Evenley, Rannulf le Gras of Astwick.*

*A*. MCA, Aynho 48. Endorsed: T. Newman. Croulton' (s.xv). Dimensions: 196 × 105 + 11 mm. Sealed *sur double queue*, parchment tag through one slit. Seal: pointed oval, white wax painted brown: 34 × 21 mm. A fleur-de-lis. Legend: ✠ S' TOME NEWMAN (very indistinct). The scribe of this act also wrote no. **A11**.

Sciant presentes et futuri quod ego Thomas *le Nyeuman* consessi, dedi et hac presenti carta mea confir-|1|-mavi pro me et heredibus meis Iohanni de *Graham* magistro hospitalis sanctorum Iacobi et Iohannis de |2| Eynho et eiusdem loci fratribus ibidem Deo servientibus duas acras terre mee arabilis inperpetuam |3| elemosinam quarum una acra iacet in campo australi de *Crouletone*, videlicet inter terram Galfridi |4| *Skilleman* versus aquilonem et terram Hosberni *Giffard* versus austrum cuius unum caput abuttat super |5| terram domini Willelmi *le Turvile* versus occidentem, et alia acra iacet in predicta villa de *Crouletone* silicet |6| in campo aquilonali, videlicet inter viam que ducit de *Crouletone* aput *Brackele* versus austrum et terram |7| Galfridi de Cruce versus aquilonem, cuius unum caput abuttat super terram Willelmi *Wakelin* que vocatur |8| *Otindene* versus orientem, habendas et tenedas predictas acras terre de me et heredibus meis sibi dictis |9| Iohanni et f[ratrib]us et successoribus eorum, libere, quiete et in elemosina pura et perpetua. Et ego predictus |10| Thom[a]s [*le Nyeuman*] de *Crouletune* et heredes mei warantizabimus, acquietabimus et def[ende]-|11|-mus predictas ac[ras] [terr]e sibi dictis Iohanni et fratribus et successoribus, contra omnes gentes |12| inperpetuum. In cuius rei testimonium presenti carte sigillum

[4] This is almost certainly the same person as Geoffrey at Cross mentioned in **A15**.

meum apposui. His testibus: domino Willelmo |[13]| *le Turvile*, domino Reginaldo *le Byeuchaumpe*, militibus, Willelmo de *le Haye*, Huberto de Eynho, Roberto |[14]| de *Syringe*, Ricardo *le Byeumund*, Tebaudo de *Evinle*, Ranulfo *le Gras* de *Hastwik*, et aliis.

## A18

[*c.*1270 × 1280]

*Act by which Thomas Newman of Croughton gives, concedes, and confirms to John of Gra(nt)ham, master of Aynho Hospital, in consideration of the receipt of one mark, one acre of his land in the fields of Croughton, of which one half acre lies above* Smalebrokeill' *between the land of* la Hyde *and that of the hospital, and of which the other half acre is above* Stanille *between the land of Geoffrey the clerk and that of the hospital in the southern field. Witnesses: William de la Haye, William Wakelin, Ralph of Weedon [Lois], Robert Sheering, Richard de Beaumont.*

*A*. MCA, Aynho 70. Endorsed: T. Newman. Crowltō. I acram cum prato (s.xv). Dimensions: 101 × 128 + 19 mm. Sealed *sur double queue*, parchment tag through one slit, seal impression missing. The scribe of this act also wrote nos. **52**, **A13–A14**.

Sciant presentes et futuri quod ego Thomas *le Neuman* de *Crowelthon'* |[1]| dedi, concessi et hac presenti carta mea confirmavi Iohanni de *Graham* dicto |[2]| magistro hospitalis de Eyno unam acram terre mee in campis de *Crowelthon'* iacen-|[3]|-tem, videlicet unam dimidiam acram iacentem super *Smalebrokeill'* inter terram *la Hy*-|[4]|-*de* et terram dicti hospitalis, et aliam dimidiam acram super *Stanille* inter terram Galfridi |[5]| clerici et terram dicti hospitalis in campo australi, habendam et tenendam dictis magistro et |[6]| fratribus et eorum successoribus in perpetuum de me et heredibus meis libere, quiete, bene ab omni |[7]| exactione et demanda. Pro hac vero donatione, concessione et presentis carte confirma-|[8]|-cione dederunt mihi predictus magister et fratres unam marcam argenti in gersum-|[9]|-ma. Et ego predictus Thomas et heredes mei predictam acram terre cum prato et pastura |[10]| adiacente et cum omnibus pertin(entiis) predictis magistro et fratribus et eorum successoribus in perpetu-|[11]|-m [w]arantizabimus et defendemus et ab omnibus serviciis secularibus, demandis, |[12]| salvo forinseco servicio, adquietabimus. In huius rei test(imonium) presenti scripto sigillum meum |[13]| apposui. Hiis testibus: Willelmo de Haye, Willelmo Walkelino, Ra[d]-(ulfo) de Wedona, |[14]| Roberto *Sering'*, Ric(ardo) de Bellomonte.

**A19**

[*c.*1279 × 1289]

*Act by which Roger, son and heir of Adam le Goer, gives, concedes, and confirms to the master and brothers of Aynho Hospital all the right and claim that he has over a plot of land in Brackley, located between the messuage of the abbess of Godstow, on the northern side, and the house of Roger of Luton, on the south, and which extends in length from the king's way to the grove of the prior of Brackley, with all the dwellings there sited and a small meadow next to the grove, from which plot of land the hospital used to receive 7s of annual rent, now to hold from the lady Ellen la Zouche for an annual payment of 12d, to be paid at three terms, namely: 4d at the Purification of the Virgin Mary, 4d at Pentecost, and 4d at the feast of St Michael. Witnesses: lord John of Chinnor, then prior of Brackley, Roger of Luton, Richard Swet, Alexander Rich, Richard of Dunstable, Thomas Terri, Robert de Cotes of Brackley, Hubert of Aynho, John Baard of Aynho, William Wakelin of Croughton.*

*A*. MCA, Aynho 14. Endorsed: Scriptum Rog(eri) le Gower (s.xiv); Brakeley (s.xv); pertinens ad Ainhoo (s.xv). Dimensions: 194 × 175 + 16 mm. Sealed sur double queue, parchment tag through one slit. Seal: pointed oval, white wax painted brown: 35 × 22 mm. A fleur-de-lis. Legend: ✠ S' ROG(*eri*) LE GOE[R] (*angled wavy line*). The scribe of this act is the same as that of nos. **A15–A16**.

Sciant presentes et futuri quod ego Rog(erus) filius et heres Ade *le* [*G*]*oer* dedi, concessi et hac presenti |[1]| carta mea confirmavi totum ius meum et clamium quod habui vel iure hereditario habere potui in |[2]| una area terre iacente in *Brackele*, inter mesuagium abatisse de *Godestowe*, ex parte boriali, |[3]| et domum Rog(eri) de *Luton'*, ex parte australi, et extendit se in longitudine a regali via usque |[4]| ad gravam domini prioris de *Brackele*, cum omnibus domibus ibidem sitis, et cum pratello eidem adiacenti |[5]| iuxta eandem gravam, magistro hospitalis apostolorum Iacobi et Iohannis de Eynho et fratribus eiusdem domus Deo |[6]| servientibus, de qua area predicta magister et fratres consuerunt percipere septem solid(os) redditus annuatim, habendam et tenendam imperpetuum dictis magistro et fratribus et eorum successoribus de domina Helena |[7]| *la Zuche* et suis heredibus, libere, quiete, bene et in pace et iure hereditario, cum omnibus aysiamentis |[8]| suis, et libero ingressu et egressu et cum omnibus aliis libertatibus ad eandem aream spectantibus, infra villam |[9]| de *Brackele* et extra, reddendo inde dicte domine Helene et heredibus suis duodecim denar(ios) argenti |[10]| ad tres terminos anni, videlicet ad purificationem beate Marie quatuor denar(ios), et ad Pentecost(em) |[11]| quatuor den(arios), et ad festum sancti Michaelis quatuor den(arios), pro omnibus serviciis, consuetudinibus,[(a)] exactionis, et demandis, |[12]| salvo forinseco servicio domini regis, ad tantum terre pertinentibus. Pro hac autem donatione et concessione et |[13]| carte mee confirmacione dederunt mihi predicti magister et fratres qu[...] [...][(b)] argenti premanibus, |[14]| ita quod nec ego Rog(erus) nec aliquis per me in dicta area terre cum pertinentiis, de cetero aliquid ius vel clamium |[15]| vel calumpniam apponere poterimus. Set ego predictus Rog(erus) et heredes mei dictam aream cum pertinen-|[16]|-ciis sicut predictum est dictis magistro et fratribus et eorum successoribus contra omnes homines warentizabimus |[17]| et defendemus inperpetuum. In huius rei testimonium, presenti scripto sigillum meum apposui. Hiis |[18]| testibus: domino Iohanne de *Chinnore*, tunc temporis priore de *Brackele*, Rog(er)o de *Luton*', Ricardo |[19]| *Swet*, Alexandro *le Riche*, Ric(ardo) de *Dunstaple*, Thome Terri, Roberto de *Cotes* de *B(r)ackele*, |[20]| Huberto de Eynho, Iohanne *Baard* de eadem villa, Willelmo *Walkilin* de *Crowelton*', et aliis.

(a) consuetutinibus *A.* — (b) *Text missing due to parchment damage, A.*

### A20

[*c.*1280 × *c.*1285]

*Act by which Alice le Beaumont, widow of Robert Sergeant of Croughton, in her full power, concedes and quit-claims to the master of Aynho Hospital and the brothers who serve God there, in consideration of the receipt of half a mark and one half quarter of corn, four acres of land in the territory of Croughton, located in the same places as those four acres granted in no.* ***A16****. Witnesses: John le Haye, Hubert of Aynho, Richard of Bedford, John Sheering, Henry, merchant of Aynho, John the cook of Carlton.*

A. MCA, Aynho 25. Endorsed: no endorsements. Dimensions: 212 × 124 + 20 mm. Sealed *sur double queue*, parchment tag through one slit. Seal: pointed oval, white wax painted brown: 34 × 20 mm. A fleur-de-lis. Legend: ✠ S'. ALICIE BEAV(*mun*)T.

Sciant presentes et futuri quod ego Alicia *le Beumunt*, relicta Roberti *le Serjaunt* de *Croulton*', in mea ligia potestate concessi |[1]| et hac presenti carta mea quietum clamavi magistro hospitalis sanctorum Iacobi et Iohannis de Aynho et fratribus eiusdem loci ibidem Deo |[2]| servientibus quatuor acras terre mee arabilis in territorio de *Crowelton*' iacentes in talibus locis subscriptis de quibus: in |3| campo boriali dimidia acra iacet in *Foxhole-furlong* inter terram Willelmi de *la Haye* et terram Walteri *Osemund*, et alia dimidia |4| acra iacet super *Roulowe* inter terram rectoris ecclesie de *Crowelton'* et terram Willelmi de *la Haye*, et alia di<mi>dia acra iacet super *Swi-*|5|*-nestifurlong* inter terras dicti recotoris et dicti Willelmi, et una roda iacet subtus *la Blakemore* inter terram dicti Willelmi et terram Galfridi |6| prepositi, et una roda iacet iuxta viam de *Hynton'*; in campo vero australi dimidia acra iacet subtus *Alnettes Aker* inter terram |7| dicti Willelmi et dicti rectoris de *Croulton'* et dimidia acra iacet super *Alnettes Aker* iuxta terram dicti Willelmi de *la Haye* ex utraque |8| parte, et dimidia acra iacet subtus *Schorthanginge* inter terram dicti Willelmi et terram hospitalis de Aynho, et dimidia acra iacet subtus Dun-|9|-ham inter terram dicti Willelmi et terram Rad(ulfi) de *Estwelle*, et duo capita prati que pertinent ad dimidiam virgatam terre mee que |10| iacent super *Smethenhulle* et *Radewellehoke*, habendas et tenendas dictis magistro hospitalis et fratribus et eorum successoribus inp-|11|-erpetuum de heredibus dicti Ric(ardi) de Bello-monte et sine calumpnia aliqua mei vel successorum meorum vel alicuius alterius ex parte mea, li-|12|-bere, quiete, bene et in pace inperpetuum in feodo et hereditate cum omnibus pertinentiis suis et aysiamentis infra villam de *Crowel-*|13|*-ton'* et extra, pro omnibus serviciis, consuetudinibus et demandis secularibus et sectis curie, salvo forinseco servicio. Pro hac autem |14| concessione et quieta clammatione et presentis carte mee confir-matione dederunt mihi predicti magister et fratres dimidiam marcam et dimidium |15| q(u)art(erium) fr(ument)i in gersummam. In huius rei testi-monium presenti scripto sigillum meum apposui. Hiis testibus: Iohanne *le Haye*, Huberto |16| de Aynh(o), Ric(ardo) de *Bedeford*, Iohanne *Schyring'*, Henrico m(er)cator(e) de Aynho, Iohanne Coco de *Cherlton'* et aliis.

*Note*. Macray dates this act *c*.1260 × 1270, but a Robert Sergeant appears among the witnesses of no. **A21**, which was definitely issued after 12 May 1282, since it refers to William of Occold, master of Aynho Hospital, who was installed on this date. If the Robert of no. **A21** and the Robert Sergeant of Croughton named here are one and the same, then this act must post-date the one below. Even if not, the hand in which Alice's act is written would suggest it was issued in the later decades of the thirteenth century.

## A21

[*c*.1285]

*Act by which Margaret, widow of Thomas Newman of Croughton, in her free widowhood, concedes and quit-claims to William of Occold, master of Aynho Hospital, and to the brothers of that place, in consideration of the receipt of half a mark, all her right of dowry in the tenement that her late husband sold to the aforementioned master and brothers in the vill of Croughton: Witnesses: John de la Haye, John Sheering, Hubert of Aynho, Robert Sergeant, Geoffrey le Beaumont.*

*A*. MCA, Aynho 47. Endorsed: Margaret' Newman. Crowlto' (s.xv). Dimensions: 177 × 64 + 11 mm. Sealed *sur double queue*, parchment tag through three slits. Seal: pointed oval, white wax painted brown: 30 × 15 mm. A pelican in her piety. Legend: ✶ SVM PELLICAN[VS D]EI.

Notum sit omnibus Christi fidelibus presens scriptum visuris vel audituris quod ego Margareta relicta |1| Thome *le Neuman* de *Crouletone* in libera viduitate mea concessi et quietum clamavi Willelmo |2| de *Acolt* magistro hospitalis sanctorum Iacobi et Iohannis de Eynho et eiusdem loci fratribus totum ius et |3| clameum quod habui vel habere potui nomine dotis in totum tenementum quod predictus Thomas ma-|4|-ritus meus quondam vendidit predictis magistro et fratribus in predicta villa de *Crouletone*. Pro hac autem |5| concessione et quiete clamacione predicti magister et fratres dederunt michi dimidiam marcam stere-|6|-lingorum premanibus. Et ut hec concessio et quieta clamacio rata maneat et stabilis huic scrip-|7|-to sigillum meum apposui. Hiis testibus: Iohanne de *la Aye*, Iohanne *Schiring'*, Huberto de Eynho, Roberto *le* |8| *Serjaunt'*, Galfrido *le Beumund*, et aliis.

# BIBLIOGRAPHY

## MANUSCRIPTS AND ARCHIVAL SOURCES


Avranches, Bibliothèque patrimoniale, MS 210.
Birmingham, Archives and Heritage Service, 403957 [IIR.33].
Brighton, East Sussex and Brighton and Hove Record Office, GLY/1139.
Cambrai, Le Labo/Archives hospitalières, IX B 55–56.
Cambridge, Christ's College, Muniments, Bourn E.
Cambridge, Corpus Christi College,
  MS 2II.
  MS 16II.
Chicago, Newberry Library, MS Greenlee 39.
Durham, University Library–Archives and Special Collections,
  1.1.Spec.50.
  2.4.Spec.8.
  4.3.Sacr.3.
  Loc. III: 6.
Évreux, Archives départementales de l'Eure, H-dépôt Évreux G7.
Exeter, Devon Record Office,
  ECA/MR 64.
  ECA/MAG 69.
  ECA/MAG 99.
Kew, The National Archives,
  C 47/9/7.
  C 241/18/114.
  DL 41/125.
  E 326/309.
  PRO C52/29.
Lichfield, Cathedral Library, QQ.1.
Limoges, Archives départementales de la Haute-Vienne/Archives hospitalières, A 2–3.
Lincoln, Lincolnshire Archives, Add. Reg. 6.
London, British Library,
  Add. Roll 15895.
  Add. Roll 17121.
  Add. Roll 19631.
  Add. Roll 24879.
  Add. Roll 47398.
  Cotton Roll XIII.6.
  Cotton Roll XVI.51–52.

Harley Roll A.28.
Harley Roll A.29.
Harley Roll G.21.
Harley Roll L.20.
Harley Roll O.5.
MS Add. 49996.
MS Add. 52729.
MS Cotton Claudius E IV.
MS Cotton Vespasian A XIX.
MS Cotton Vespasian E XVIII.
MS Egerton 3033.
MS Harley 259.
MS Harley 6951.
MS Lansdowne 259.
Northampton, Northamptonshire Archives, CA/9/1/4; *olim* 6268.
Norwich, Norfolk Record Office,
BRA 833/14/1, 669X1.
Hare 624 188 x 1.
Oxford, Bodleian Libraries,
MS Dodsworth 49.
MS Dodsworth 157.
MS Norfolk Rolls.
Oxford, Lincoln College, EL/OXF/D/5.
Oxford, Magdalen College,
All Saints 51.
All Saints 52.
Astwick and Evenley 2.
Astwick and Evenley 4.
Astwick and Evenley 8.
Astwick and Evenley 11.
Astwick and Evenley 13.
Astwick and Evenley 46.
Astwick and Evenley 47.
Astwick and Evenley 50.
Astwick and Evenley 51.
Astwick and Evenley 52A.
Astwick and Evenley 56.
Astwick and Evenley 61.
Astwick and Evenley 63A.
Astwick and Evenley 64A.
Astwick and Evenley 68A.
Astwick and Evenley 77A.
Astwick and Evenley 80A.
Astwick and Evenley 83A.
Astwick and Evenley 84A.
Astwick and Evenley 85A.
Astwick and Evenley 86A.
Astwick and Evenley 91A.

Astwick and Evenley 95A.
Astwick and Evenley 101A.
Astwick and Evenley 102A.
Astwick and Evenley 106A.
Astwick and Evenley 107A.
Astwick and Evenley 108A.
Astwick and Evenley 129A.
Aynho 5.
Aynho 8.
Aynho 11.
Aynho 13.
Aynho 14.
Aynho 16.
Aynho 18.
Aynho 19.
Aynho 21.
Aynho 22.
Aynho 24.
Aynho 25.
Aynho 26.
Aynho 27.
Aynho 28.
Aynho 30.
Aynho 31.
Aynho 32.
Aynho 34.
Aynho 36.
Aynho 37.
Aynho 38.
Aynho 39.
Aynho 40.
Aynho 41.
Aynho 42.
Aynho 43.
Aynho 44.
Aynho 45.
Aynho 46.
Aynho 47.
Aynho 48.
Aynho 49.
Aynho 50.
Aynho 51.
Aynho 52.
Aynho 53.
Aynho 54.
Aynho 55.
Aynho 56.
Aynho 58.

Aynho 59.
Aynho 60.
Aynho 61.
Aynho 62.
Aynho 63.
Aynho 64.
Aynho 65.
Aynho 66.
Aynho 67.
Aynho 68.
Aynho 70.
Aynho 71.
Aynho 77.
Aynho 80.
Aynho 81.
Aynho 82.
Aynho 83.
Aynho 84.
Aynho 85.
Aynho 86.
Aynho 87.
Aynho 88.
Brackley 2A.
Brackley 4A.
Brackley 5.
Brackley 6A.
Brackley 9A.
Brackley 10.
Brackley 13.
Brackley 23A.
Brackley 25.
Brackley 36A.
Brackley 39.
Brackley 47A.
Brackley 49A.
Brackley 51.
Brackley 52.
Brackley 52A.
Brackley 54.
Brackley 57.
Brackley 58.
Brackley 59.
Brackley 63.
Brackley 63A.
Brackley 70A.
Brackley 76A.
Brackley 82.
Brackley 85A.

Brackley 87A.
Brackley 88A.
Brackley 89A.
Brackley 94A.
Brackley 97A.
Brackley 116.
Brackley 127.
Brackley 131(a).
Brackley 132A.
Brackley 135.
Brackley 136.
Brackley 137.
Brackley 138.
Brackley 141.
Brackley 142.
Brackley 150.
Brackley 152.
Brackley 155.
Brackley 161.
Brackley 163.
Brackley 165.
Brackley 169.
Brackley 170.
Brackley 171.
Brackley 174.
Brackley 179.
Brackley 184.
Brackley 203.
Brackley B20.
Brackley B23.
Brackley B50.
Brackley B63.
Brackley B67.
Brackley B92.
Brackley B93.
Brackley B98.
Brackley B106.
Brackley B108.
Brackley B110.
Brackley B130.
Brackley B131.
Brackley B152.
Brackley B154.
Brackley B178.
Brackley B182.
Brackley B189.
Brackley B233.
Brackley B237.

Brackley B239.
Brackley B243.
Brackley B184.
Brackley B201.
Brackley C2.
Brackley C5.
Brackley C6.
Brackley C9.
Brackley C11.
Brackley C20.
Brackley C33.
Brackley C36.
Brackley C40.
Brackley C43.
Brackley C46.
Brackley C52.
Brackley C57.
Brackley C74.
Brackley C84.
Brackley C108.
Brackley C109.
Brackley C114.
Brackley C133.
Brackley C134.
Brackley C135.
Brackley D4.
Brackley D7.
Brackley D10.
Brackley D17.
Brackley D20.
Brackley D21.
Brackley D22.
Brackley D24.
Brackley D37.
Brackley D40.
Brackley D89.
Brackley D90.
Brackley D91.
Brackley D98.
Brackley D102.
Brackley D133.
Brackley D141.
Brackley D142.
Brackley D161.
Brackley D163.
Brackley D182.
Brackley D190.
Brackley D193.

Brackley D194.
Brackley D196.
Brackley D201.
Brackley D202.
Brackley D203.
Brackley D205.
Brackley D218.
Brackley D239.
Brackley D243.
Brackley D247.
Brackley D248.
Chartae Regiae 50.5
Chipping Norton 2.
Chipping Norton 4.
Cowley 2.
Cowley 7.
CP/3/31.
EP/76/30.
EP/137/1.
Garsington 22.
Holywell 9.
MP/1/54(i).
MS 275.
Oddington 1A.
Oddington 5A.
Oddington 28A.
Oddington 31A.
Oddington 41.
South Newington 2A.
South Newington 11A.
South Newington 12A.
St Giles 9.
St Martin's 7.
St Martin's 8.
St Mary Magdalene 3
St Mary the Virgin 8.
St Peter's in the East 7A.
St Peter's in the East 20B.
St Peter's in the East 46A.
St Peter's in the East 47.
St Peter's in the East 50.
St Peter's in the East 51D.
St Peter's in the East 62C.
St Peter's in the East 74.
St Peter's in the East 76.
Syresham 11.
Syresham 28.
Syresham 37.

Syresham 42.
Syresham 52.
Thornborough 19.
Thornborough 40.
Thornborough 85.
Westbury 34A.
Westbury 35A.
Westcote 6.
Westcote 7.
Westcote 33.
Westcote 87.
Whitfield 2.
Whitfield 3.
Whitfield 4.
Whitfield 5.
Whitfield 12.
Whitfield 18.
Whitfield 16.
Whitfield 17.
Whitfield 21.
Whitfield 23.
Whitfield 24.
Whitfield 26.
Whitfield 32.
Whitfield 36.
Whitfield 40.
Whitfield 41.
Whitfield 47.
Whitfield 48.
Whitfield 61.
Whitfield 73.
Whitfield 79.
Whitfield 80.
Whitfield 91.
Whitfield 100.
Whitfield 104.
Whitfield 106.
Whitfield 107.
Whitfield 108.
Whitfield 109.
Whitfield 110.
Whitfield 122.
Whitfield 123.
Whitfield 126.
Whitfield 135.
Whitfield 144.
Whitfield 155.
Whitfield 161.

Whitfield 166.
Willoughby 3A.
Willoughby 56.
Preston, Lancashire Record Office, DDTO/box AA.
Sheffield, City Archives and Local Studies Library, CD433.
Stafford, William Salt Library, MS 539.
The Hague, Museum Meermanno, MS 10 B 23.
Tournai, Bibliothèque de la Ville, Cod. 4A.
Vatican, Biblioteca Apostolica Vaticana, MS Vat. lat. 2639.
York, University of York–Borthwick Institute for Archives, CP.F.112.
York Minster Library and Archives, P 1/1/9.

## PRINTED PRIMARY SOURCES

Bain, J., G. Simpson, and J. Galbraith (eds), *Calendar of Documents Relating to Scotland preserved in Her Majesty's Public Record Office, London* (5 vols, Edinburgh, 1881–6).
Barraclough, G. (ed.), *Facsimiles of Early Cheshire Charters* (Preston, 1957).
Barraclough, G. (ed.), *The Charters of the Anglo-Norman Earls of Chester, c. 1071–1237* (Chester, 1988).
Bates, D. (ed.), *Regesta regum Anglo-Normannorum: The Acta of William I (1066–1087)* (Oxford, 1998).
Bouchard, C.B. (ed.), *The Cartulary-Chronicle of St-Pierre of Bèze* (Toronto, ON, 2020).
Brown, V. (ed.), *Eye Priory Cartulary and Charters* (2 vols, Woodbridge, 1992–94).
Brown Davis, W. (ed.), *Cartularium prioratus de Gyseburne* (2 vols, Durham, 1889–94).
Burton, J. (ed.), *The Cartulary of Byland Abbey* (Woodbridge, 2004).
Büttner, A. et al. (eds), *Kopialbuch der Zisterzienserabtei Schönau (Generallandesarchiv Karlsruhe 67/1302)* (Heidelberg, 2020).
*Calendar of Charter Rolls preserved in the Public Record Office* (6 vols, London, 1903–27).
*Calendar of Entries in the Papal Register Relating to Great Britain and Ireland: Papal Letters* (23 vols, London, 1893–).
*Calendar of Inquisitions Post Mortem and other analogous Documents, 1236–1307* (4 vols, London, 1904–13).
*Calendar of the Close Rolls preserved in the Public Record Office. Henry III* (14 vols, London, 1902–38).
*Calendar of the Close Rolls preserved in the Public Record Office. Edward I* (5 vols, London, 1900–08).
*Calendar of the Fine Rolls preserved in the Public Record Office* (22 vols, London, 1911–62).
Camps, H.P.H. et al. (eds), *Oorkondenboek van Noord-Brabant tot 1312* (4 vols in 2, 's-Gravenhage, 1979–2000).
Carlin, M. and D. Crouch (eds and trans.), *Lost Letters of Medieval Life. English Society, 1200–1250* (Philadelphia, PA, 2013).

Carpenter, D.X. (ed.), *The Cartulary of St Leonard's Hospital, York* (2 vols, Woodbridge, 2015).
Clark, A. (ed.), *The English Register of Godstow Nunnery, Near Oxford, Written About 1450* (London, 1911).
Clay, C.T. (ed.), *Early Yorkshire Charters* (10 vols, York, 1935–65).
*Close Rolls of the Reign of Henry III preserved in the Public Record Office, 1227–1272* (14 vols, London, 1902–38).
Conway Davies, J. (ed.), *The Cartae Antiquae, Rolls 11–20* (London, 1960).
*Curia regis rolls ... preserved in the Public Record Office* (20 vols, London, 1920–2006).
Davis, F.N. et al. (eds), *Rotuli Ricardi Gravesend diocesis Lincolniensis* (Oxford, 1925).
Dalby, A. (ed. and trans.), *The Treatise of Walter of Bibbesworth* (Totnes, 2012)
Dugdale, William, *Monasticon Anglicanum*, new edn by H. Ellise and B. Bandinel (6 vols, London, 1817–30).
*English Episcopal Acta* (47 vols, Oxford, 1980–).
English Place-Name Society, *Survey of English Place-Names* (151 vols, Cambridge, 1924–).
Everard, J. (ed.), *The Charters of Duchess Constance of Brittany and her Family, 1171–1221* (Woodbridge, 1999).
Fauroux, M. (ed.), *Recueil des actes des ducs de Normandie de 911 à 1066* (Caen, 1961).
Gibbons A. (ed.), *Liber antiquus de ordinationibus vicariarum tempore Hugonis Wells, Lincolniensis Episcopi, 1209–1235* (Lincoln, 1888).
Hall, H. (ed.), *The Red Book of the Exchequer* (3 vols, London, 1986).
Hardy, T.D. (ed.), *Rotuli chartarum in Turri londinensi asservati* (London, 1837).
—— (ed.), *Rotuli de oblatis et finibus in Turri Londinensi asservati, tempore regis Johannis* (London, 1835).
—— (ed.), *Rotuli litterarum clausarum in turri Londinensi asservati* (2 vols, London, 1833–4).
—— (ed.), *Rotuli litterarum patentium in turri londinensi asservati* (London, 1835).
Harper-Bill, C. (ed.), *Blythburgh Priory Cartulary* (2 vols, Woodbridge, 1980–1).
Hill, R.M.T. (ed.), *The Rolls and Register of Bishop Oliver Sutton* (8 vols, Woodbridge, 1948–).
Hoskin, P. (ed.), *Robert Grosseteste as Bishop of Lincoln: The Episcopal Rolls, 1235–1253* (Woodbridge, 2015).
Howard, J.J. (ed.), *Miscellanea genealogica et heraldica*, 2nd ser (5 vols, London, 1884–94).
Hunter, J. (ed.), *Fines, sive pedes finium ... A.D. 1195–A.D. 1214* (2 vols, London, 1835–44).
Illingworth, W. (ed.), *Placita de quo warranto temporibus Edw. I. II. & III. In curia receptæ scaccarij Westm. asservata* (London, 1818).
Johnston, R.C. (ed.), *Jordan Fantosme's Chronicle* (Oxford, 1981).
Kerling, N.J.M. (ed.), *Cartulary of St Bartholomew's Hospital, Founded 1123: A Calendar* (London, 1973).
Landon, L. (ed.), *The Cartae Antiquae, Rolls 1–10* (London, 1939).
Le Neve, J., *Fasti Ecclesiae Anglicanae 1066–1300*, new edn D.E. Greenway (11 vols, London, 1968–).

Luard, H.R. (ed.), *Matthæi Parisiensis, monachi Sancti Albani, Chronica majora* (7 vols, London, 1872–83).

Madden, F. (ed.), *Matthæi Parisiensis, monachi Sancti Albani, Historia anglorum* (3 vols, London 1866–9).

Maitland, F.W. (ed.), *Bracton's Note Book: A Collection of Cases decided in the King's Courts during the Reign of Henry III* (3 vols, London, 1887).

Mansi, J.D. (ed.), *Miscellanea nova ordine digesta* (4 vols, Lucca, 1761–4).

Maxwell-Lyte, H.C. (ed.), *Calendar of the Patent Rolls preserved in the Public Record Office. Henry III* (6 vols, London, 1901–13); H.C. Maxwell-Lyte (ed.), *Calendar of the Patent Rolls preserved in the Public Record Office. Edward I* (4 vols, London, 1893–1901).

Maxwell-Lyte, H.C. (ed.), *Liber Feodorum. The Book of Fees, Commonly Called Testa de Nevill. Reformed from the Earliest MSS. by the Deputy keeper of the Records* (3 vols, London, 1920–31).

Morris, J. (ed.), *Domesday Book* (35 vols, Chichester, 1973–86).

Mortimer, R. (ed.), *Leiston Abbey Cartulary and Butley Priory Charters* (Ipswich, 1979).

Oliver, A.M. (ed.), *Northumberland and Durham Deeds: From the Dodsworth MSS. in Bodley's Library, Oxford* (Newcastle upon Tyne, 1929).

Palgrave, F. (ed.), *Rotuli Curiæ Regis: Rolls and Records of the Court held before the King's Justiciars or Justices* (2 vols, London, 1835).

Phillimore, W. and F.N. Davis (eds), *Rotuli Hugonis de Welles, Episcopi Lincolniensis A.D. MCCIX-MCCXXXV* (3 vols, Lincoln, 1912–14).

Ramsay, N. and J.M. Willoughby (eds), *Hospitals, Towns, and the Professions* [= *CBMLC* XIV] (London, 2009).

Richardson, H.G. (ed.), *The Memoranda Roll for the Michaelmas Term of the First Year of the Reign of King John, 1199–1200* (London, 1943).

Roberts, C. (ed.), *Excerpta è rotulis finium in Turri londinensi asservatis, Henrico Tertio rege, A.D. 1216–1272* (2 vols, London, 1835–6).

Roger of Howden, *Gesta regis Henrici secundi Benedicti abbatis: The Chronicle of the Reigns of Henry II and Richard I, A.D. 1169–1192*, ed. W. Stubbs (2 vols, London, 1867).

Ross, C.D. (ed.), *Cartulary of St Mark's Hospital, Bristol* (Bristol, 1959).

Round, J.H. (ed.), *Rotuli de dominabus et pueris et puellis de XII comitatibus (1185)* (London, 1913).

Salter, H.E. (ed.), *A Cartulary of the Hospital of St John the Baptist* (3 vols, Oxford, 1914–17).

Seale, Y. and H. Wacha (eds), *The Cartulary of Prémontré* (Toronto, ON, 2023).

Sharpe, R. et al. (eds), *Corpus of British Medieval Library Catalogues* (16 vols, London, 1990–).

Smith D. (ed.) *The Acta of Hugh of Wells, Bishop of Lincoln, 1209–1235* (Woodbridge, 2000).

Stapelton, T. (ed.) *Magni rotuli Scaccarii Normanniae sub regibus Angliae* (2 vols, London, 1840–4).

Stenton, D. (ed.), *The Chancellor's Roll for the Eighth Year of the Reign of King Richard I Michaelmas 1196* (London, 1930).

Tabuteau, B. (ed.), *Le Cartulaire de la léproserie d'Évreux* (Compiègne, 2021).

Toulmin Smith, L. (ed.), *The Itinerary of John Leland in or About the Years 1535–1543* (5 vols, London, 1906–10).
Treharne, I.F. and I.J. Sanders (eds), *Documents of the Baronial Movement of Reform and Rebellion* (Oxford, 1973).
Underwood, M.G. (ed.), *The Cartulary of the Hospital of St John the Evangelist, Cambridge* (Cambridge, 2008).
Viaut, L. (ed.), *Le cartulaire de l'abbaye du Palais Notre-Dame (XIIe et XIIIe siècles): Édition critique* (Pessac, 2021).
Vincent, N. (ed.), *The Letters and Charters of Henry II, King of England, 1154–1189* (7 vols, Oxford, 2021–4).
Watkiss, L. and D. Greenway (eds and trans.), *The Book of the Foundation of Walden Monastery* (Oxford, 1999).
Wordsworth, C. (ed.), *The Fifteenth-Century Cartulary of St Nicholas' Hospital: With Other Records* (Salisbury, 1902).

## SECONDARY WORKS

Agúndez San Miguel, L. and F. Tinti, 'Introduction: New Perspectives after Thirty Years of Cartulary Studies', *Studia Historica. Historia Medieval*, 42 (2024), 3–8.
Allen, R. and B. Pohl, 'Mills, Manuscripts, and Monastic Archives: The Phillipps Charters of Mont Saint-Michel', *Bulletin of the John Rylands Library*, 100 (2024), 1–37.
Allen, R., 'À la recherche d'un atelier d'écriture de la Normandie cistercienne: le scriptorium de l'abbaye de Savigny (XII^e^–XIII^e^ siècles)', in A. Baudin and L. Morelle (eds), *Les pratiques de l'écrit dans les abbayes cisterciennes (XII^e^–milieu du XVI^e^ s.): Produire, échanger, contrôler, conserver* (Paris, 2016), pp. 31–54.
——, 'Les chartes originales de Savigny des origines jusqu'au XIII^e^ siècle (1112–1202)', in V. Gazeau and B. Galbrun (eds), *L'abbaye de Savigny (1112–2012): Un chef d'ordre anglo-normand* (Rennes, 2019), pp. 55–82.
——, 'Episcopal *Acta* in Normandy, 911–1204: The Charters of the Bishops of Avranches, Coutances and Sées', *ANS*, 37 (2015), 25–32.
——, 'La production diplomatique des évêques de Bayeux et de Coutances (XI^e^–XIII^e^ siècles)', in G. Combalbert and C. Senséby (eds), *Écrire à l'ombre des cathédrales. Pratiques de l'écrit en milieu cathédral (espace anglo-normand et France de l'Ouest, XI^e^-XIII^e^ siècle)* (Actes du colloque de Cerisy-la-Salle, 8–12 juin 2016) (Rennes, 2024), pp. 25–41
——, '"*Qui scripsit hanc cartam*": Charters and their Scribes through the Archives of Magdalen College, Oxford (*c*.1100–*c*.1300), *ANS*, forthcoming.
Ambler, S.T., *The Song of Simon de Montfort: England's First Revolutionary and the Death of Chivalry* (London, 2019).
*An Inventory of the Historical Monuments in the County of Northampton* (6 vols, London, 1975–).
Angenendt, A., '*Donationes pro anima*: Gift and Countergift in the Early Medieval Liturgy', in J.R. Davis and M. McCormick (eds), *The Long Morning of Medieval Europe: New Directions in Early Medieval Studies* (Aldershot, 2008), pp. 131–54.
Armstrong, A., *The Materiality of Medieval Administration in Northern England* (Turnhout, 2024).

Assmann, A., 'Four Formats of Memory: From Individual to Collective Constructions of the Past', in C. Emden and D. Midgley (eds), *Cultural Memory and Historical Consciousness in the German-Speaking World since 1500* (Oxford, 2004), pp. 19–38.
Assmann, A., *Zeit und Tradition: Kulturelle Strategien der Dauer* (Cologne, 1999).
Assmann, J. and J. Czaplicka, 'Collective Memory and Cultural Identity', *New German Critique*, 65 (1995), 125–33.
Assmann, J., 'Communicative and Cultural Memory', in A. Erll at al. (eds), *Cultural Memory Studies: An International and Interdisciplinary Handbook* (Berlin, 2008), pp. 109–18.
——, 'Introduction: What Is Cultural Memory?', in J. Assmann and R. Livingstone (eds), *Religion and Cultural Memory: Ten Studies* (Stanford, CA, 2006), pp. 1–30.
Baker, G., *The History and Antiquities of the County of Northampton* (2 vols, London, 1822–41).
Barker, J., *The Tournament in England, 1100–1400* (Woodbridge, 1986).
Barrow, J., *The Clergy in the Medieval World: Secular Clerics, their Families and Careers in North-Western Europe, c.800–c.1200* (Cambridge, 2015).
Bäuml, F.H., 'Varieties and Consequences of Medieval Literacy and Illiteracy', *Speculum*, 55 (1980), 237–65.
Beam, A., *The Balliol Dynasty 1210–1364* (Edinburgh, 2008).
Bennett, S., *Elite Participation in the Third Crusade* (Martlesham, 2021).
Berkhofer, R.F. III, *Day of Reckoning: Power and Accountability in Medieval France* (Philadelphia, PA, 2004).
——, *Forgeries and Historical Writing in England, France, and Flanders, 900–1200* (Woodbridge, 2022).
——, 'Interpreting Monastic Cartularies in Northwest Europe, 900–1200: Thirty Years of Scholarship', *Studia Historica. Historia Medieval*, 42 (2024), 25–46.
Bertrand, P., *Documenting the Everyday in Medieval Europe: The Social Dimensions of a Writing Revolution, 1250–1350* (Turnhout, 2019).
——, *Les écritures ordinaires: Sociologie d'un temps de révolution documentaire (1250–1350)* (Paris, 2015).
Bisson, T.N., 'A Micro-Economy of Salvation: Further Thoughts on the "Annuary" of Robert of Torigni', *ANS*, 40 (2018), 213–19.
Blanton, T.R. IV, *A Spiritual Economy: Gift Exchange in the Letters of Paul of Tarsus* (New Haven, CT, 2017).
Bond, S., 'The Attestation of Medieval Private Charters Relating to New Windsor', *Journal of the Society of Archivists*, 4 (1971), 278–84.
Bouchard, C.B., 'Review of J. Tucker, *Reading and Shaping Medieval Cartularies*', *TMR* (2021), <https://scholarworks.iu.edu/journals/index.php/tmr/article/view/32128/35956>.
Bridbury, A.R., 'Thirteenth-Century Prices and the Money Supply', *The Agricultural History Review*, 33 (1985), 1–21.
Brown, M.P., *A Guide to Western Historical Scripts from Antiquity to 1600* (London, 1990).
Burke, J., *A Genealogical and Heraldic History of the Commoners of Great Britain and Ireland* (4 vols, London, 1835–8).
Burton, J.E., 'A Roll of Charters for Lenton Priory', *Borthwick Institute Bulletin*, 2 (1979), 13–26.

Carlin, M., 'Medieval English Hospitals', in L. Granshaw and R. Porter (eds), *The Hospital in History* (London, 1989), pp. 21–39.
Carpenter, D., *Henry III: Reform, Rebellion, Civil War, Settlement, 1258–1272* (New Haven, CT, 2023).
——, *Henry III: The Rise to Power and Personal Rule, 1207–1258* (New Haven, CT, 2021).
——, *The Minority of Henry III* (Berkeley, CA, 1990).
Cassidy, R., *Approaching Pipe Rolls: The Thirteenth Century* (Abingdon, 2023).
Chastang, P., 'Cartulaires, cartularisation et scripturalité médiévale: La structuration d'un nouveau champ de recherche', *Cahiers de civilisation médiévale*, 49 (2006), 21–31.
——, 'Des archives au codex: Les cartulaires comme collections (XIe–XIVe siècle)', in B. Grévin and A. Mairey (eds), *Le Moyen Âge dans le texte: Cinq ans d'histoire textuelle au Laboratoire de médiévistique occidentale de Paris* (Paris, 2016), pp. 25–44.
Cheney, C.R., *English Bishops' Chanceries, 1100–1250* (Manchester, 1950).
Church, S.D., *The Household Knights of King John* (Cambridge, 1999).
Clanchy, M.T., *From Memory to Written Record: England 1066–1307*, 3rd edn (Malden, 2013).
Clay, C.T., 'The Ancestry of the Early Lords of Warkworth', *Archaeologia Aeliana*, 32 (1954), 65–71.
Clay, R.M., *The Mediæval Hospitals of England* (London, 1909).
Cleaver, L., 'From Codex to Roll: Illustrating History in the Anglo-Norman World in the Twelfth and Thirteenth Centuries', *ANS*, 36 (2014), 69–90.
Clemens, R. and T. Graham, *Introduction to Manuscript Studies* (Ithaca, NY, 2007).
Colvin, H., *The White Canons in England* (Oxford, 1951).
Cooper, N., *Aynho: A Northamptonshire Village* (Banbury, 1984).
Coss, P., 'Identity and Gentry c. 1200-c. 1340', *Thirteenth-Century England*, 6 (1997), pp. 49–60.
Craster, H.H.E., *A History of Northumberland* (15 vols, Newcastle upon Tyne, 1914).
Cuenca, E., 'Town Clerks and the Authorship of Custumals in Medieval England', *Urban History*, 46 (2019), 180–201.
Cunningham, I.C., 'Medieval Cartularies of Great Britain: Amendments and Additions to the Scottish Section of Davis', *MRB*, 3 (1997), 1–6.
Dalton, P., 'Eustace Fitz John and the Politics of Twelfth-Century England: The Rise and Survival of a Twelfth-Century Royal Servant', *Speculum*, 71 (1996), 358–83.
Davis, A.J., *The Medieval Economy of Salvation: Charity, Commerce, and the Rise of the Hospital*, rev. pb. edn (Ithaca, NY, 2021).
Davis, G.R.C., *Medieval Cartularies of Great Britain and Ireland*, rev. C. Breay et al. (London, 2010).
Davis, V., *William Waynflete, Bishop and Educationalist* (Woodbridge, 1993).
De G. Birch, W., *Catalogue of Seals in the Department of Manuscripts in the British Museum* (6 vols, London, 1887–1900).
De Sturler, J., *Les relations politiques et les échanges commerciaux entre le duché de Brabant et l'Angleterre au moyen âge* (Paris, 1936).
Delafield, J.R., *Delafield, the Family History* (2 vols, New York, 1945).
Denholm-Young, N., *Collected Papers on Mediaeval Subjects* (Oxford, 1946).

Dewez, H. and L. Tryoen (eds), *Administrer par l'écrit au Moyen Âge (XIIe–XVe siècle)* (Paris, 2019).

Dewez, H. (ed.), *Du nouveau en archives: Pratiques documentaires et innovations administratives (XIIIe–XVe siècle)* (Saint-Denis, 2019).

——, 'Le Rouleau comme support des comptes manoriaux au prieuré cathédral de Norwich (mi-XIIIe–mi-XIVe siècles)', *Comptabilités*, (2011), <https://journals.openedition.org/comptabilites/400>.

Drexler, M., 'Dervorguilla of Galloway', *Transactions of the Dumfriesshire and Galloway Natural History and Antiquarian Society*, 79 (2005), 101–46.

Drimmer, S., 'The Shapes of History: Houghton Library, MS Richardson 35 and Chronicles of England in Codex and Roll', in J.F. Hamburger et al. (eds), *Beyond Words: Illuminated Manuscripts in Boston Collections* (Toronto, ON, 2021), pp. 253–68.

Dugdale, W., *The Baronage of England* (2 vols, London, 1675–6).

Durham, B. et al., 'The Infirmary and Hall of the Medieval Hospital of St John the Baptist at Oxford', *Oxoniensia*, 56 (1991), 17–75.

Dutton, K., 'The Cartulary of the Cistercian Abbey of Kirkstead, Lincolnshire: The Landscape Realities and Documentary Defences of an Abbey Site in the Thirteenth and Fourteenth Centuries', *Journal of Medieval Monastic Studies*, 12 (2023), 77–121.

——, 'The Cistercian Abbey of Kirkstead, Lincolnshire: Rethinking a Twelfth-Century Foundation and its Thirteenth-Century Cartulary', *ANS*, 46 (2023), 161–83.

Eyton, R., 'Robert Fitz Wimarch and his Descendants', *Transactions of the Shropshire Archaeological and Natural History Society*, 2 (1879), 1–34.

Flachenecker, H. et al. (eds), *Urkundenbücher, Chroniken, Amtsbücher: Alte und neue Editionsmethoden* (Torún, 2019).

Fleming, P., 'Review of Sheila Sweetinburgh, *The Role of the Hospital in Medieval England: Gift-Giving and the Spiritual Economy*', *EHR*, 122 (2007), 471–3.

Florea, C., 'Beyond the Late Medieval Economy of Salvation: The Material Running of the Transylvanian Mendicant Convents', *Hereditas monasteriorum*, 3 (2013), 97–110.

Fowler, G.H. and M.W. Hughes, 'A Calendar of the Pipe Rolls of the Reign of Richard I for Buckinghamshire and Bedfordshire, 1189–1199', *Publications of the Bedfordshire Historical Record Society*, 7 (1923), 204–7.

Furtado, R. and M. Moscone (eds), *From Charters to Codex: Studies on Cartularies and Archival Memory in the Middle Ages* (Turnhout, 2019).

Gasper, G.E.M., 'Bernard of Clairvaux, Material and Spiritual Order, and the Economy of Salvation', *JMH*, 45 (2019), 580–96.

——, 'Economy Distorted, Economy Restored: Order, Economy and Salvation in Anglo-Norman Monastic Writing', *ANS*, 38 (2016), 51–66.

Gazeau, V., *Normannia monastica* (2 vols, Caen, 2007).

Goodfellow, P., 'Medieval Bridges in Northamptonshire', *Northamptonshire Past and Present*, 7 (1986), 143–58.

——, 'Medieval Markets in Northamptonshire', *Northamptonshire Past and Present*, 7 (1987–8), 305–23.

Grant, L., 'The Chapel of the Hospital of Saint-Jean at Angers: *Acta*, Statutes, Architecture and Interpretation', in J.A. Franklin et al. (eds), *Architecture and Interpretation: Essays for Eric Fernie* (Woodbridge, 2012), pp. 306–14.

Green, J., 'Aristocratic Loyalties on the Northern Frontier of England, circa 1100–1174', in D. Williams (ed.), *England in the Twelfth Century: Proceedings of the 1988 Harlaxton Symposium* (Woodbridge, 1990), pp. 83–100.

——, *English Sheriffs to 1154* (London, 1990).

——, *The Aristocracy of Norman England* (Cambridge, 1997).

Gullick, M., 'How Fast Did Scribes Write? Evidence from Romanesque Manuscripts', in L.L. Brownrigg (ed.), *Making the Medieval Book: Techniques of Production* (London, 1995), pp. 39–58.

——, 'Professional Scribes in Eleventh- and Twelfth-Century England', *English Manuscript Studies 1100–1700*, 7 (1998), 1–24.

Gumbert, J.P., 'The Speed of Scribes', in E. Condello and G. de Gregorio (eds), *Scribi e colofoni: Le sottoscrizioni di copisti dalle origini all'avvento della stampa* (Spoleto, 1995), pp. 57–69.

Gussone, M. and M.B. Rössner-Richarz, 'Kopiare als Arbeitsinstrumente', in M. Gussone et al. (eds), *Adelige Lebenswelten im Rheinland: Kommentierte Quellen der Frühen Neuzeit* (Cologne, 2009), p. 96–100.

Guyotjeannin, O. et al. (eds), *Les Cartulaires: Actes de la table ronde organisée par l'École nationale des chartes et le G.D.R. 121 du C.N.R.S* (Paris, 1993).

Guyotjeannin, O., 'Écrire en chancellerie', in M. Zimmermann (ed.), *Auctor et auctoritas: invention et conformisme dans l'écriture médiévale. Actes du colloque tenu à l'Université de Versailles-Saint-Quentin-en-Yvelines, 14–16 juin 1999* (Paris, 2001), pp. 17–35.

Hall, D., 'Aynho Fields, Open and Enclosed', *Northamptonshire Past and Present*, 59 (2006), 7–22.

Hammond, M., 'Royal and Aristocratic Attitudes to Saints and the Virgin Mary in Twelfth- and Thirteenth-Century Scotland', in S. Boardman (ed.), *The Cult of Saints and the Virgin Mary in Medieval Scotland* (Woodbridge, 2010), pp. 61–85.

Hartshorne, C., *Feudal and Military Antiquities of Northumberland and the Scottish Borders* (London, 1858).

Hayes, R., 'The Historical Manuscripts Commission's Project on the Records of Medieval Religious Houses', *MRB*, 5 (1999), 1–26.

Heal, F., 'Good Gifts, the Household and the Politics of Exchange in Early Modern England', *Past and Present*, 199 (2008), 41–70.

Hodgson, J., *A History of Northumberland* (15 vols, Newcastle upon Tyne, 1899).

Hodson, J., 'Medieval Charters: The Last Witness', *Journal of the Society of Archivists*, 5 (1974), 71–89

Holsinger, B., *On Parchment: Animals, Archives, and the Making of Culture from Herodotus to the Digital Age* (New Haven, CT, 2022).

Holt, J.C., *Colonial England 1066–1215* (London, 1997).

——, *The Northerners: A Study in the Reign of King John* (Oxford, 1992).

Holz, S.G., 'The *Onus Scaccarii* Rolls Under Edward I (1272–1307)', in J. Peltzer et al. (eds), *The Roll in England and France in the Late Middle Ages: Form and Content* (Berlin, 2020), pp. 167–96.

Hoskin, P., 'Medieval Cartularies of Great Britain: Amendments and Additions to the Davis Catalogue', *MRB*, 2 (1996), 1–12.

Howell, M.C., 'Documenting the Ordinary: The "Actes de la Pratique" of Late Medieval Douai', in A.J. Kosto and A. Winroth (eds), *Charters, Cartularies, and*

*Archives: The Preservation and Transmission of Documents in the Medieval West* (Toronto, ON, 2002), pp. 151–73.

Hui, R. et al., 'Medieval Social Landscape through the Genetic History of Cambridgeshire before and after the Black Death', *BioRxiv* (2023), <https://doi.org/10.1101/2023.03.03.531048>.

Hunt, T., 'Bibbesworth, Walter of', in *ODNB*, vol. 5, p. 639.

Inskip, S. et al., 'Pathways to the Medieval Hospital: Collective Osteobiographies of Poverty and Charity', *Antiquity*, 97 (2023), 1581–97.

Jahner, J.A., 'The Poetry of the Second Barons' War: Some Manuscript Contexts', in A.S.G. Edwards and O. Da Rold (eds), *English Manuscripts before 1400* (London, 2012), pp. 200–22.

Jarry, T., 'Évaluer, inventorier, exploiter: Le *Rotulus de denariis* de l'abbaye Saint-Étienne de Caen (XIIIe siècle)', *Tabularia* (2006), <https://doi.org/10.4000/tabularia.876>.

Johnston, M., *The Middle English Book: Scribes and Readers, 1350–1500* (Oxford, 2023).

Keats-Rohan, K.S.B. (ed.), *Domesday People: A Prosopography of Persons occurring in English Documents, 1066–1166. 1: Domesday Book* (Woodbridge, 1999).

—— (ed.), *Domesday Descendants: A prosopography of Persons occurring in English Documents 1066–1166. 2. Pipe Rolls to Cartae Baronum* (Woodbridge, 2002).

Kennedy, K.E., 'Aging Artists and Impairment in Fifteenth-Century England', *Different Visions: New Perspectives on Medieval Art*, 10 (2023), 1–30.

Ker, N.R., 'Hemming's Cartulary: A Description of the Two Worcester Cartularies in Cotton Tiberius A. XIII', in R.W. Hunt (ed.), *Studies in Medieval History, Presented to Frederick Maurice Powicke* (Oxford, 1948), pp. 49–75.

Kjær, L. and G. Strenga (eds), *Gift-Giving and Materiality in Europe, 1300–1600: Gifts as Objects* (London, 2022).

Kjær, L., *The Medieval Gift and the Classical Tradition: Ideals and the Performance of Generosity in Medieval England, 1100–1300* (Cambridge, 2019).

Knowles, D. and R. Hadcock, *Medieval Religious Houses: England and Wales* (London, 1953).

——, *Medieval Religious Houses: England and Wales*, rev. edn (London, 1971).

Kössinger, N., 'Gerollte Schrift: Mittelalterliche Texte auf Rotuli', in A. Kehnel and D. Panagiotopoulos (eds), *Schriftträger–Textträger: Zur materialen Präsenz des Geschriebenen in frühen Gesellschaften* (Berlin, 2015), pp. 151–68.

Kosto, A.J. and A. Winroth (eds), *Charters, Cartularies and Archives: The Preservation and Transmission of Documents in the Medieval West* (Toronto, ON, 2002).

Krausman Ben-Amos, I., *The Culture of Giving: Informal Support and Gift-Exchange in Early Modern England* (Cambridge, 2008).

Lamazou-Duplan, V. and E. Ramirez Vaquero (eds), *Les cartulaires médiévaux: Écrire et conserver la mémoire du pouvoir, le pouvoir de la mémoire* (Pau, 2013).

Latham, R., D. Howlett and R. Ashdowne (eds), *Dictionary of Medieval Latin from British Sources* (London, 1975–2013).

Latham, R.E. (ed.), *Revised Medieval Latin Word-List from British and Irish Sources* (London, 1965).

Letouzey-Réty, C., 'Administrer par l'écrit dans une grande abbaye de femmes anglo-normand: La Sainte-Trinité de Caen (XIIe–XIIIe siècles)', in H. Dewez and L. Tryoen (eds), *Administrer par l'écrit au Moyen Âge (XIIe–XVe siècle)* (Paris, 2019), pp. 23–40.

——, 'Le cartulaire de l'abbaye de la Trinité de Caen (fin XIIe–début XIIIe siècle)', *Tabularia* (2009), <https://doi.org/10.4000/tabularia.482>.

Levelt, S. and A. Putter, *North-Sea Crossings: The Literary Heritage of Anglo-Dutch Relations 1066–1688* (Oxford, 2021).

Lewis, B.J., 'St Mechyll of Anglesey, St Maughold of Man and St Malo of Brittany', *Studia Celtica Fennica*, 11 (2014), 24–38.

Lutter, C. et al., 'Kinship, Gender and the Spiritual Economy in Medieval Central European Towns', *History and Anthropology*, 32 (2021), 249–70.

MacEwen, A., 'A Clarification of the Dunbar Pedigree', *The Genealogist*, 9 (1988), 229–41.

MacKenzie, E., *An Historical, Topographical, and Descriptive View of the County of Northumberland*, 2nd edn (2 vols, Newcastle upon Tyne, 1825).

Macray, W.D., *Notes from the Muniments of St Mary Magdalen College, Oxford, from the Twelfth to the Seventeenth Century* (Oxford, 1882).

——, 'St Mary Magdalen College', *Appendix to The Eighth Report of the Historical Manuscripts Commission* (London, 1881), pp. 262–69.

——, 'The Manuscripts of St Mary Magdalene College, Oxford', *Appendix to The Fourth Report of the Historical Manuscripts Commission* (London, 1874), pp. 458–65.

——, *Fourth Report of the Royal Commission on Historical Manuscripts. Part I. Report and Appendix* (London, 1874)

Magnani, E., 'Almsgiving, Donatio Pro Anima and Eucharistic Offering in the Early Middle Ages of Western Europe (4th–9th century)', in M. Frenkel and Y. Lev (eds), *Charity and Giving in Monotheistic Religions* (Berlin, 2009), pp. 111–24.

Mersiowsky, M., 'Urkunden, Kopiare, Zinsbücher: Die Esslinger Bettelordensklöster und ihre pragmatische Schriftlichkeit im Spätmittelalter', in M. Mersiowsky et al. (eds), *Schreiben–Verwalten–Aufbewahren: Neue Forschungen zur Schriftlichkeit im spätmittelalterlichen Esslingen* (Ostfildern, 2018), pp. 251–328.

Metzler, I., *Disability in Medieval Europe: Thinking about Physical Impairment during the High Middle Ages, c.1100–1400* (London: 2006).

Mills, A.D., *A Dictionary of British Place Names* (Oxford, 2003).

Molitor, S., 'Das Traditionsbuch: Zur Forschungsgeschichte einer Quellengattung und zu einem Beispiel aus Südwestdeutschland', *Archiv für Diplomatik*, 36 (1990), 61–92.

Mooney, L.R., 'Professional Scribes? Identifying English Scribes who had a Hand in More than One Manuscript', in D. Pearsall (ed.), *New Directions in Later Medieval Manuscript Studies: Essays from the 1998 Harvard Conference* (York, 2000), pp. 131–42.

Müller, M., *Childhood, Orphans and Underage Heirs in Medieval Rural England: Growing Up in the Village* (London, 2019).

Niederkorn-Bruck, M., 'Prosopographisches in Martyrologien', in R. Berndt (ed.), *"Eure Namen sind im Buch des Lebens geschrieben": Antike und mittelalterliche Quellen als Grundlage moderner prosopographischer Forschung* (Münster, 2014), pp. 205–28.

Niermeyer, J.F. and C. van de Kieft (eds), *Mediae Latinitatis lexicon minus*, rev. edn (2 vols, Leiden, 2002).

Norgate, K., *England under the Angevin Kings* (2 vols, London, 1887).
Oksanen, E., *Flanders and the Anglo-Norman World, 1066–1216* (Cambridge, 2012), pp. 178–213.
Olney, R., *English Archives: An Historical Survey* (Liverpool, 2023).
Oram, R., 'Quincy, Roger de, earl of Winchester (c. 1195–1264)', *ODNB* 2004.
Orme, N. and M. Webster, *The English Hospital,* c.*1070–1570* (New Haven, CT, 1995).
Orme, N., 'Lay Literacy in England, 1100–1300', in A. Haverkamp and H. Vollrath (eds), *England and Germany in the High Middle Ages* (Oxford, 1996), pp. 35–56.
Ormerod, G., *The History of the County Palatine and City of Chester* (3 vols, London, 1819).
Overgaauw, E.A., 'Fast or Slow, Professional or Monastic: The Writing Speed of Some Late-Medieval Scribes', *Scriptorium*, 49 (1995), 211–27.
Painter, S., *The Reign of King John* (Baltimore, 1949).
Papin, É., 'Les cartulaires de l'abbaye de Margam: Le processus de cartularisation et l'administration des biens monastiques au pays de Galles au XIIIe siècle', *Médiévales*, 76 (2019), 11–24.
——, 'Les cartulaires-rouleaux de l'abbaye de Margam: Matérialité et fonctions des rouleaux cisterciens au pays de Galles au XIIIe siècle', in J. Peltzer et al. (eds), *The Roll in England and France in the Late Middle Ages: Form and Content* (Berlin, 2020), pp. 197–215.
Parkes, M.B., *English Cursive Book Hands, 1250–1500*, rev. edn (Ilkley, 1979).
——, *Their Hands before Our Eyes: A Closer Look at Scribes* (Aldershot, 2008).
——, 'The Provision of Books', in J. Catto et al. (eds), *The History of the University of Oxford* (8 vols, Oxford, 1984–2000), vol. 2, pp. 407–83.
Patterson, R.B., *The Scriptorium of Margam Abbey and the Scribes of Early Angevin Glamorgan: Secretarial Administration in a Welsh Marcher Barony,* c.*1150*–c.*1225* (Woodbridge, 2001).
Paxton, F.S., 'The Early Growth of the Medieval Economy of Salvation in Latin Christianity', in S.C. Reif et al. (eds), *Death in Jewish Life: Burial and Mourning Customs Among Jews* (Berlin, 2014), pp. 17–42.
Peacham, H., *The Compleat Gentleman* (London, 1622).
Peacock, E., 'A Mutilated Roll of Instruments Relating to the Hospital of St Edmund, at Sprotborough, near Doncaster', *Archaeologia*, 42 (1870), 398–404.
Peltzer, J., 'The Roll in England and France in the Late Middle Ages: Introductory Remarks', in J. Peltzer et al. (eds), *The Roll in England and France in the Late Middle Ages: Form and Content* (Berlin, 2020), pp. 1–19.
Perkins, N., *The Gift of Narrative in Medieval England* (Manchester, 2021).
Pohl, B., 'A Reluctant Historian and His Craft: The Scribal Work of Andreas of Marchiennes Reconsidered', *ANS*, 45 (2023), 141–62.
——, *Abbatial Authority and the Writing of History in the Middle Ages* (Oxford, 2023).
——, *Dudo of Saint-Quentin's* Historia Normannorum*: Tradition, Innovation and Memory* (York, 2015).
——, *Publishing in a Medieval Monastery. The View from Twelfth-Century Engelberg* (Cambridge, 2023).
——, 'Robert of Torigni's "Pragmatic Literacy": Some Theoretical Considerations', *Tabularia* (2022), <http://journals.openedition.org/tabularia/5576>.

——, 'Who Wrote MS Lat. 2342? The Identity of the *Anonymus Beccensis* Revisited', in F. Siri et al. (eds), *France et Angleterre: Manuscrits médiévaux entre 700 et 1200* (Turnhout, 2020), pp. 153–89.

Pollard, G., 'The Medieval Town Clerks of Oxford', *Oxoniensia*, 43 (1966), 44–76.

——, 'The University and the Book Trade in Medieval Oxford', *Beiträge zum Berufsbewusstsein des mittelalterlichen Menschen. Miscellanea Medievalia*, 3 (1964), pp. 336–44.

Pollock, M.A., *Scotland, England and France after the Loss of Normandy, 1204–1296: 'Auld Amitie'* (Woodbridge, 2015).

Power, D., *The Norman Frontier in the Twelfth and Early Thirteenth Centuries* (Cambridge, 2004).

Prestwich, M., *The Place of War in English History, 1066–1214* (Woodbridge, 2004).

Rawcliffe, C., 'Communities of the Living and of the Dead: Hospital Confraternities in the Later Middle Ages', in C.N. Bonfield et al. (eds), *Hospitals and Communities, 1100–1960* (Bern, 2013), pp. 125–54.

——, '"Gret criynge and joly chauntynge": Life, Death and Liturgy at St Giles's Hospital, Norwich, in the Thirteenth and Fourteenth Centuries', in C. Rawcliffe et al. (eds), *Counties and Communities: Essays on East Anglian History Presented to Hassell Smith* (Norwich, 1996), pp. 37–55.

——, 'Isolating the Medieval Leper: Ideas—and Misconceptions—about Segregation in the Middle Ages', in P. Horden (ed.), *Freedom of Movement in the Middle Ages* (Donington, 2007), pp. 229–48.

——, 'Learning to Love the Leper: Aspects of Institutional Charity in Anglo-Norman England', *ANS*, 23 (2001), 231–50.

——, *Leprosy in Medieval England* (Woodbridge, 2006).

——, 'Passports to Paradise: How English Medieval Hospitals and Almshouses Kept Their Archives', *Archives*, 27 (2002), 2–22.

——, 'The Cartulary of St Mary's Hospital, Great Yarmouth', in C. Rawcliffe et al. (eds), *Poverty and Wealth: Sheep, Taxation and Charity in Late Medieval Norfolk* (Norwich, 2007), pp. 157–230.

——, '"Written in the Book of Life": Building the Libraries of Medieval English Hospitals and Almshouses', *The Library*, 3 (2002), 127–62.

Reif, S.C., 'A Response to Professor Paxton's Paper', in S.C. Reif et al. (eds), *Death in Jewish Life: Burial and Mourning Customs Among Jews* (Berlin, 2014), pp. 43–50.

Rice, N.R., *The Medieval Hospital: Literary Culture and Community in England, 1350–1550* (Notre Dame, IN, 2023).

Richardson, D., *Magna Carta Ancestry: A Study in Colonial and Medieval Families*, 2nd edn (Salt Lake City, UT, 2011).

Ridgeway, H., 'An English Cartulary Roll of Peter of Savoy, Lord of Richmond (1240–1268): Archives, Interests and Servants of an Alien Favourite of King Henry III', in N. Saul and N. Vincent (eds), *English Medieval Government and Administration: Essays in Honour of J.R. Maddicott* (Woodbridge, 2023), pp. 203–28.

Robinson, P., 'The Format of Books: Books, Booklets and Rolls', in N.J. Morgan and R.M. Thomson (eds), *The Cambridge History of the Book in Britain. Vol. 2: 1100–1400* (Cambridge, 2008), pp. 41–54.

Rosand, D., 'Style and the Ageing Artist', *Art Journal*, 46 (1987), 91–3.

Rosenthal, J.T., *The Purchase of Paradise: Gift Giving and the Aristocracy, 1307–1485* (London, 1972).

Round, J.H., 'A Charter of William, Earl of Essex (1170)', *EHR*, 6 (1891), 364–7.

——, 'The Early Sheriffs of Norfolk', *EHR*, 35 (1920), 481–96.

——, 'Who was Alice of Essex?', *Transactions of the Essex Archaeological Society*, n.s. 3 (1889), 243–51.

Rubin, M., *Charity and Community in Medieval Cambridge* (Cambridge, 1987).

——, 'Development and Change in English Hospitals, 1000–1500', in L. Granshaw and R. Porter (eds), *The Hospital in History* (London, 1989), pp. 41–59.

——, 'Imagining Medieval Hospitals: Considerations on the Cultural Meaning of Institutional Change', in J. Barry and C. Jones (eds), *Medicine and Charity Before the Welfare State* (London, 1991), pp. 14–25.

Ruffini-Ronzani, N., 'The Counts of Louvain and the Anglo-Norman World' (*c.*1100–*c.*1215), *ANS*, 42 (2020), 135–54.

Ryley, H., *Re-using Manuscripts in Late Medieval England: Repairing, Recycling, Sharing* (York, 2022).

Sadler, J., *The Second Barons' War: Simon de Montfort and the Battles of Lewes and Evesham* (Barnsley, 2008).

Sanders, I.J., *English Baronies: A Study of Their Origin and Descent, 1086–1327* (Oxford, 1960).

Satchell, M., 'Towards a Landscape History of the Rural Hospital in England', in J. Henderson, P. Horden, and A. Pastore (eds), *The Impact of Hospitals 300–2000* (Oxford, 2007), pp. 237–56.

Sayers, J.E., *Papal Government and England During the Pontificate of Honorius III (1216–1227)* (Cambridge, 1984).

Scott, I.R., *College Farm, Aynho, Northamptonshire. Archaeological Evaluation Report* (Oxford, 1999).

Sharpe, R., *Libraries and Books in Medieval England: The Role of Libraries in a Changing Book Economy (The Lyell Lectures for 2018–19)*, ed. J. Willoughby (Oxford, 2023).

Smith, R.J., 'Henry II's Heir: The *Acta* and Seal of Henry the Young King, 1170–83', *EHR*, 116 (2001), 297–326.

Soden, I. and D.J. Leigh, 'The Hospital Chapel of St John, Northampton', *Northamptonshire Archaeology*, 34 (2006), 125–38.

Stein, H., *Bibliographie générale des cartulaires français, ou relatifs à l'histoire de France* (Paris, 1907).

Stock, B., *The Implications of Literacy: Written Language and Models of Interpretation in the Eleventh and Twelfth Centuries* (Princeton, NJ, 1983).

Stokes, P., 'Scribal Attribution Across Multiple Scripts: A Digitally Aided Approach', *Speculum*, 92 (2017), 65–85.

Strickland, M., *Henry the Young King, 1155–1183* (New Haven, CT, 2016).

Sweetinburgh, S., *The Role of the Hospital in Medieval England: Gift-Giving and the Spiritual Economy* (Dublin, 2004).

Szirmai, J.A., *The Archaeology of Medieval Bookbinding* (Farnham, 1999).

Tabuteau, B. and F. Epaud, 'Le prieuré-léproserie de Saint-Nicolas d'Évreux: Dossier historique et patrimonial', *Bulletin des Amis des Monuments et Sites de l'Eure*, 138 (2011), 11–50.

Talbot, D., 'Review of Charles C. Rozier, *Writing History in the Community of St Cuthbert, c.700–1130: From Bede to Symeon of Durham*', *History*, 106 (2021), 477–8.

Thomson, R.M. et al., 'Technology of Production of the Manuscript Book', in N.J. Morgan and R.M. Thomson (eds), *The Cambridge History of the Book in Britain. Vol. 2: 1100–1400* (Cambridge, 2008), pp. 75–109.

Thomson R.M., 'Scribes and Scriptoria', in E. Kwakkel and R.M. Thomson (eds), *The European Book in the Twelfth Century* (Cambridge, 2018), pp. 68–84.

Thorpe, D.E. and J.E. Alty, 'What Type of Tremor Did the Medieval "Tremulous Hand of Worcester" Have?', *Brain: A Journal of Neurology*, 138 (2015), 23–31.

Thorpe, D.E., 'Tracing Neurological Disorders in the Handwriting of Medieval Scribes: Using the Past to Inform the Future', *Journal of the Early Book Society for the Study of Manuscripts and Printing History*, 18 (2015), 241–48.

Tock, B.-M., *Une chancellerie épiscopale au XII^e^ siècle: le cas d'Arras* (Louvain-la-Neuve, 1991).

Tomkinson, A., 'Retinues at the Tournament of Dunstable, 1309', *EHR*, 74 (1959), 70–89.

Tucker, J., *Reading and Shaping Medieval Cartularies: Multi-Scribe Manuscripts and their Patterns of Growth* (Woodbridge, 2020).

——, 'Recognising Cartulary Studies Thirty Years after *Les Cartulaires*', *Studia Historica. Historia Medieval*, 42 (2024), 9–24.

——, 'Understanding Scotland's Medieval Cartularies', *Innes Review*, 70 (2019), 135–70.

Turner, R.V., 'The Mandeville Inheritance, 1189–1236: Its Legal, Political and Social Context', *Haskins Society Journal*, 1 (1989), 147–72.

Van Houts, E.M.C., *Married Life in the Middle Ages, 900–1300* (Oxford, 2019).

——, *Memory and Gender in Medieval Europe, 900–1200* (Basingstoke, 1999).

Vanwijnsberghe, D., 'Cartulaire de l'hôpital Saint-Jacques de Tournai [Tournai, Bibliothèque de la Ville, Cod. 4A (conservé n° 27)]', in M. Smeyers and J. Vander Stock (eds), *Manuscrits à peintures en Flandre, 1475–1550* (Ghent, 1997): pp. 186–87 (= no. 30).

——, 'Cartulaire de l'hôpital Saint-Jacques de Tournai: Description commentée des images', *Art de l'enluminure*, 73 (2020), 31–61.

Vincent, N., 'Enrolment in Medieval English Government: Sickness or Cure?', in J. Peltzer et al. (eds), *The Roll in England and France in the Late Middle Ages: Form and Content* (Berlin, 2020), pp. 103–45.

——, 'Medieval Cartularies: Additions and Corrections', *MRB*, 3 (1997), 7–38.

——, 'Medieval Cartularies: Further Additions II', *MRB*, 5 (1999), 26–28.

——, 'Medieval Cartularies: Further Additions', *MRB*, 4 (1998), 6–12.

——, 'Some Pardoners' Tales: The Earliest English Indulgences', *Transactions of the Royal Historical Society*, 12 (2002), 23–58.

——, 'Why 1199? Bureaucracy and Enrolment under John and His Contemporaries', in A. Jobson (ed.), *English Government in the Thirteenth Century* (Woodbridge, 2004), pp. 17–48.

Vogeler, G., 'Digitale Urkundenbücher: Eine Bestandsaufnahme', *Archiv für Diplomatik*, 56 (2010), 363–92.

Ward, J., *Women of the English Nobility and Gentry, 1066–1500* (Manchester, 2013).

Ward, W.H., *A History of the Manor and Parish of Iver* (London, 1933).

Wareham, A., *Lords and Communities in Early Medieval East Anglia* (Woodbridge, 2005).
——, 'The Motives and Politics of the Bigod Family, *c.*1066–1177', *ANS*, 17 (1995), 223–42.
Watson, S., 'A Mother's Past and her Children's Futures: Female Inheritance, Family and Dynastic Hospitals in the Thirteenth Century', in C. Leyser and L. Smith (eds), *Motherhood, Religion, and Society in Medieval Europe, 400–1400: Essays Presented to Henrietta Leyser* (London, 2016), pp. 213–49.
——, 'City as Charter: Charity and the Lordship of English Towns, 1170–1250', in C.J. Goodson et al. (eds), *Cities, Texts, and Social Networks, 400–1500: Experiences and Perceptions of Medieval Urban Space* (Farnham, 2010), pp. 235–62.
——, *On Hospitals: Welfare, Law, and Christianity in Western Europe, 400–1320* (Oxford, 2020).
——, 'Responding to Leprosy in the Twelfth and Thirteenth Centuries', in A. Medcalf et al. (eds), *Leprosy: A Short History* (Hyderabad, 2016), pp. 29–38.
——, 'The Origins of the English Hospital', *Transactions of the Royal Historical Society*, 16 (2006), 75–94.
——, 'The Sources for English Hospitals 1100 to 1400', in M. Scheutz et al. (eds), *Quellen zur europäischen Spitalgeschichte in Mittelalter und Früher Neuzeit / Sources for the History of Hospitals in Medieval and Early Modern Europe* (Vienna, 2010), pp. 65–104.
Wattenbach, W., *Das Schriftwesen im Mittelalter*, 3rd edn (Leipzig, 1896).
Weever, J., *Antient Funeral Monuments, of Great-Britain, Ireland, and the Islands Adjacent* (London, 1767).
Whalley, P. (ed.), *The History and Antiquities of Northamptonshire. Compiled from the Manuscript Collections of the Late Learned Antiquary John Bridges, Esq* (2 vols, Oxford, 1791).
Williams, A., 'Asgar the Staller (d. after 1066)', in *ODNB*, vol. 2, pp. 596–7.
Willoughby, J., 'The Chronicle of Ralph of Coggeshall: Publication and Censorship in Angevin England', in S. Niskanen and V. Rovere, *The Art of Publication from the Ninth to the Sixteenth Century* (Turnhout, 2023), pp. 131–66.
Woolgar, C.M., 'Two Cartularies at Magdalen College, Oxford', *Journal of the Society of Archivists*, 6 (1981), 498–9.
Yarrow, S., *Saints and Their Communities: Miracle Stories in Twelfth-Century England* (Oxford, 2006).

## UNPUBLISHED WORKS

Bevan, K., 'Clerks and Scriveners: Legal Literacy and Access to Justice in Late Medieval England', unpublished PhD dissertation, University of Exeter, 2013.
Fry, C., '"Hospitality, Chantries, and Other Works of Piety": A Select Study of the Functions and Longevity of Hospitals in Small Towns and Villages in Medieval England, *c.*1150–*c.*1450', unpublished PhD dissertation, University of Oxford, 2020.
Keyser, R.L., 'Gift, Dispute, and Contract: Gift Exchange and Legalism in Monastic Property Dealings, Montier-la-Celle, France, 1100–1350', unpublished PhD dissertation, Johns Hopkins University, 2001.

Macray, W.D., ['A Descriptive Calendar of the Muniments of St Mary Magdalen College, Oxford'], 48 vols, unpublished manuscript and typescript (1864–78).

Partida, T., 'Drawing the Lines: A GIS Study of Enclosure and Landscape in Northamptonshire', unpublished PhD dissertation, University of Huddersfield, 2014.

Satchell M., 'The Emergence of Leper-houses in Medieval England, 1100-1250', unpublished PhD dissertation, University of Oxford, 1998.

Watson, S., '*Fundatio*, *ordinatio*, and *statuta*: The Statues and Constitutional Documents of English Hospitals to 1300', unpublished PhD dissertation, University of Oxford, 2004.

Woolgar, C.M., 'A Catalogue of the Estate Archives of St Mary Magdalen College, Oxford', 10 vols, unpublished typescript (1981).

# INDEX OF PERSONS AND PLACES

Arabic numerals in roman type indicate pages. Arabic numerals in boldface indicate the acts of the cartulary or those edited in the Appendix if preceded by the letter A. The letter W following a boldface number indicates a witness. Except for major towns/cities, English placenames are followed by their county and, when further precision is necessary/possible, their hundred. French placenames are followed by their department and canton, and Belgian placenames by their province and arrondissement or municipality. The following abbreviations are used for English counties:

| | | | |
|---|---|---|---|
| Bedfordshire | Bd. | Leicestershire | Lei. |
| Berkshire | Brk. | Lincolnshire | Li. |
| Buckinghamshire | Bk. | Norfolk | Nf. |
| Cambridgeshire | Ca. | Northamptonshire | Np. |
| Cheshire | Chs. | Northumberland | Nd. |
| Cumbria | Cum. | Nottinghamshire | Nt. |
| Derbyshire | Dy. | Oxfordshire | Ox. |
| Essex | Ess. | Staffordshire | St. |
| Dorset | Do. | Suffolk | Sf. |
| Gloucestershire | Gl. | Surrey | Su. |
| Hertfordshire | Hrt. | Sussex | Sx. |
| Huntingdonshire | Hu. | Warwickshire | Wa. |
| Kent | Kt. | Wiltshire | Wi. |
| Lancashire | Lan. | Yorkshire | Yk. |

The following abbreviations are also used:

| | | | |
|---|---|---|---|
| archbishop(s) | abp(s). | canon(s) | can(s). |
| archdeacon(s) | archd(s). | church | ch. |
| bishop(s) | bp(s). | hospital | hosp. |

# INDEX OF SUBJECTS

Roman or Arabic numerals in roman type indicate pages. Arabic numerals in boldface indicate the acts of the cartulary or those edited in the Appendix if preceded by the letter A.

abbess (*abbatissa*), **A19**; *see also names under* Pontécoulant, Marie VI de
abbot, *see names under* Geoffrey; Osbern; Richard; Suppo
acre (*acra*), xiv, 56–58, 65, 74, 80–82; **29, 32–33, 40, 44, 49–51, 55–56, A6–A7, A11–A20**
advocate (*advocator*), *see* church
advowson, 16–17, 26 n. 59, 84–85
alms (*elemosina*), grant in free, pure, or perpetual, 15, 30, 43, 46, 50, 74, 139; **2, 4, 7–9, 11, 20–24, 26–27, 29, 31–37, 41–43, 45–46, 56–58, A1, A7, A10–A11, A15, A17**
altar (*altare*), **32, A7**; *see also*, lamp
animals (*averia*), **58**
draught (*affri*), pasture for, **9**
anniversary celebrations for the dead (*anniversarium*), 66, 70, 73–74; **33, 56, A10**; *see also*, obit book
archbishop (*archiepiscopus*); *see names under* Canterbury
archdeacon (*archidiaconus*); *see names under* Gloucester; Huntingdon; Leicester; Stow
archives, 3, 8–9, 17, 48 n. 5, 83–86, 121, 130
  record storage, 8, 122 n. 29, 123, 130
assignee (*assignatus*), **32, 52, A5–A6, A11–A12**
authority (*auctoritas*), **2, 11**
  apostolic, **1**
  episcopal, **47–48**
  *see also*, church

beams (*trabes*), **30**
bells (*campanae*), ringing of, **1**
benefit (*beneficium*), **2**
bishop (*episcopus*); *see names under* Hugh; Richard; Cheney; Grosseteste; Lexington; Lincoln; Montbray; Sutton; Vere; Waynflete; Wells; Winchester
boundary (*meta*), **28**
brothers (w. ref. to religious of hosp.) (*fratres*), 18, 32, 46–47, 50, 74, 76, 96, 120 n. 22; **1–2, 4–5, 12–14, 17–18, 20–27, 29–34, 44, 49–50, 52, 55–58, A7–A21**
burgage (*burgagium*), **1**
burial (*sepultura*), 70, 73
  right of, 76; **1**

candles (*cerei*), **31**
cartularies,
  examples of, 115–17, 136–137
  roll cartularies, 114–115, 121–122, 142
  studies of, 3, 5–8, 133–135
cemetery (*cimiterium*), **1, 26–27**
  wall of, **26–27**
chapels (*capellae*), 18, 40, 55–56, 70, 74, 76–77, 80, 90, 120; **1, 22–24, 31, 40–48, A2–A4**
  patron of, **47–48, A2**
chaplains (*capellani*), **A10**; *see names under* Adderbury; Alan; Aynho; Deddington; Ernald; Hasculph; Hinton in the Hedges; Hugh; Ingelram; Jordan; Newbottle; Robert; Roger; Steane; Stuchbury; Turbert/Turbern; Walter; Weedon Lois; Woodford Halse
  activities of, 32, 89, 93–94, 97 n. 46, 120
  pledging faith in hands of, **20**

charity (*caritas*), 9–11, 46–47, 53, 64, 67–68, 76, 78, 140; **1**, **8**, **14**, **18**, **25**
cheese (*caseum*), **40**
church (*ecclesia*), 16–18, 42, 65, 76; **2**, **32–33**, **55**
  advocate of, **40**
  authority (*dignitas*) of, **47–48**
  chapter (*capitulum*) of, **48**
  mother, rights of, **1**, **40**
claim (*clameum*), 17, 30, 36; **A19**, **A21**
clerks, (*clerici*), **3**
  scribal activities of, 94–112
codex, codices, 4 n. 2, 8, 12, 114, 118–119, 121, 137
coronation (*coronatio*), **A9**
cottage (*cotagium*), 79; **31**
cottager (*cotarius*), 63; **8**
count, *see names under* Fitz Count; Philip I; Robert
countess (*comitissa*), *see names under* Euphemia; Margaret
court (*curia*), *see* obligations
courtyard (*curia*), 54, 79, 81; **22–23**, **26–27**, **A5**
croft (*croftum*), 56, 79; **15**, **17**, **19**
curtilage (*curtilagium*), **A8**
customs (*consuetudines*), **3–4**, **9**, **14–15**, **18**, **31–33**, **36–37**, **56–57**, **A7**, **A11**, **A16**, **A19–A20**
  episcopal, **47–48**

demand (*demanda*) (for service or payment), **32–34**, **50–51**, **55–57**, **A6–A8**, **A11–A12**, **A15–A16**, **A18–A20**
demesne (*dominicus*, *dominium*), 16 n. 6, 40, 49, 79; **5**, **7**, **9**, **11**, **20**, **29**, **40**, **48**, **55**
document (*pagina*, *scriptum*), **1–2**, **11**, **17**, **40**, **44**, **A1**, **A7**, **A9–A10**, **A13**, **A21**
Domesday Book, 16, 49, 55, 58
donation, 10, 40, 48, 50–53, 56–57, 70, 90, 134
  *in elemosinam*, 50, 70–72, 75
  *pro anima*, 70–72, 75
doors (*ianuae*), *see also* marriage
closing of, **1**
dower, 22, 24, 31, 33, 35, 36 n. 128, 49, 51, 139
dowry (*dos*), **A21**

duke, *see names under* Alan IV; Conan IV; Henry I; William

earl (*comes*); *see names under*, Essex; Leicester; Richmond; Winchester; *see also* service
easements (*aisiamenta*), **15**, **A12–A13**, **A16**, **A19–A20**
envoys (*nuntii*), **2**
exaction (*exactio*), **3**, **9**, **14**, **18**, **22–24**, **29**, **34**, **36–37**, **A8–A9**, **A11–A12**, **A14–A15**, **A19**

fee/fief (*feodum*), 21, 36 n. 128, 40–41, 141; **25**, **40**, **51**
  land held in, **3**, **15**, **A5**, **A9**, **A13**, **A16**, **A20**
fields (*campi*), **17**, **21**, **24**, **32–33**, **48–51**, **55**, **A6**, **A11–A12**, **A14–A18**, **A20**
  organisation of, 52, 58, 63–64
fleece (*vellus*), **40**
foreign (*extrinsecum*, *forinsecum*), *see* service
freedoms (*libertates*), **3–4**, **14**, **18**, **21**, **24**, **57**, **A5**, **A12–A13**
frank-marriage (*maritagium*), **13**
friend, *amicus*, **3**, **6**

gable (*gabla*), **30**
Gospel book (*sacrosanctus*), grant made on, **20**
gifts, gift-giving, 10, 42, 47, 49, 56, 67–68, 70, 72–73, 76–77, 139
grain (*annona*, *frumentum*), 16 n. 6; **35**
grove (*grava*), **A19**
guests (*hospites*), 76, **1**

handwriting, 86–87, 127–130
headland (*capitalis*, *forera*), **55**, **A6**
heir(s) (*heres*, *heredes*), 21, 24–26, 28, 31, 36, 40, 51, 53, 71; **3–4**, **14**, **17–18**, **20–27**, **30–32**, **35**, **48–52**, **55**, **A6–A7**, **A9–A10**, **A12**, **A16–A20**
  rent due to, **17**
hereditary (*hereditarius*), right, **A19**
hide (unit of arable land) (*hida*), xiv, 17, 49–50, 53, 79; **1**, **4–7**, **10–11**
homage (*homagium*), **15–17**, **48**
hospitality (*hospitium*), **4**, **7**, **11**
hospitals,
  functions and endowment of, 34–35, 47–38, 51–52, 66–77, 120–121

studies of, 9–10, 13, 43
house (of religion or sim.) (*domus*), **1–2**
residential, rental of, 54, 56, 80, 99; **30–31, 34, A8, A18**

inheritance (*hereditas*), 24, 26, 30, 51; **A2**
land held in, **3, 15–16, A5, A13, A16, A20**
inspeximus, **48**

king (*rex*), scutage of, **A11**; *see also*, road; service; *see names under* Alexander II; Edward I; Henry I; Henry II; Henry III; Henry VI; John; Richard I; William; William I

lamb (*agnus*), **40**
lamp (*lampas*), before altar, **32, A7**
layperson (*laicus*), **3**
letters (*litterae*), **52, A9**
license (*licencia*), *see* parson
literacy, 93, 117, 120, 130
pragmatic literacy, 126

Magna Carta, 28
marriage, 20–21, 26, 29, 31, 40, 72; *see also* dower; frank-marriage
mass (liturgy) (*missa*), **1, 31**
master (w. ref. to head of hosp.) (*magister*), **12–13, 17, 22, 26–27, 30–34, 52, 55–57, A7–A9, A11–A21**; *see also names under* Aynho; Castref'; Chester; Croughton; Fingest; Gerard; Gra(nt)ham; Graveley; Halse; Jordan; Leicester; Lincoln; Maldon; Norwich; Occold; Rolleston; Salomon; Simon; St Martin; Stephen; Stuchbury; Swalecliffe; Walensi; Windsor
meadow(land) (*pratum*), 49–50, 52, 58, 79–82; **1, 3–4, 8–9, 20–21, 24, 32, 36–37, 57, A7, A14**
outlying (*forinsecum*), 54; **32, A7**
small (*pratellum*), **A19**
messuage (*masagium*), 40, 50, 52, 54–55, 79–82; **3, 7, 11–12, 22–24, 31, 57–58, A5, A8, A19**
mill (*molendinum*), 19 n. 24, 49, 55; **4, A10**
miller (*mollendinarius*), **51, A6**
tithes of, **40**
mowing (*falcatio*), **32, A7**

needle (*acus*), **A12**
needy (of persons) (*indigens*), **1**

obit book (*martilogium*), **33**
obligation (*secta*), of court **32, 50–51, 55–57, A6–A9, A11–A12, A14, A16, A20**
open land (*planus*), 53; **4, 8**
oxen (*boves*), pasture for, 53, 119; **9**

parchment, 12, 118–119, 124, 126–127
parson (*persona*), 16–17, 36; **33, 40, A11**
license of (*licencia*), **40**
pasture (*pascuum, pastura*), 50, 52–53, 79, 119; **3–4, 8–9, 14, 18, 20–21, 24, 36–37, 57, A14**
path(s) (*semita*), 53; **4, 8, 14, 18, 21, 24, 57**
patron (*patronus*), *see* chapel
patronage (*patronatus*), right of, 18, 40, 84; **A2**
penance (*penitentia*), 47; **2**
piglet (*porcellus*), **40**
pit (*fovea*), **A11**
pittance (*pitantia*), **56**
plot (*area*), **A19**
ploughland (*campus, cultura*), 49, 55, 63–64; **51, A6, A11**
poor (of persons) (*pauper, pauperes*), 10, 35, 50, 53, 65, 68, 76, 138; **1–2, 4–7, 11**
pope, *see under name* Innocent III; John XXII
prior (w. ref. to religious house) (*prior*), 36, 46–47; **2, A19**
privilege (*privilegium*), 47; **1**
proctor (*procurator*), 36, 120; **1–2**
province (eccl.) (*provincia*), **2**

quitclaim (*quieta clamatio*), **34, 52, A5, A9, A20–A21**

rebellion, 22–23, 28–29, 40
rector (*rector*), 16–17, 36, 90; **1, A1, A16, A20**
rent (*redditus*), 31; **52, A19**; *see also*, heir(s)
of mill, **A10**
of the lord of the manor, **12–13**
road (*via*), **4, 8, 14, 21, 24, 57, A16–A17, A20**
of the king (king's way), **57, A8, A18**

rood (of land) (*roda*), 57, 74, 80; **56**, **A13**, **A16**, **A20**

sacrament (*sacramentum*), **1**
scribes,
of Aynho Cartulary, 120–121, 127–131, 135–136
of Aynho charters, 88–97
scribal milieux, 86–88, 93–112
scutage (*scutagium*), *see* king
servant (*serviens*), 49 n. 7; 52 n. 15; **3**, **A10**
service (obligation) (*servitium*), 26, 30, 42; **3–8**, **11**, **14–16**, **18**, **22–23**, **31**, **33–34**, **48–51**, **55–57**, **A6**, **A8**, **A11–A12**, **A14–A16**, **A18–A20**
due to earl, **3**, **10**
due to king, **3**, **12–13**, **21**, **24**
foreign (*extrinsecum*, *forinsecum*), **15**, **17**, **20–21**, **24**, **42–44**, **51**, **A6**, **A13**, **A16**, **A18–A20**
silver (*argentum*), **14–16**, **18**, **27**, **49–50**, **55**, **A5–A6**, **A9**, **A18–A19**
sin (*peccatum*), **2**
soul (*anima*), grant made for wellbeing of, 70–72, 75; **4–9**, **12–13**, **17**, **20–21**, **25–27**, **29–37**, **41–42**, **44–46**, **56–57**, **A3–A4**, **A7**, **A11**
*spiritualia*, **40**
spiritual economy, 10–11, 13, 45, 51, 66–77

tenement (*tenementum*), 57, 82; **6–7**
territory (*territorium*), **52**, **A13–A16**, **A20**
timberwork (*meirinum*), **30**
tithes (*decima*), 16, 64–65, 67; **40**
toft (*tofta*), **31**
tournaments, 15 n. 1, 23, 31, 42–44, 139

vicars, perpetual, 16–17
violence (*violentia*), **1**
virgate (*virgata*), xiv, 40, 50, 53–56, 79–80, 82; **1**, **3**, **8**, **12–21**, **24**, **36–39**, **57–58**, **A16**, **A20**

wall (*murus*), **28**; *see also*, cemetery
warranty (act of) (*warantizare*), **15**, **18**, **20–23**, **25–27**, **30–33**, **36–37**, **48–51**, **55–57**, **A6–A19**
widow (*relicta*), 17, 21 n. 36, 22, 24, 26, 30, 33; **A20**
widowhood (*viduitas*), **21**, **25**, **A20–A21**
will (*testamentum*), **31**
woodland (*boscus*, *boscum*), 53, 64; **4**, **8**

Printed in the United States
by Baker & Taylor Publisher Services